APPROACHES TO
CROSS-CULTURAL
PSYCHIATRY

APPROACHES TO CROSS-CULTURAL PSYCHIATRY

Edited by

Jane M. Murphy *and*

Alexander H. Leighton

Cornell University Press

ITHACA, NEW YORK

CORNELL UNIVERSITY PRESS

First published 1965

Second printing 1966

Library of Congress Catalog Card Number: 65-13631

PRINTED IN THE UNITED STATES OF AMERICA

BY VALLEY OFFSET, INC.

Preface

THIS work, reporting on methods and concepts for comparative studies of mental illness in different cultural groups, is the outgrowth of efforts sponsored by the Cornell Program in Social Psychiatry to explore and understand the nature of some of the problems confronting research in this field. The contributors have approached this topic through reviews of the literature, seminar discussions, and trial investigations. The exploratory field studies were carried out among Eskimos, Navahos, and Mexicans, as well as British and Acadian French in Nova Scotia.

In the early 1950's, two epidemiological studies were undertaken in northeastern America. One study was concerned with a rural county in Maritime Canada. This, the Stirling County Study, was formulated and directed by Alexander H. Leighton.* The research was conducted through Cornell's Department of Sociology and Anthropology on the campus at Ithaca, New York. The other epidemiological study, the Midtown Manhattan Study, concerned an area in metropolitan New York. Instituted by Thomas A. C. Rennie,† who directed it until his death in

* Other chief investigators in the Stirling Study were B. P. Dohrenwend, J. S. Harding, C. C. Hughes, D. C. Leighton, D. B. Macklin, the late A. M. Macmillan, the late G. E. McCreary, J. M. Murphy, A. L. Nangeroni, R. N. Rapoport, and M.-A. Tremblay.

† For the Midtown Study, the other main investigators were P. Kirkpatrick, T. S. Langner, S. T. Michael, M. K. Opler, V. Rubin, L. Srole, and A. Weider.

1956, it was based at the Cornell University Medical College in New York City. The main results of the two studies have been reported in a series of volumes which give detailed presentations of theoretical orientations, methods employed, and analysis of findings.* After Rennie's death, the Stirling and Midtown Studies were joined under the directorship of Alexander H. Leighton and the name "Cornell Program in Social Psychiatry" was adopted.

The two investigations of populations in Western culture were conceived with somewhat similar frames of reference. Although each faced unique problems and pursued a separate course of data gathering and analysis, the exchange of ideas in defining concepts and developing methods of research gave a measure of comparability to the two studies. In both there was interest in the full range of psychiatric disorders from psychoses and mental deficiency to psychoneuroses and behavior disturbances. From the theoretical viewpoint, however, it seems probable that psychoneurotic and psychophysiologic symptoms are the kinds most directly under the influence of different sociocultural experiences and most likely to be found with significant distribution in nonhospitalized and noninstitutionalized groups. The investigators determined, therefore, to pay special attention to discovering the mild as well as the severe forms of mental illness. To accomplish this, questionnaire interviewing was employed as one means of case-finding in each of the studies.

In Stirling County, a fishing, lumbering, and subsistence-

* *Stirling County Study:* A. H. Leighton, *My Name Is Legion* (New York: Basic Books, 1959); C. C. Hughes, M.-A. Tremblay, R. N. Rapoport, and A. H. Leighton, *People of Cove and Woodlot* (New York: Basic Books, 1960); D. C. Leighton, J. S. Harding, D. B. Macklin, A. M. Macmillan, and A. H. Leighton, *The Character of Danger* (New York: Basic Books, 1963).

Midtown Study: L. Srole, T. S. Langner, S. T. Michael, M. K. Opler, and T. A. C. Rennie, *Mental Health in the Metropolis* (New York: McGraw-Hill, 1962); T. S. Langner and S. T. Michael, *Life Stress and Mental Health* (New York: The Free Press of Glencoe, 1963).

farming region inhabited by two main ethnic groups, English and French Acadian, the research program was concerned with studying community life in its total impact upon individuals. The analysis of sociocultural environment focused on contrasts in cultural background as well as on differences in degree of "social integration" and "disintegration." The concepts of integration and disintegration provided a framework for selecting communities displaying both adequate and inadequate functioning, the features of which were predicted to have differential effect on mental health and mental illness. Hence social disintegration was considered to be a pattern or combination of a number of noxious conditions. The criteria by which this process was identified included such factors as poverty, secularization, cultural confusion, fractured social relationships, and rapid sociocultural change. Other components of the process are inadequacies in leadership, recreation, associations, communication, and control of crime and delinquency.

The aim was to find out whether there are important correlations between the prevalence of psychiatric symptoms and residence in integrated or disintegrated communities. Other aspects of life experience, such as age, sex, and ethnic identity, were also investigated. A probability sample of 1,010 adults was surveyed to elicit sociocultural information and data on health of both a physical and psychiatric nature. The county's local physicians were also interviewed about the members of the statistically selected sample, and mental and other hospital records were considered when they pertained to the sample members.

The Midtown Study, as already noted, dealt with a section of Manhattan in the city of New York. In contrast to the rural study area, Midtown is a much more complex and heterogeneous society with several ethnic groups represented: Irish, Italian, German-Austrian, Hungarian, Czechoslovakian, Polish, British, Old American, and others. Broad diversity exists in the occupations and professions present, and the span of economic levels is extremely wide. In this study the concept of "socioeconomic status" was employed as a way of quartering the environment in order to uncover sociocultural patterns which correlate with the distribution of psychiatric symptoms. A number of the elements of social disintegration used in the Stirling Study were given attention in the Midtown Study. For example, "life stress" was analyzed in terms of components such as broken homes, economic deprivation, ill health, and so on. The prevalence survey in Midtown was carried out with a probability sample of 1,660 adults.

Allowing for the many limitations to comparison and generalization imposed by the differences of procedure in the two studies, some tentative conclusions are nevertheless possible. The differences in environment encompassed by the terms "urban" and "rural" and by the divisions of Western society into ethnic groups such as French, English, Irish, and Italian did not parallel major differences in the prevalence of psychiatric disorder in the two sample populations. Psychoneurotic symptomatology formed an overwhelming part of the total picture of disorders among these nonhospitalized people, and it was much more prevalent than had been suspected. In the Stirling Study the factors of advancing age, of being a woman, and of low occupational position, as well as the experiences of living in a disintegrated environment were correlated with high rates of symptoms. Among the Midtown adults, advancing age and low economic position had similar relationships.

This platform of trends, as well as general interest in non-Western and developing countries, raised several questions for exploration in contrasting groups:

1. What kinds of psychiatric disorders are there and what is the actual prevalence in groups that practice life-ways very different from those of the West? That is to say, will greater cultural contrasts than those found in Midtown and Stirling bring to light significant qualitative and quantitative differences?

2. Do the apparent influences of age, sex, and occupational position hold up cross-culturally? What effects do rural or urban residence have when looked at in cross-cultural perspective?

3. How may sociocultural disintegration be defined cross-culturally, and does it continue to have the same association with prevalence of psychiatric disorders?

4. What is the effect of cultural change, so rapid and extensive all around the world, on these interrelated factors? In other words, do the patterns of social disintegration, rapid acculturation, and low socioeconomic position have similar relevance for the epidemiology of disorders in non-Western populations?

As a start toward investigating cross-cultural problems of this type, many questions of concepts, theory, methods, and feasibility had to be reviewed by members of the Cornell Program. According to interests and opportunities, the contributors chose particular topics and decided on various ways of exploring them. The approaches entailed field studies as well as work in clinics and libraries; and this book is one result.

The volume has been organized so that chapters with a common theme are grouped together. In order to link the chapters to the overall purpose of the book, the editors have prepared an introductory comment preceding all but two of the chapters. These two chapters, the first and the eighth, are general orientations written by one or both of the editors. The first chapter, "Cross-cultural Psychiatry," concerns history of the field, definition of terms, and a map of the problems to be approached. It opens Part One, which focuses predominantly on questions of identifying and surveying for psychiatric disorders. Chapter VIII, "Social Science Concepts and Cross-cultural Methods for Psychiatric Research," begins Part Two, which deals mainly with sociocultural approaches useful to cross-cultural psychiatric research.

Following the first chapter in Part One are two chapters

concerning identification of disorders in societies with cultures very different from that of the West. They complement each other in that Chapter II is devoted to disorder as defined in Western psychiatric terms, while Chapter III is addressed to indigenous conceptions of illness and deviance. The next two chapters take up questions about certain indicators that might be employed to estimate the prevalence of disorder in different cultures. Chapter IV discusses a questionnaire, which is largely concerned with psychophysiologic symptoms. Chapter V deals with the possibility of employing physiological tests that might indicate psychiatric disorder. The next chapters, VI and VII, also deal with a common theme. They concern the special problems of establishing criteria of disorder among adolescents and children. Their interest is heightened by the fact that most of the work done so far has dealt with adults.

Part Two consists of four chapters. The first, Chapter VIII, has been mentioned above. Chapter IX concerns the life story as an instrument for intensive studies of ill and well individuals with a focus on analysis of cultural roles. Chapter X gives consideration to the socially shared sentiments characteristic of different groups of people and discusses what meaning they may have for mental health and mental illness. Chapter XI is the report of an exploratory field study in which certain of the previously described techniques were given trial and in which correlations are pointed up between some kinds of psychiatric symptoms and some kinds of social experiences.

The work described in this volume was carried out between 1956 and 1960. In 1961 some of the investigators began a comprehensive epidemiological study of a rural area in Nigeria. Dr. T. Adeoye Lambo, who was at that time Medical Superintendent of the Aro Hospital for Nervous Diseases in the Western Region of Nigeria, was co-director of this study, which was called the Cornell-Aro Mental Health Research Project. Many of the methods of data gathering and analysis discussed in this book were applied in the Nigerian study, and further effort was made to substantiate their validity and reliability.*

Our coverage of the field in this volume is, of course, partial and selective. Taken together, however, the chapters deal with a number of technical questions both conceptual and methodological that are germane to a wide variety of problems regarding the relationship of sociocultural environment to psychiatric disorder. Our hope is that they will be useful to others approaching cross-cultural psychiatry.

JANE M. MURPHY

New York, New York
April, 1965

* A. H. Leighton, T. A. Lambo, C. C. Hughes, D. C. Leighton, J. M. Murphy, and D. B. Macklin, *Psychiatric Disorder among the Yoruba: A Report from the Cornell-Aro Mental Health Research Project* (Ithaca, N.Y.: Cornell University Press, 1963).

Acknowledgments

ALTHOUGH this volume comprises the individual work of fourteen contributors, it represents a common enterprise largely undertaken within one framework. This general acknowledgment therefore supplements the specific acknowledgments that appear in the notes appended to the separate chapters.

The research reported in this book has been sponsored by the Cornell Program in Social Psychiatry, which, in turn, is administratively attached to the Department of Psychiatry in the Cornell University Medical College and to the Department of Sociology of the College of Arts and Sciences in Cornell University. During most of the time when this volume was being developed and written, the Program was also attached to the Department of Anthropology.

The Cornell Program in Social Psychiatry has received financial aid from a number of institutions. The work herein has been mainly supported by a program grant from the Ford Foundation's Behavioral Science Division. The Cornell Program is, however, an outgrowth of the Stirling County Study and the Midtown Manhattan Study. Both these Studies constitute a fundamental background for the projects described in this book. The Stirling County Study was carried out with funds derived primarily from four sources: the Milbank Memorial Fund, the Carnegie Corporation of New York, the Department of National Health and Welfare of Canada, and the Department of Public Health of the Province of Nova Scotia. The Midtown Manhattan Study was given financial aid from the National Institute of Mental Health in the United States Public Health Service, the Milbank Memorial Fund, the Grant Foundation, the Rockefeller Brothers Fund, and the Corporation Trust Company. These foundations are not, of course, the authors, owners, publishers, or proprietors of this book and are not to be understood as approving, by virtue of their grants, any of the statements made or views expressed therein.

In addition to this general support, the following is to be noted. The work represented in Chapter II was made possible by fellowships granted to Charles Savage and Alexander H. Leighton from the Center for Advanced Study in the Behavioral Sciences. A study of Eskimos on St. Lawrence Island, Alaska, is referred to throughout this book and specifically in Chapters II, III, IV, VII, and IX. The 1954–1955 investigation of this population was conducted by Charles C. Hughes and Jane M. Murphy from funds supplied by the Social Science Research Center of Cornell University and by Dr. and Mrs. Rex Murphy. The 1940 study was carried out by Alexander H. Leighton and Dorothea C. Leighton on a joint fellowship from the Social Science Research Council. The study of adolescent symptoms reported in Chapter VI was supported by a grant from the Health Research Council of the City of New York and the Foundations Fund. The Health Research Council is also giving financial backing to the study of childhood symptoms described in Chapter VII. Chapter X reports a comparative analysis of materials gathered in the Stirling County Study and the Cornell-Navaho Southwest Project. Funds for the latter project were given by the Carnegie Corporation of New York.

Several chapters of this book have been written in the light of statistical guidance given by consultants to the Cornell Program in Social Psychiatry. Special acknowledgment is therefore given to Melvin S. Schwartz, David B. Macklin, and John S. Harding.

This book has been reviewed in whole or in part by a number of colleagues. Some of these reviews have been by authors of one chapter for authors of other chapters. Outside the list of contributors and statistical consultants, grateful acknowledgment is made especially to Dr. William T. Lhamon, Professor and Chairman, Department of Psychiatry, Cornell University Medical College, and Dr. Robin M. Williams, Jr., Professor of Sociology, Cornell University, who serve as members of an editorial board for the Cornell Program in Social Psychiatry. Dr. Allan R. Holmberg, Professor and Chairman of the Department of Anthropology, and Dr. Gordon Streib, Professor and Chairman of the Department of Sociology, both of Cornell University, have also reviewed the manuscript. For reading and commenting on particular chapters, appreciation is expressed to Robert Ascher, Charlotte Babcock, David V. Becker, Laurel H. Hodgden, Alice L. Nangeroni, and Peter Stokes.

Technical assistance has been given by Veronica A. Shaw and Marlene Mandel. Administrative and secretarial help has come from Amorita Suarez, Dee Watt, Norma Bain, and Donna Hamilton.

For all this aid and assistance, the editors and the authors express sincere thanks.

Biographical Notes on Contributors

GLORIA J. BERK is presently a psychotherapist in private practice. Mrs. Berk received a master's degree from the Smith College School for Social Work. Before joining the staff of the Payne Whitney Adolescent Psychiatric Out-Patient Clinic of the New York Hospital, she participated in the work of the Bureau of Mental Hygiene in Hartford, Connecticut, and the Co-ordinated Community Mental Health Clinics of Brooklyn.

CHARLES C. HUGHES, Professor of Anthropology and Director of the African Studies Center at Michigan State University, received his Ph.D. degree in anthropology from Cornell University. Dr. Hughes has been a Fellow at the Center for Advanced Study in the Behavioral Sciences and has done field research in Nova Scotia, Alaska, Liberia, and Nigeria. His publications include *An Eskimo Village in the Modern World* (Cornell University Press, 1960) and co-authorship of *People of Cove and Woodlot* (Basic Books, 1960) and *Psychiatric Disorder among the Yoruba* (Cornell University Press, 1963). He has published articles on Eskimo culture, cultural change and social psychiatry in such journals as the *American Anthropologist, Current Anthropology*, and the *Journal of Social Issues*.

THOMAS S. LANGNER, Assistant Professor of Psychiatry (Sociology) at the New York University School of Medicine, received his Ph.D. in sociology from Columbia University. Dr. Langner has done anthropological research in Mexico and the American Southwest; race relations research for the Anti-Defamation League; propaganda analysis for the Voice of America, and studies of the aged. He is currently engaged in a program of interdisciplinary research at New York University, Department of Psychiatry. His publications include contributions to many scholarly journals as well as co-authorship of *Five Hundred Over Sixty* (Russell Sage, 1956), *Mental Health in the Metropolis* (McGraw-Hill, 1962), and *Life Stress and Mental Health* (The Free Press of Glencoe, 1963).

ALEXANDER H. LEIGHTON, Director of the Cornell Program in Social Psychiatry, is Professor of Psychiatry (Social Psychiatry) at the Cornell University Medical College and Professor of Sociology and Professor of Anthropology at the College of Arts and Sciences, Cornell University. Dr. Leighton received his medical degree from Johns Hopkins Medical School. He has been a Fellow at the Center for Advanced Study in the Behavioral Sciences and the holder of a Reflective Fellowship from the Carnegie Corporation of New York. His publications include *The Governing of Men* (Princeton University Press, 1945), *Human Relations in a Changing World* (E. P. Dutton, 1949), *My Name Is Legion* (Basic Books, 1959), *An Introduction to Social Psychiatry* (Charles C. Thomas, 1960), and co-authorship of *People of Cove and Woodlot* (Basic Books, 1960), *The Character of Danger* (Basic Books, 1963), and *Psychiatric Disorder among the Yoruba* (Cornell University Press, 1963).

DOROTHEA C. LEIGHTON is Clinical Associate Professor of Psychiatry (Social Psychiatry) at the Cornell University Medical College and Senior Research Associate and Lecturer in the Department of Sociology and in the Department of Anthropology of the College of Arts and Sciences, Cornell University. Dr. Leighton received her medical degree from Johns Hopkins Medical School and has done field research among the Navaho, Zuñi,

St. Lawrence Eskimos, and Yoruba. She has been doing epidemiological research in the Stirling County Study, now a part of the Cornell Program in Social Psychiatry. Her publications include co-authorship of *The Navaho Door* (Harvard University Press, 1944), *The Navaho* (Harvard University Press, 1946), *Children of the People* (Harvard University Press, 1947), *The Character of Danger* (Basic Books, 1963), and *Psychiatric Disorder among the Yoruba* (Cornell University Press, 1963).

EDWARD LLEWELLYN THOMAS is Associate Professor of Pharmacology at the University of Toronto and Medical Research Associate at Ontario Hospital, New Toronto. He received his medical training at McGill University. Before the war, he trained as an engineer at the University of London and is at present carrying on his research at the Institute of Bio-medical Electronics, a joint project between the Faculty of Medicine and the Faculty of Engineering at the University of Toronto. Dr. Thomas is also a part-time Professor of Psychology at the University of Waterloo, where he has been teaching a course in Human Factors Engineering in Canada. He has contributed articles to *Science, Canadian Medical Association Journal, Canadian Psychiatric Association Journal, Radiology, Canadian Journal of Psychology, Journal of Aerospace Medicine,* and the *Journal of Projective Techniques.*

JAMES F. MASTERSON, Clinical Associate Professor of Psychiatry at the Cornell University Medical College, is Director of the Research Project on Psychiatric Disorder in Adolescents and is in charge of the Adolescent Division of the Payne Whitney Out-Patient Department. Dr. Masterson received his medical degree from Jefferson Medical College and combines his research interests with part-time practice in psychiatry. He has contributed to journals such as *Psychiatry, Journal of Nervous and Mental Disease, American Journal of Psychiatry,* and *The Medical Clinics of North America.*

JANE M. MURPHY is Assistant Professor of Anthropology in the Department of Psychiatry of the Cornell University Medical College and Research Associate in the Department of Sociology and in the Department of Anthropology, College of Arts and Sciences in Cornell University. Dr. Murphy received her Ph.D. degree in anthropology from Cornell University and has done field work in Alaska, Nova Scotia, and Nigeria. She contributed to the research of the Stirling County Study and is currently with the Cornell Program in Social Psychiatry. Her publications include collaboration on *An Eskimo Village in the Modern World* (Cornell University Press, 1960), co-authorship of *Psychiatric Disorder among the Yoruba* (Cornell University Press, 1963), and articles on cross-cultural psychiatry and psychotherapy in *World Mental Health*, the *Milbank Memorial Fund Quarterly*, and *Magic, Faith, and Healing*, edited by Ari Kiev (The Free Press at Glencoe, 1964).

SEYMOUR PARKER, Associate Professor of Anthropology and Associate Professor of Social Science at Michigan State University, was formerly a cultural anthropologist in the Department of Psychiatry of the Jefferson Medical College. He received his Ph.D. degree in anthropology from Cornell University, and his field work includes research in Nova Scotia, New Mexico, and Alaska. He has also participated in studying the social structure of a mental hospital in England, and is currently working on a study of mental health among Negroes in Philadelphia. Dr. Parker has contributed to many journals such as the *American Anthropologist, American Sociological Review, Psychiatry, Ethnology,* and *Human Relations*.

TOM T. SASAKI is Associate Professor in the Department of Sociology, University of New Mexico. His Ph.D. degree in sociology was received from Cornell University. He has done field work among the Navaho and the Jicarilla Apache and has served as a social science consultant to the Navaho Indian

Tribe as well as to various training and extension programs in the American Southwest. Dr. Sasaki was formerly Field Director of the Cornell-Navaho Project in Technological Change. He is the author of *Fruitland, New Mexico: A Navaho Community in Transition* (Cornell University Press, 1960) and has published articles about the American Indians in the *American Anthropologist, Journal of Social Issues, Rural Sociology, New Mexico Business,* and other journals.

CHARLES SAVAGE is Director of Research, Spring Grove State Hospital, Baltimore, Maryland. Dr. Savage received his medical degree from the University of Chicago and is a graduate of the Washington School of Psychiatry and a member of the American Psychoanalytic Association. He has been a Fellow at the Center for Advanced Study in the Behavioral Sciences; earlier he was Acting Chief of the Adult Psychiatric Branch of the National Institute of Mental Health. He has had field experience among the Navahos in New Mexico and the Yoruba of Nigeria and has contributed papers to numerous journals such as *American Journal of Psychiatry, Journal of Nervous and Mental Disease, Archives of Psychiatry and Neurology, Psychoanalytic Review, Diseases of the Nervous System,* and *Psychiatry.*

MARIE-LOUISE SCHOELLY is Clinical Assistant Professor of Psychiatry in the Division of Child Psychiatry of the Cornell University Medical College. She received her medical education at the University of Zurich, Switzerland, and took her psychiatric residency at the Psychiatric University Clinic in Basel, Switzerland. She is currently engaged in research concerning psychiatric symptoms in childhood and also practices psychiatry in New York City. Dr. Schoelly has written on the use of curare in electroshock therapy and on psychosis associated with tetany in such journals as the *Journal of American Physical Medicine* and the *Monthly Review of Psychiatry and Neurology.*

ALBERT C. SHERWIN is Clinical Associate Professor of Psychiatry in the Department of Psychiatry and Director of the Division of Child Psychiatry in the Cornell University Medical College. He received his medical degree from Columbia University Medical College of Physicians and Surgeons. In addition to a part-time practice, Dr. Sherwin is doing research on childhood symptoms. He has published articles on the relationship between psychopathology and music as well as papers on various psychiatric disorders found in children in journals such as the *American Journal of Psychiatry, Journal of Nervous and Mental Disease, Bulletin of the New York Academy of Medicine,* and the *Journal of Chronic Diseases.*

KENNETH F. TUCKER, who received his medical degree from Cornell University Medical College, is a Clinical Instructor in Psychiatry at that institution. Currently he devotes the major part of his time to the private practice of psychiatry. He has participated in the research on adolescence conducted at the Payne Whitney Clinic. He has contributed to the *American Journal of Psychiatry.*

Contents

Part Two. Assessing the Sociocultural Environment

Charts

Figures

Tables

Part One

IDENTIFYING AND SURVEYING PSYCHIATRIC DISORDERS

I: Cross-cultural Psychiatry

By Alexander H. Leighton and Jane M. Murphy

IF one takes a broad definition of social psychiatry, then it is appropriate to regard cross-cultural psychiatry as occupying a position within this field and as focusing on certain aspects in certain ways.[1] The point of attention is the relationship between two orders of phenomena: psychiatric disorders and sociocultural environment. As areas of interest, the fields of social and cross-cultural psychiatry rest on the assumption that there *is* an interdependence between psychiatric and sociocultural processes that is in some measure distinct from the relationships between psychiatric processes and organic experiences or heredity.

It is well recognized, however, that such compartmentalizations are as false to phenomena in psychiatry as they are in other fields of human science. The old arguments about heredity versus environment and body versus mind have been set aside if not settled in the twentieth century, and it is generally accepted that human functioning cannot be adequately comprehended if viewed from one orientation to the exclusion of others. Nonetheless, a division of the total problem into subfields such as cross-cultural psychiatry facilitates the organization of ideas along lines that are amenable to research and that utilize the concepts and skills of different disciplines. Current specialization of focus is thus justified by the intention of achieving an ultimate convergence in which fuller understanding of psychiatric phenomena will be reached through a number of perspectives.

Within the broad framework of interest in causes of psychiatric disorder it is not only permissible but useful to ask what is more and what less important. The goal may be heuristic understanding or it may be a desire to modify and control. In the latter case the investigator is concerned with the major obstacles to be overcome and opportune points at which to initiate change in the process. Those that promise the most effect for the least effort can be considered the most important whether the phenomenon in question be considered part of genetics, physiology, psychology, cultural processes, or some division or overlapping area in one or more of these.

The purposes of this chapter are, therefore, to explain what we mean by cross-cultural psychiatry, trace briefly its history as a body of thought and investigation, define terms, and list some of the important problem areas.

Nature and History of Cross-cultural Psychiatry

Cross-cultural psychiatry, as conceived here, is a way of observing and ordering facts about the processes of psychiatric disorders by studying people in numbers rather than as individual patients and by comparing the sociocultural processes of different groups of people. There are, as it happens, many groups that can be isolated for comparative analysis within Western society. Thus comparisons can be made between ethnic enclaves that have been transplanted into complex societies.[2] Nonetheless, the full scope of interest in cross-cultural psychiatry is worldwide. It includes concern with people in their native habitats and deals with maximal cultural contrasts, identified (though probably misnamed) by such differentiating terms as "Western" and "non-Western"; "underdeveloped," "developing," and "industrialized"; "primitive" and "civilized."

One problem of basic research is to discover what factors or combinations of factors in the environment produce, encourage, or perpetuate what kinds of psychiatric disorders. A first step toward this end is to sort apart universals and variables. How do the patterning, frequency, and duration of psychiatric disorders vary in the light of sociocultural differences? What psychiatric disorders appear in more or less the same form in many populations—perhaps all—regardless of culture? In view of what is already known, conditions such as mental deficiency, chronic brain syndrome, and some types of schizophrenia appear to exist in all human groups.

A further interest is to discover what relationships various kinds of psychiatric disorders bear (when looked at in cross-cultural perspective) to the universal categories of the human situation—being male, being female, or being at different points in the life-arc of childhood, adolescence, maturity, and senescence. Since there is wide variation in the way cultural groups employ age and sex in defining rights and obligations, the patterning of cultural roles may exert a major influence on the development and distribution of psychiatric symptoms. It follows, therefore, that questions about human universals and cultural differences are fundamental.

Although by no means a new field, cross-cultural psychiatry is still in a formative stage. There is considerable fluidity in defining its problems and a great deal of variability in the terms used to denote its character. In an early phase it was referred to as "primitive psychiatry," and it has also been called "anthropological psychiatry" and "ethnopsychiatry." These designations have usually been employed in connection with studies of various exotic types of psychopathology found in specific cultural groups.

Among anthropologists the field is sometimes known as "psychiatric anthropology," but more commonly it is subsumed under "culture and personality." These titles tend to emphasize an interest in what psychiatry can offer to an understanding of cultural processes and focus attention on the relatively normal development and functioning of personality in different cultural contexts rather than on psychiatric disorders *per se*.

By the welfare-minded and among those involved in the administration of psychiatric services, the field has been included under "public health psychiatry" and "psychiatry for developing countries." These labels clearly indicate a major interest in treatment, control, and—where possible—prevention.

Finally and more specifically the field has been called "cultural psychiatry," "transcultural psychiatry," and, as here, "cross-cultural psychiatry."

This multiplicity of names makes difficult the task of communication and choice of words. The problem indicates the interdisciplinary nature of the topic and the consequent necessity to talk in several languages at once—at a minimum the languages of psychiatry, social science, and public health. It also indicates that the people interested in this subject see the pertinent phenomena from many points of view and may refer to similar ideas by several different terms.

We have selected the term "cross-cultural psychiatry" for two reasons: (1) the phrase adequately conveys the fact that in this field the main conceptual and methodological tool for inquiry is comparative analysis, and (2) "cross-cultural" research is a familiar idea to social scientists in the United States; its use allows us to identify with and draw on the efforts of those who have concerned themselves with cross-cultural research methods.*

Modern scientific endeavor in cross-cultural psychiatry is said to have begun with Kraepelin. He traveled extensively to see whether the "disease" types he had specified could be found in places other than Europe. His attention was primarily, though

---

* It should be noted here that our approach to cross-cultural psychiatry has much in common at a general level with the transcultural psychiatric research being carried out by Wittkower, Fried, and their colleagues in Canada.

not exclusively, directed toward heredity and "racial" tendencies.

Freud [3] was also interested in culture and cultural differences, influenced in this area by such anthropological contemporaries as Tylor, Frazer, and Lang as well as by the Lamarckian tradition in Europe regarding the inheritance of acquired characteristics. He concerned himself with the possibility that racial experience is transmitted through the unconscious to succeeding generations. At root, his ideas were primarily within the framework of evolutional biology as this was conceived at the turn of the century.

Meyer's psychobiological approach [4] included attention to the probable effects of social and cultural factors in personality development and to subsequent patterns of adaptation all along the course of life. Impelled by this interest, he sought out and made himself familiar with the ideas of such men as George Herbert Mead, W. I. Thomas, and William McDougall. He went on later to exchanges with anthropologists such as Edward Sapir, Ruth Benedict, Bronislaw Malinowski, and others.

As the names above reflect, there was considerable expansion of interest in the relationships between personality patterns and cultural milieu from some time in the twenties up through World War II—especially in the United States. By 1950 widespread concern for this field had tapered off somewhat—probably because of the ending of the war. At that time the urgency for seeking the causes of human conflict, especially as they might hinge on cultural differences, began to lessen. In the sixties, however, there are noticeable evidences of some revival.

Before and during the war period, the widened scope of interest was perhaps due more to anthropologists' delving into psychiatric ideas than to psychiatrists' becoming interested in cultural anthropology.[5] The union of the two disciplines for the sake of inquiry is marked by a number of collaborative efforts beginning with the Kardiner and Linton seminars at Columbia University which started in the mid-thirties.[6] Today there is a sizable roster of joint anthropological and psychiatric studies as well as an expanding number of books specifically on this topic.[7]

When at its height the combined approach had a stimulating influence which suffused much of American anthropology. This was not limited exclusively to an interest in mental and emotional problems but appeared in a broadened view of the "whole man" and of human relations in cultural situations. During this period the subfield of "culture and personality" achieved considerable popularity. It acquired academic standing as an area of specialization in the graduate programs of anthropology departments. A number of field investigations were designed for the collection of Rorschach and dream materials. The Oedipal theme and various hypotheses from psychoanalytic theory were taken into field work for examination in different nonliterate cultures. One major effort involved national character studies.

Up until mid-century two trends of thought had been evident in cross-cultural psychiatry. Much of the early psychiatric interest in non-Western groups had been dominated by biological and racial determinism. Later the field of "culture and personality," and with it much of the thinking about psychiatric disorder, was pervaded by cultural determinism. Although acknowledgment was often made to "biological factors," the written and even more the spoken words of many anthropological investigators did not seem to treat these as real. More than this, there was often a feeling that there is something reprehensible about giving credence to hereditary factors as controlling human behavior in any important way. No doubt the reasons for this are manifold, but beyond the myopia common to most specialized interests and resistance to anything that might detract from the feeling of working on the central complex of causes, there were also matters of moral and political belief. At a time when racist ideas were a focus of world struggle, liberal-minded people were reluctant to do anything that might appear to strengthen such a framework for injustice and crime.

The rational basis for cultural determinism rested largely on assumptions of psychological determinism, and this in turn drew heavily on dynamic psychiatry, particularly psychoanalysis. This reliance was, however, somewhat selective, overlooking Freud's fundamental ideas about constitutional factors as well as the more diffuse conceptions of multiple biological influences which permeate much of the rest of psychiatry.

Since World War II there has been a dropping away of insistence on cultural determinism, owing in part to "culture and personality" losing ground as an area of interest. This in turn followed on the realization that a great deal more work was needed in developing and validating research methods. It also stemmed from the growing awareness that quick answers to world problems were not yet on the horizon.

The influence of cultural determinism has also diminished through the advance of knowledge on many relevant fronts. Expanding anthropological field work has clarified both cultural variation and cultural similarities. The early spectacular theories of the relationship between culturally defined child-rearing practices and basic personality patterns have been progressively modified as more solid information about peoples of different backgrounds has accumulated. Equally, demonstrated progress in the fields of genetics and biological determinants is such that it is more difficult for students of personality to ignore. On all these accounts, a fairly balanced cognizance is now given both to cultural and biological considerations and to the interplay between them.

It is obvious, of course, that anthropology and psychiatry have not been the sole contributors to the development of ideas regarding the relationships between sociocultural and psychiatric phenomena. From other branches of behavioral science have come general semantics, communication theory, the concept of role, the concept of class structure, field theory, and reference group concepts. Names such as Alfred Korzybski, Gregory Bateson, Leonard S. Cottrell, Kurt Lewin, Jurgen Ruesch, Robert Merton, and Lloyd Warner help illustrate the point. Learning and conditioned reflex theory have long been potentially important but have had, in fact, relatively little influence in studies of culture and psychiatric disorder except through Dollard and Miller.[8] The ideas from these various fields tend to emphasize *situations* as of etiological importance and, hence, at least indirectly refer to culture.

We have attempted in a recent article to present some of the ideas that have emerged over the last fifty years as to how culture and cultural situations might exert causal or determining influences on psychiatric disorders.[9] These can be summarized by saying that culture has been conceived as:

1. Determining the pattern of certain specific disorders, such as *lâtah* (in Malaya), *koro* (in China), and *witiko* (in the Indian cultures of Northeast America);

2. Producing basic personality types, some of which are especially vulnerable to psychiatric disorder;

3. Producing psychiatric disorders (usually considered latent for a time) through certain child-rearing practices;

4. Having a selective influence on a population's potential for psychiatric disorder as well as the pattern of disorder through types of sanctions and whether "shame" or "guilt" is engendered;

5. Precipitating disorder in an otherwise adequately functioning personality by confrontation with stressful roles;

6. Perpetuating disorder by rewarding it in prestigeful roles such as holy man, witch doctor, or shaman;

7. Precipitating disorder by changing more rapidly than personality systems are able to tolerate;

8. Producing disorder through the inculcation of sentiments (beliefs and values) that produce emotional states damaging to personality, such as fears, jealousies, and unrealistic aspirations;

9. Affecting the distribution of some kinds of disorder through breeding patterns;

10. Influencing the amount and distribution of disorder through patterns of poor hygiene and nutrition.

The above are all couched in terms of possible variations between sociocultural groups such as would result in different frequencies and kinds of disorder. There is also one overarching idea, namely that culture *per se*—that is, any and all cultures—produces a certain amount of psychiatric disorder. This arises because regulation of the basic natural urges in the growing human organism is conceived to be both universal and psychologically injurious. Although sociocultural factors may vary in the degree and extent of their effects from group to group, they have been thought to produce some damage and some disorder in all.

It is apparent that the point in current cross-cultural psychiatry is no longer to prove that culture is a major cause, but rather to ask what kind of a cause it is. So far as the total process in the development of psychiatric disorder is concerned, it would seem best to assume that hereditary, biological, and psychological factors are all three engaged. To claim dominance for one, or for any subarea within one, *as a matter of general theory*, is to express a linear conception of cause and effect which is out of keeping with what we know about all the processes in the world around us. More germane is an approach to the topic that aims to discover and map out the interrelated factors and the nature of their interrelationships.

Definition of Terms

It is appropriate at this point to define "psychiatric disorders" and "sociocultural environment" more precisely.

I. By *psychiatric disorders* we mean all those behaviors, emotions, attitudes, and beliefs commonly regarded as proper for the attention of a psychiatrist.[10] More specifically the term includes brain syndromes, mental deficiency, the functional psychoses, psychophysiological disorders, psychoneuroses, personality trait disturbances, sociopathic behavior, and acute situational reactions. In our use, then, "psychiatric disorder" has a somewhat broader connotation than "mental illness," which is often restricted to the functional psychoses and severe psychoneuroses.

All of these patterns of psychiatric disorder are conceived as process phenomena having origin, course, and outcome which can be fully understood only in relation to the total life history of the individual. We hazard the guess that the disorders most thoroughly affected by sociocultural experiences and therefore most likely to vary according to different sociocultural factors are symptoms of a psychoneurotic and psychophysiologic nature. On the other hand, it is apparent that tendencies toward these symptoms can be part of a person's genetic and constitutional heritage and may be precipitated, maintained, or inhibited by such physiological events as a long illness or sustained malnutrition.

In the predominantly hereditary or organic disturbances, sociocultural factors may be related to cause (and hence influence the prevalence of such disorders) through breeding patterns or patterns of physical hygiene. Furthermore the *functioning* of people with psychiatric disorders which are chiefly of hereditary or physiological origin may relate significantly to the sociocultural setting in which they find themselves. If the sociocultural environment offers protection, makes fewer demands, or has the resources for therapy, the course and outcome of the process may be very different from that in an environment which lacks these properties.

What has been said thus far about psychiatric disorders refers to the province of psychiatry in Western culture. At several points in this volume (especially Chapters II and III) the problems of cultural relativity and variable conceptions of disorder and deviance will be taken up. For the most part this involves comparing Western views with those found in other groups in order to discover the areas of overlap and divergence. As an underlying principle we take an attitude of inclusiveness in these regards just as we do in dealing with the range of psychiatric phenomena as defined in Western thought.

While systematic studies are needed to reveal the kinds of

behavior that are considered normal and abnormal in different cultural groups, it seems unnecessary to waver in the face of cultural relativism as though we completely lacked valid standards of functioning. As a beginning there is evidence that some disorders are so impairing as to command recognition in any society no matter what its cultural patterning.

We do not mean to imply that all beliefs and knowledge about the causes and cures of psychiatric disorders can be put on the same plane. The distinction between magical and scientific explanations obviously remains a necessary and fruitful one. But the fact that they are quite different orders of explanation, and involve contrasting ways of dealing with events, is not reason for ignoring either one. The belief that one has been "hexed" through witchcraft is clearly apposite as a background feature in some kinds of psychiatric disorders just as is the fact that magic-oriented therapy is apparently effective in some instances.

Our concern for the moment, however, is less with ideas of cause and methods of cure than with the question of what forms of emotion, belief, and behavior are considered psychiatric in other cultural streams of thought. For basic research it is unwise, we believe, to allow the definition of the phenomena to be colored by etiological assumptions and views of treatment emerging from our own tradition *or* other traditions. To *discover* further information about causal factors, which can then be employed in developing methods of prevention and therapy, is the major reason for conducting the kinds of research that constitute the topic of this book. This very fact argues strongly against building preconceptions of cause into the definition of the phenomena about which we are making inquiry in order to avoid a later situation in which real findings would be obscured by dazzling correlations we ourselves inserted.

II. In using the phrase *sociocultural environment* we employ a combination of concepts thought to be advantageous for the kinds of studies discussed here. It is a combination that provides a way of talking about the total configuration of what is going on outside the individual organism whose psychiatric character-istics are of concern.

Certain important distinctions between "society" and "cul-ture" need to be emphasized in studies focusing strictly on social structure or strictly on cultural processes. In a recent paper Kroeber and Parsons point to a confusion about what is social and what cultural that has not yet been clarified and that "is frequently glossed over by the use of the term socio-cultural with full awareness that the hyphen is no symbol of integra-tion." [11] It is equally to be recognized, however, that in any empirical situation the two are intertwined and that many times the differences cannot be fully specified. For the purpose of investigating the relationships between psychiatric phenomena as characteristic of individual personalities and the many environ-mental factors that impinge upon them, we have found it more appropriate to combine than to separate the two components.

Following customary usage, "society" is defined as a group of human beings who live together in a system of social relation-ships. Except for a minuscule and presumably diminishing num-ber of hermits, all human beings live in social groups. Although this definition and generalization are widely accepted, it is not immediately evident just what kinds of groups or what aspects of groups should be studied for characteristics that may have significance in psychiatric disorder. There are short-lived groups and long-lived (a committee or task force as compared to a town). There are small groups and large (families as compared to national units). There are artificial and institutional as well as natural groups (a mental hospital as compared to a community). And there are homogeneous and heterogeneous groups (a tribe as compared to a city). These different characteristics influence the degree and kind of system of relationships by which the group operates, but all, at one or another level of generalization, can be said to exhibit the structural and functional qualities of a social system.

Psychiatric studies are currently going on in nearly all these contexts. In cross-cultural psychiatry we have elected to focus on perduring and culturally cohesive groups localized in natural geographic habitats. There are, however, several questions about choosing a group and setting analytic boundaries around it for study purposes, which together with the problem of population mobility will be taken up in Chapter VIII.

"Culture" is an abstraction which encompasses the total way of life of a society. It is a precipitate of the group's history and expresses its adaptation to the physical environment. It is characterized especially by what A. I. Hallowell has called a "psychological reality." [12] That is, it refers to the shared patterns of belief, feeling, and knowledge—the basic values, axioms, and assumptions—that members of the group carry in their minds as guides for conduct and the definition of reality. Along these lines C. P. Snow has observed: "Without thinking about it, they respond alike. That is what a culture means." [13] And Ruth Benedict has spoken of "the unconscious canons of choice" that characterize one group in contrast to another. [14]

Besides social relationships, technology, economics, religion, and other aspects of human life, culture refers to the interconnections and interdependencies that bind part to part to make a whole. Culture is constantly changing; it is learned; it is transmitted from one generation to the next; and all societies have it. The style, however, varies from one group to another. When the variation between groups is marked it is appropriate to speak of different cultures.

Combining "sociocultural" with "environment" emphasizes that the milieu for any given individual is composed of other individuals who share similar or reciprocal sociocultural experiences. This usage of terms also underscores the fact that the group as a whole exists in particular physical circumstances of climate, altitude, natural resources, and the presence or absence of noxious agents, such as the tsetse fly, which produce endemic disease. That these factors may be relevant to cross-cultural psychiatry is demonstrated in localizations of psychiatrically important diseases such as trypanosomiasis in Africa.[15] In the same way, one must also consider theories such as those that propose a relationship, for example, between the inclemency of the arctic environment, and the various manifestations called "arctic hysteria." [16] Thus, similar to the definition of psychiatric disorders, our view of environment is made broad enough to include multiple types of sociocultural factors that may be causally related to different kinds of disorders.

Problem Areas in Cross-cultural Psychiatry

This volume makes no attempt at being comprehensive. However, underlying the various approaches three main problem areas may be noted.

1. COMPARATIVE STUDY OF DIAGNOSTIC ENTITIES

Within Western culture we are accustomed to comparing patients with each other. The results of psychiatric examinations, history-taking, and continuing observation of various cases are laid side by side in clinical analysis. Groups of cases with similarities and differences may thus be assembled with further comparative analysis and tests, all aimed at elucidating the character of the underlying psychological processes. It is through this method of essentially qualitative analysis that most of what we understand about psychiatric disorder has been derived.

What happens when this procedure is extended between cultures? Can it be rendered more objective and susceptible to quantitative treatment? What can be learned as to the potentialities and limitations of cultural influence? These problems of diagnostic entities are taken up mainly in Chapters II and III.

2. COMPARATIVE EPIDEMIOLOGY

As applied to psychiatry, comparative epidemiology refers to the study of prevalence or incidence of disorder in different populations. Such study has several uses.

First, it helps in the planning of services, both as to kind and as to distribution.

Second, it helps add to scientific knowledge. In cross-cultural studies we are at the edge of a virtually unknown continent; and hence there is a primary need for observation and information collecting. Epidemiology is one systematic way of doing this. If done successfully, it will lay a quantitative baseline from which all manner of other studies can be carried out, for it deals with one of the first questions that has to be asked in comparing psychiatric disorder in two or more cultures, more or less regardless of what the ultimate aim may be.

Third, epidemiology may be used as an instrument for exploring causes. By studying populations with different cultures we may find associations between certain cultures or subcultures on the one hand and the distribution of certain types of psychiatric disorder on the other. The demonstration of such associations is then a basis for additional comparative studies, designed to elucidate reasons, together with longitudinal and experimental investigations. We can clarify theories of cause by making them a basis for predicting findings and then checking prediction by means of epidemiological surveys.

Discussions of the problems connected with comparative epidemiology thread throughout this book but are especially prominent in Chapters IV, V, VI, VII, and XI.

3. COMPARATIVE STUDIES OF PERSONALITY
AND PERSONALITY FORMATION

While the first two problem areas concern the frankly pathological or at least deviant, comparative study of personality in different cultural settings implies an interest in normal processes. What can be learned about personality from comparative studies of "nature's experiments" through data collecting and analysis?

Attacks on this question have led in the past to a wealth of ideas and the development of theory, but, as noted earlier, effort has dwindled since the war. One reason is probably the difficulty of making studies in a variety of cultural contexts that are sufficiently explicit and factual to permit a satisfying comparative analysis for checking theories. It is plain that we need operative theories that can be more easily converted into research practice, better systems by which to identify and classify the phenomena of interest, and better instruments with which to detect and count. Dealing with these needs would seem to be the next steps beyond present work with projective tests, symbolic interpretations, descriptions of child-rearing practices, and the reporting of isolated life histories.

These topics will be discussed chiefly in Chapters IX and X, although the chapters on children and adolescents (VI and VII) are indirectly pertinent.

Approaches to all the problem areas just outlined are closely related. Quantitative information about the distribution of disorders and their trends in time is necessary for an understanding of the meaning of personality studies as well as for comparative case analysis. One may regard the personality studies and the clinical case studies as being at the intensive end of a series of related problems that has epidemiology at the extensive end. The intensive studies leave unanswered questions as to how far one can generalize. The extensive studies, on the other hand, leave us unsatisfied about underlying meaning. When the intensive can be set in the context of the extensive, and both in a knowledge of the relevant sociocultural systems, areas of doubt may be reduced and sets of findings mutually illuminated.

Notes

1. A. H. Leighton, J. S. Clausen, and R. N. Wilson, eds., *Explorations in Social Psychiatry* (New York: Basic Books, 1957); see also A. H. Leighton, *An Introduction to Social Psychiatry* (Springfield, Ill.: Charles C. Thomas, 1960); and "Culture and Mental Health," in *Trends in Modern American Society*, C. Morris, ed. (Philadelphia: University of Pennsylvania Press, 1962).

2. E. D. Wittkower, and J. Fried, "Some Problems of Transcultural

Psychiatry," in *Culture and Mental Health*, M. K. Opler, ed. (New York: Macmillan, 1959).

3. S. Freud, *Totem and Taboo* (New York: New Republic, Inc., 1931).

4. A. Meyer, *Psychobiology: A Science of Man*, compiled and edited by E. E. Winters and A. M. Bowers (Springfield, Ill.: Charles C. Thomas, 1957).

5. C. Kluckhohn, "The Influence of Psychiatry on Anthropology in America during the Past One Hundred Years," in *Personal Character and Cultural Milieu*, D. G. Haring, ed. (Syracuse: Syracuse University Press, 1956), pp. 485–533.

6. A. Kardiner, *The Individual and His Society* (New York: Columbia University Press, 1939); see also Kardiner, R. Linton, C. Du Bois, and J. West, *The Psychological Frontiers of Society* (New York: Columbia University Press, 1945).

7. The literature on psychiatric problems in different cultures is reflected in numerous articles published in professional journals as well as a number of books. The following is a selection of books that indicate part of the coverage of world areas or that deal with problems in cross-cultural psychiatry and have bibliographies that might be useful: R. Linton, *Culture and Mental Disorders* (Springfield, Ill.: Charles C. Thomas, 1956); J. W. Eaton, and R. J. Weil, *Culture and Mental Disorders: A Comparative Study of the Hutterites and Other Populations* (New York: The Free Press of Glencoe, 1955); M. K. Opler, ed., *Culture and Mental Health* (New York: Macmillan, 1959); J. C. Carothers, *The African Mind in Health and Disease* [Monograph Series No. 17 (Geneva: World Health Organization, 1953)]; M. K. Opler, *Culture, Psychiatry, and Human Values: The Methods and Values of a Social Psychiatry* (Springfield, Ill.: Charles C. Thomas, 1956); N. Kline, ed., *Psychiatry in the Underdeveloped Countries*, Report of Roundtable Meetings, Atlantic City, N.J., 116th Annual Meeting of the American Psychiatric Association (Washington, D.C.: American Psychiatric Association, 1960); E. A. Weinstein, *Cultural Aspects of Delusion: A Psychiatric Study of the Virgin Islands* (New York: The Free Press of Glencoe, 1962); M. J. Field, *Search for Security: An Ethno-Psychiatric Study of Rural Ghana* (Evanston, Ill.: Northwestern University Press, 1960); P. M. Yap, *Suicide in Hong Kong*, with special reference to attempted suicide (New York: Oxford University Press, 1958); G. M. Carstairs, *Twice Born: A Study of a Community of High-Caste Hindus* (London: Hogarth Press, Ltd., 1957).

8. J. Dollard, and N. E. Miller, *Personality and Psychotherapy* (New York: McGraw-Hill, 1950).

9. A. H. Leighton, and J. M. Murphy (formerly Hughes), "Cultures as Causative of Mental Disorder," *Milbank Memorial Fund Quarterly*, vol. 39 (July 1961).

10. A. H. Leighton, *My Name Is Legion: Foundations for a Theory of Man in Relation to Culture* [Vol. I, The Stirling County Study of Psychiatric Disorder and Sociocultural Environment (New York: Basic Books, 1959)].

11. A. L. Kroeber, and T. Parsons, "The Concepts of Culture and of Social System," *American Sociological Review*, vol. 23, no. 5 (Oct. 1958).

12. A. I. Hallowell, *Culture and Experience* (Philadelphia: University of Pennsylvania Press, 1955).

13. C. P. Snow, *The Two Cultures and the Scientific Revolution* [The Rede Lecture, 1959 (New York: Cambridge University Press, 1959)], p. 11.

14. R. Benedict, *Patterns of Culture* (Boston: Houghton Mifflin, 1934).

15. J. C. Carothers, *op. cit.*

16. S. Novakovsky, "Arctic or Siberian Hysteria as a Reflex of the Geographic Environment," *Ecology*, vol. 5 (1924), pp. 113–127.

II: The Problem of Cross-cultural Identification of Psychiatric Disorders

By Charles Savage, Alexander H. Leighton, and Dorothea C. Leighton

EDITORIAL NOTES

The questions posed in the present chapter arise from the relationship of psychiatric disorder to culture. Psychiatric activities and ideas form a subpattern within the family of Western cultures, and the definitions of psychiatric disorders have their base in Western views about what human nature is or ought to be. As phenomena, the disorders are patterns of behavior and feeling that are out of keeping with cultural expectations and that bother the person who acts and feels them, or bother others around him, or both. Since, however, different cultures are by definition different systems of standards and expectation, it follows that what may be disturbing in one culture may be regarded as desirable in another. Thus the man or woman who in America is hospitalized for hearing voices or jailed for his sexual activities might have this behavior ignored, accepted, or even venerated in some other cultural group.

An extreme proponent of cultural relativity, using this line of argument, could deny the possibility of identifying and enumerating the same kinds of psychiatric disorder in markedly different cultures. Any pattern of behavior, so the argument might run, is healthy or sick only to the extent that it is so defined by a given culture. Certain patterns of behavior may be defined as psychiatric disorder in the West, but it does not follow that they will be so defined in another culture. Conversely, behavior patterns that we regard as normal or admirable may be defined in other cultures as abnormal. The greater the contrast, furthermore, between cultures, the more radical these discrepancies are apt to be. To speak, then, of "the same psychiatric disorder in two different cultures," is virtually self-contradictory.

Such an extreme view with regard to cultural relativity embodies two rather doubtful assumptions. One is that the possibilities for variation among cultures is limitless. The second, which is more or less necessary to the first, is that personality is infinitely plastic, that all of us as we begin life are capable of every form of human behavior and feeling. With regard to the first, despite the considerable variation evident among known cultures the range does not appear to be boundless. On the contrary, the evidence suggests that there are denominators and limitations common to all sociocultural systems. This applies not only to certain specific patterns such as the incest taboo, but also to larger functional attributes. There are, for instance, no cultural groups known that lack patterns of leadership and followership, or that have no set of rules regarding what is right and what is wrong.

In a similar way one may argue that the evidence available is against a theory of infinite plasticity in personality. It would seem more probable that there are some biological factors at work that influence the norms and deviations of personality found in any sociocultural group. Hence, from the point of view of psychiatry we may say that although cultures differ, there are some characteristics common to all cultures and hence also universal forms of deviance. The mentally deficient, the person who kills *indiscriminately*, and the person who exhibits *uncontrolled* excitement are possible examples.

If, however, one rejects an extreme view with regard to cultural relativity, he must also on the basis of available anthropological evidence reject a corresponding extreme of biological determinism. Some behavior pertinent to psychiatry is relative to culture, and cultural differences must enter to some extent into the definitions and perceptions of psychiatric disorders. The problem then is: If we start with our traditional Western definitions of disorder and the criteria by which we recognize them, how far can we go with these into other cultures with some hope of being able to identify comparable phenomena?

THIS chapter attempts to point out a lattice of criteria whereby psychiatric disorders as they occur among adults may be recognized outside the European family of cultures. As noted in the first chapter of this book, a reason for this interest is the hope of discovering something about etiology. We want to use prevalence and incidence studies as a way of gathering evidence about what kinds of sociocultural factors influence the origin, the course, and the outcome of psychiatric disorders.

As soon as one begins to define the criteria of disorder, however, he becomes aware of an enormous number of difficult questions. They buzz about in the mind and in the air of discussion, coming and going from here and there, disturbing, insistent, and unconnected—or perhaps connected only dimly by unclear premises.

In part the problem arises from the language of psychiatry itself, which, although technical, is often neither precise nor consistent. Moreover, many of the terms for disorders and even symptoms imply theories of cause, so that it is difficult to separate reference to phenomena from reference to etiological ideas.

This distinction is, of course, of fundamental importance when you wish to examine the phenomena in order to develop and check the ideas.

Another set of questions hovers around the matter of deviance and conformity. Deviance from cultural expectation is a characteristic common to most behavior recognized in our society as psychiatric disorder, and it would seem desirable as one criterion in any definition of disorder in another culture. By itself, however, deviance is far from being an adequate guide. The comment of Sapir [1] on the Indian, Two Crows, who denied that two and two make four was: "We suspect that he is crazy." On the other hand, perhaps Two Crows was a mathematical genius who had transcended the ordinary rules of counting. A person may also be considered as deviant by members of his cultural group as a result of accidental events; in some tribes, for instance, a man who had the bad luck to lose two wives and six children through sickness might be regarded finally as a witch, and hence deviant.

Turning the coin over, we must also observe that just as deviance from cultural standards is not sufficient evidence of psychiatric disorder, so conformity and adaptation are not sufficient evidence of its absence. It is possible for roles to be filled by persons whom we as clinicians would say were psychoneurotic or schizophrenic. In talking with Navahos we have noted that impairment from senility was not perceived as either illness or deviance, but rather a part of the expected behavior (role) of older people.

A similar problem arises from the fact that in the diagnosis of psychiatric cases there are sociological, biological, and psychological parameters, any one of which may predominate. This makes it impossible to describe psychiatric disorder in unitary terms and leads the diagnostician to jump from one level of discourse to another. For example, in defining illness we find ourselves with two different and divergent models, the one more or less traditional in clinical medicine, the other statistical.

According to the medical view, if a person has *treponema pallidum* in his system he has syphilis and he is ill. Even if he is not contagious, and is not in any way impaired, he still has syphilis. Furthermore, if everyone else in the community has it so that deviance consists in not having syphilis, he is still considered ill.

This viewpoint also applies to conditions in which there is no recognized specific causal agent—for instance in diabetes, coronary thrombosis, and cancer. The center of disorder in conditions of this sort is considered to be the malfunctioning of some organ or set of organs. In cancer the disorder is in the growth characteristics of cells. It is thought probable, of course, that unknown factors are at work producing these malfunctions, and in some instances there may even be fairly well-founded theories. Cause in this sense, however, is not part of the diagnosis as it is in syphilis and tuberculosis. The agent as a critical factor in diagnosis is replaced by criteria for recognizing the pathology —blood sugar level, electrocardiogram reading, microscopic cell characteristics, and so on.

If we carry this model over into psychiatry then we would say with Knight [2] that a "touch of schizophrenia is like a touch of syphilis," or, if not syphilis, at least like diabetes. But to do this we must have criteria that point infallibly to pathology; they can be more complicated than the blood sugar or electrocardiogram but they must have at least a comparable degree of specificity. At times it almost seems that we have such criteria, but on closer scrutiny they tend to melt away.

A clinical example will serve as illustration. A young woman calls a psychiatrist, asking for an appointment. She complains of backache. She calls again and breaks the appointment, saying she is going south to see her doctor. She shows up for the broken appointment fifteen minutes early. She enters the office furtively. She wears dark glasses. Her hair is slicked back. She sits tensely on the couch and then moves over to a chair by the window. A dark flush creeps up over her neck and face. Even before she has said a word the conviction has formed in the psychiatrist's mind that she is an acute paranoid schizophrenic. She then relates that she has violated a taboo. She has been intimate with a piano salesman. She complains that he was a Communist, that the police are watching her, and that the doctors in a hospital where she was examined for ulcer symptoms have planted a radio in her stomach.

Even if she vomited a radio, many of us would still be inclined to cling to our original diagnosis. Are there not sufficient critical points evident so that one can say: this is schizophrenia, regardless? Yet all the immediate signs and symptoms which we interpret as schizophrenia could point just as well to panic. As a matter of fact, in this patient after two weeks of tranquilizers and psychotherapy all the schizophrenic indicators disappeared and have not returned over a period of several years. They could still recur, and the natural history of the case might eventually establish the patient as schizophrenic, but with periods of remission in symptoms. We know, however, from other cases that it is also possible that the symptoms will never return, or if they do they will again be of brief duration and related to stressful events.

We can go further and say that in some situations her behavior would not be regarded as symptomatic even of panic, but rather as realistic fear—if, for example, she lived in a police state in the midst of a stringent campaign against communism. The "radio in her stomach" might turn out to be an uneducated person's version of some medical maneuver involving the use of radioactive isotopes.

This example demonstrates how illusive the clinical model can be. The same problem occurs, of course, with diagnosis in other branches of medicine, and the difference is one of degree—but the degree in psychiatry is considerable. If psychoneurosis rather than schizophrenia were chosen for illustration, the problem would appear even greater. The idea of disease as a type of malfunction works well so long as the agent causing the malfunction, or a central aspect of the malfunction, or both, can be detected with a high degree of accuracy and reliability. In psychiatry we have difficulty meeting these criteria except where there is an organic condition. Usually what we have to deal with is malfunctional behavior. This immediately raises the question: "Malfunctional according to whom?" There are two broad types of possible answers: those according to cultural expectations, and those according to dynamic theories of psychiatry. If we lean heavily on the first of these, we are back again to the problem of deviance. If we lean on the other, we are building answers into the questions we wish to investigate.

The statistical definition of *normal* and *deviance* is easily explained and easily applied, but if employed independently of concepts about function and malfunction, it brings its own share of difficulties. Strictly applied, it would rule out the possibility of finding the majority of any cultural group to be neurotic. If it were utilized in this manner in other branches of medicine, tonsilitis, sinus trouble, and tooth decay would be obliterated as types of illness because most people have them. In some parts of the world malaria, hookworm, and vitamin deficiency would be similarly eliminated.

We have given here only a bare indication of the questions that can be raised. They are numerous, complex, and entangling; they are also slippery as to foundations and full of hidden premises. It is notable, too, that they cut across each other with introductory expressions such as "But if . . . ," "Suppose you should find that . . . ," "How about a case such as . . . ?"

Now, there are many possible "supposes" and "ifs" that do not exist in nature, and it occurred to us in due time that perhaps some of these were wrong questions. We turned from them, consequently, for the time being and took up a different approach.

What we did was to select one by one each entity recognized as a psychiatric disorder and then we tried to answer two questions: (1) By what criteria would I as a psychiatrist diagnose this condition in a person in our own society and culture? (2) Which of these criteria would I expect to remain employable in most other cultures as well? We did not seek general criteria that would distinguish all disorder from nondisorder, but only criteria for each recognized clinical entity such as mental deficiency, psychoneurosis, and obsessive-compulsive personality. Attention was concentrated on observable phenomena and, to the greatest extent possible, all definitions based on theories of psychological and sociocultural cause were avoided.

The review of criteria was conducted in the autumn of 1957 at the Center for Advanced Studies in the Behavioral Sciences in a series of weekly seminars. Four psychiatrists participated: the authors and Dr. David Hamburg. The guide employed in the deliberations was the 1952 *Diagnostic and Statistical Manual of Mental Disorders*, issued by the American Psychiatric Association. By January 1958 a set of criteria had been developed upon which the four psychiatrists could agree. Hamburg left the Center at this time, but the authors moved on to invite a group of anthropologists to participate in a continuation of the seminar, reviewing the criteria in the light of the cultural group with which each anthropologist was most familiar. The participants were Ethel Albert, Ward Goodenough, Dell Hymes, David Mandelbaum, Milton Singer, and Charles Wagley. The cultural groups that served as the main points of reference were the Rundi of Burundi (Africa), the Eskimos of St. Lawrence Island (Alaska), the Gilbert Islanders (Micronesia), the Navahos (American Southwest), the Tapirepé (Brazil), and the peoples of India.

In June 1958 the criteria were taken by Savage and A. Leighton to Many Farms, Arizona, and reviewed during a two-day session with Dr. Walsh McDermott and his staff, who had run an experimental clinic for Navahos during the preceding three years. Although the Many Farms Clinic was not concerned with psychiatric disorder as such, it had inevitably encountered some cases. The Navaho assistants, particularly the "health visitors," were a valuable source of comment.[3] The criteria offered in the following pages are the upshot of these several steps.

Criteria for Identifying Psychiatric Disorder in Non-Western Cultures

BRAIN SYNDROME

The APA *Manual* divides psychiatric disorder into two major groups: the brain syndromes, which compose mental disturbances resulting from or precipitated by lesions of the brain; and everything else, including mental disturbances in which brain damage is secondary, absent, or never yet demonstrated. The number of categories in each major group is about the same, but the number of cases occurring in nature is far different. The brain syndromes are much fewer. The main reason for their having so many subdivisions is that the causal agents and associated organic malfunctions make it therapeutically useful, interesting, and easy to frame numerous differentiations.

So far as behavior goes, the brain syndrome has the following main components, which are seen in a variety of organic contexts: impairment of orientation, memory, comprehension, ability to learn, and judgment, and manifest lability and shallowness of affect. The latter may take the form of easily provoked crying, unwarranted agitation, irritability, and "corny" joking.

To list all the subcategories of brain syndrome and to discuss their cross-cultural criteria would be lengthy, repetitive, and concerned with only a small proportion of the total instances of psychiatric disorder likely to be found in any general population. We shall therefore handle the matter by taking the commonest subcategory—senile disorders—for more or less detailed discussion and treat selected others in a summary fashion. The remainder will be omitted.

1. SENILE DISORDERS

Within the senile disorders we include the cerebral-cardiovascular difficulties as well as disturbances from the direct aging of the brain. Below are given the items that require consideration in making a diagnosis of senility. The first two are matters of background or contextual evidence. The remaining three are components of senile behavior itself. Since each of these can also occur as a part of other patterns of disturbed behavior, and no single one is essential, it is evident why this disorder is called a syndrome. Its diagnosis consists in eliciting plural evidences and then judging whether these are sufficient to warrant stating that the condition is present.

A. *Age.* For operational purposes, we suggest that a person should be at least fifty years old to be placed in this classification.

The degree to which determination of age is a problem varies from culture to culture. With some peoples, such as the Gilbert Islanders and the St. Lawrence Island Eskimo, birth dates are known and so there is no difficulty. Among others such as the Rundi, the Navaho, and the Tapirepé, nobody is apt to know when he or anyone else in his group was born. In this case approximations can be achieved by finding out the dates of well-known events (great storms, famines, accession of a chief, etc.) and then asking which of these was closest to the birth of the person in question. This method has been used considerably by anthropologists and others in compiling life histories.

In the interpretations of responses about age, one must also be aware that in some cultural groups answers of "young," "old," "middle-aged," or even answers in terms of years such as "about thirty," refer to appearance and status rather than chronological age. We were once told by a Navaho, for instance, that a certain individual five years previously had been "about the same age he is now."

B. *Signs of age.* Usually with senility there is indication of physical wearing out: muscular wasting, general feebleness, dryness and atrophy of the skin, and tortuous, pipe-stem systemic and retinal arteries.

Evidence of this sort is not likely to be difficult to ascertain. Its evaluation, however, may require taking into account particular characteristics of the population under study due to prevailing conditions of diet, disease, climate, and type of work. As is well known, some groups show physical changes earlier than others, and within any group there is also considerable individual variation. In other words, this suggestive concomitant of senility varies as to age of onset, and the syndrome itself may or may not be parallel.

C. *Loss of recent memory with retention of remote memory.* This is an exceedingly characteristic and early manifestation of the senile syndrome.

Standards of memory and ways of checking both recent and remote recall, must, however, be worked out for each culture. The crucial items to employ are those things in which people are customarily interested. A common practice in our own society is for the psychiatrist to learn privately from a family member what the person he is examining had for lunch that day and then ask him. This procedure loses its usefulness in a culture where all meals are the same or in which lunch is not taken. We believe, however, that substitute questions can be devised that will reveal this type of memory impairment.

D. *Habit deterioration.* This refers particularly to matters of personal care, neatness, and cleanliness. It may manifest itself in lack of sphincter control, in sloppiness of dress, care of hair and fingernails, and in eating.

While the standards of proper care must be known for a given culture in order to detect this kind of personal deterioration, there are few if any cultures in the world that do not have such standards. The Tapirepé, for instance, go about nearly naked, yet if a man exposes his glans penis, he is considered to have something wrong with him, and women must be attentive to maintaining proper bodily postures.

E. *Transient confusion.* Here we are concerned with misperception, misidentification of people, and misinterpretation of the environment. The condition is frequently intermittent and brief. During the daytime senile persons may be normal yet during the night wander about, fail to recognize the people they encounter and confuse them with those known in youth. Thurber's grandfather may have been an example of this sort of thing when during the night he shot a policeman, thinking he was a deserter from Meade's army, and then the next day asked his grandson: "What was the idee of all them cops taryhootin' around the house last night?" [4]

There can be little doubt that transient confusion would be noted by the people of virtually any culture, and it seems probable that a history-taking psychiatrist could learn of it if his informants were willing to tell him.

Let us pause a moment to take stock, after this first example, of criteria that might be employed cross-culturally. Within our own society it is perhaps evident that senility is easy to recognize when the condition is advanced and information is available. The criteria are clear enough for that. The diagnosis can be difficult and uncertain in cases where impairment is slight and in situations in which information is withheld, or in which special features conspire to obscure the picture. This latter occurs from time to time with people who through remote memory and habit continue to perform roles they have been carrying out the greater part of their lives. For a long time no one may suspect that they are disoriented for time, place, and person. Thomas [5] mentions this sort of thing among older fishermen, and one of us recalls the case of a professor who lectured so well to his classes that an advanced state of senility was not discovered until he moved to a new house and thereafter could never find his way home. His lectures, it was said, remained for a time unimpaired.

The existence of many borderline cases and the occurrence of the odd one that is obscured by special circumstances do not require that the senile category be written off as too nebulous. If one were to insist on such standards, he would also have to insist on the uselessness of virtually every disease entity and all epidemiology. The point is rather to recognize the limits of precision that are attainable in trying to "count every case" and to focus on research problems that are workable within this level of approximation.

When we turn to the application of the senile criteria to another culture, our expectations must not be higher than the attainable in our own. The same difficulties and risks of error are bound to occur. The question is: Are there more of them, or is there a new and different order of difficulty such as to suggest much greater, or a particular kind of, error?

We cannot generalize to all the cultures of the world, but we can say that for the cultural groups reviewed by our seminar, the answer was no. We do not assert that cultural problems are absent, or that differences in the total count obtained in two different groups might not be due to cultural factors rather than to differences of true prevalence. However, the criteria do have a measure of cross-cultural applicability, and if one wished to identify and count cases in two or more different cultural groups, it is reasonable to believe that through careful study of the particular conditions in each, adaptations could be made such as to yield a useful degree of comparability. One would not, furthermore, need to be in the dark as to the likely sources of error, and ways could be found for evaluating their extent. It would remain true that minor differences could be due to cultural factors just as they could to chance and to variation in technique. Major differences, however, that stood up under repeated surveys and cross-checks on methods and sources of bias, would command serious attention as genuine differences between the populations with respect to senility.

To summarize, it seems that although cultural difference adds to rather than subtracts from an already complex set of problems, it does not appear to present insuperable difficulties, and many of the theoretical problems noted in the introduction to this chapter lose their importance when actual groups are considered. We have not been seriously bothered with questions of clinical versus statistical concepts of normal, of deviance, or of cultural relativity.

It must be admitted, however, that we have begun with one of the easiest syndromes for which to propose cross-cultural criteria. As progress is made to other categories, especially those that have no known organic etiology, it can be expected that the outlook will not remain so comfortable.

2. SOME ADDITIONAL TYPES OF BRAIN SYNDROMES

The conditions to be mentioned here are those due to toxic agents, infections, trauma, nutritional deficiency, disorders of metabolism, and tumor. In all of these, diagnosis depends on discovering and noting the characteristics of behavioral disturbance and identifying the underlying organic condition or agent.

Acute disorders of the brain such as from high fever or the ingestion of some poisons may produce delirium, a fairly clear-cut pattern of behavior. It involves rapid onset, disorientation for place, time, and people, delusions, hallucinations and, outstandingly, fear. When this occurs in the setting of an infection, especially with a high fever, the presumptive evidence of a brain syndrome is so strong that any instances of mistaken diagnosis could hardly have statistical significance. It is reasonable to expect that the same situation would obtain in another culture, the symptoms being what they are and the physical signs of acute infection presenting no particular characteristics apt to be masked by cultural differences.

Delirium without evidence of a concurrent infection is a far different matter diagnostically. There are a wide variety of possible organic causes, and there are nonorganic syndromes such as psychoneurotic dissociation and the acute onset of schizophrenia that may for a time at least be indistinguishable from delirium. The brain syndrome diagnosis then depends on finding the organic cause, or some concomitant neurological evidence of brain damage. Accomplishing this is very difficult among patients of our own culture, and the results are often exceedingly doubtful. With people of other cultural groups there is little ground for expecting it would be either worse or better. The best one can say is that the problem is rare.

The behavioral manifestations of other brain disorders, particularly those that are chronic, are almost infinitely manifold and varied. Here and there occur little syndrome islands of more or less clear symptoms such as the Korsakow, which presents gross memory defect combined with a remarkable capacity to fill this gap with plausible invention. On the whole, however, diagnosis depends not primarily on the identification of particular patterns of behavior, but on finding neurological signs of disturbance and evidence of having taken a known poison; of having a disease that affects the brain, such as syphilis; of having had a serious blow on the head, with some indication of cranial injury; of having physical appearance and history of nutritional deficiency; of having endocrine disturbance; and of having X-ray or electroencephalographic indication of a tumor. Since the behavioral aspects do not raise any questions that have not already been mentioned under senile disorder, or that will not be taken up later, we may pass them by.

The identification of organic trouble within the body that is affecting the brain is usually difficult, except in extreme and far-advanced cases. On the other hand, the procedures involved are objective, and the interpretation of results should not raise questions because of cultural factors. There is, however, the practical question of getting people to submit to all that is involved, and this might be affected by culture. The matter is not always easy among persons of our own society, and one could readily anticipate that it would be much more difficult among people unacquainted with the European brand of medicine.

The identification of possible toxic agents that come into the body from the outside presents a comparable set of problems. To deal with these it would obviously be desirable to learn all one could about the use of alcohol and drugs and the availability of poisons in whatever cultural groups he intended to survey. Thus, the fact that Navahos take Jimson weed (Datura) means they consume stramonium alkaloids. The Many Farms Clinic had seen a case of one severely disturbed girl with a history of eating this plant. She tried to disrobe and run out of the clinic and the doctors had difficulty restraining her. Behavior of this type has been linked with Datura intoxication ever since Captain John Smith's crew was affected at the time Jamestown was founded.

Peyote, which contains mescaline, is another example. The usual clinical picture is of people with widely dilated pupils, perspiring freely, in a trancelike state, living in an internal world from which they can be aroused to perform ordinary functions, but prefer not to.

The main problem, however, about the identification of toxic agents in peoples of other cultures is the possible use of some that are unknown to us, thus leaving the matter exceedingly open-ended. The behavioral aspects of many brain syndromes are nonspecific, and knowledge is incomplete as to the varieties of agents that can produce them. Furthermore, even in the case of those agents that are known, few reliable and valid tests for their presence exist.

These considerations do not appear very important in surveys of psychiatric disorders in general populations of North America, but we have to recognize that they might be in special groups. In approaching other cultures the possibility does exist that brain syndromes of various obscure types are statistically significant. This is a matter to have in mind as a possible research target if a number of cases are discovered which alert suspicion because they do not fit well into the other categories to be described presently, or because the prevalence of one or more categories of these other disorders seems unusually high and might contain unrecognized brain syndromes.

If we look back now at the conclusions reached after considering senile disorder, it is evident that by contrast we have here the likelihood of some major problems as a result of cultural factors. The problem is not, however, a general theoretical stumbling block and does not involve much puzzling over how to recognize abnormal behavior in groups with different standards and systems of sentiment. The problem is much more specific: it consists in the possibility that in some cultural groups it may be customary to consume foods, herbs, and extracts that affect the brain but are unknown to the fields of pharmacology and physiology. The difficulties are not diminished by the fact that some of our own modern drugs, such as iproniazid (for tuberculosis), have turned out to be able to affect brain and behavior in ways not at first realized. Since new drugs are continually coming into use and are being distributed over the world, there is the possibility that some of these may set going one or another kind of brain syndrome.

MENTAL DEFICIENCY

Following the *Manual*'s usage, we include in this classification all grades of retardation. The category as we propose to employ it has no subcategories that parallel those in brain syndrome, only groupings according to degree of impairment. In our culture and society degree is defined by statistical deviation from norms of performance, and this has been highly standardized through tests. It is often expressed as I.Q., with less than 70 being considered an indication of marked handicap, 70 to 85 borderline, and over 85 as reaching into the normal range and above.

Intelligence testing is a highly specialized field, and the problems of comparing persons brought up with different kinds of background, especially cultural, are well recognized. The definitions of normal and subnormal (and supernormal) are much more genuinely statistical than with other types of psychiatric disorder. For this reason and because of the influence of upbringing and experience, each sociocultural group does have to be a measure of itself, where the milder types of deficiency are concerned. This is not, however, necessarily true for more grossly impairing kinds of defect—that is, those where the condition approximates an I.Q. of 70 or under. In almost any culture, we think, behavioral standards could be established that would enable one to single out the grossly defective. The following criteria might be employed for identifying the more obvious degrees of impairment.

A. *History*. A story of growth and development that shows marked delay compared to other children of the same group. We have in mind particularly such matters as age of sitting up, walking, talking, recognizing people, developing commonplace manual skills, and grasping simple instructions.

One difficulty is that culture could involve radically different ways of handling children, so that cross-cultural comparison of the age when walking, talking, and so on occurred would be inappropriate. This is certainly a matter to consider, especially under some conditions, but for the kind of behavior that stands out in the history of persons who have an I.Q. of 70 or less, the issue does not seem significant from the epidemiological point of view. In the cultural groups reviewed by the seminar there were some differences in standard expectations regarding child development, but none of these was great enough to create problems of any serious proportion. The matter was also discussed at some length with a number of Navaho informants and it was evident that they considered slowness in walking and talking as good indicators of retardation ("his mind not strong enough to take care of himself") and that their standards were close to our own.

B. *Current performance*. If tests exist that are standard in the culture, they may help. The degree of retardation being considered here, however, can be detected by very simple questions aimed at checking ordinary levels of memory, counting, information, and puzzle solving. Data can also be gathered from those close to the person as to how he performs in the daily round of work, feeding, dressing, and understanding what people say to him.

One must be alert to the fact that in some cultural groups there are roles for the mentally deficient that might make it difficult to find such persons. Thus, the Buddhist Monastery in

Burma may be a refuge for retarded boys, and being a Sadhu in India could on occasion help conceal retardation.

We conclude that gross manifestations of mental retardation can be identified and that, conversely, mild forms may be very difficult to detect and distinguish from behavior that is cultural rather than the result of intellectual disability. The real problem, therefore, is not whether mental retardation can be identified and compared cross-culturally, but rather, how far upward from the gross toward the mild this identification can proceed. No general answer is likely to be forthcoming, but it does seem probable that standards could be set, at least after field trial, for any two or three particular cultural groups one desired to survey.

PSYCHOSIS WITHOUT DEMONSTRABLE ORGANIC DISEASE

1. SCHIZOPHRENIA

The diagnosis of this condition is vexatious because of the range of opinion among psychiatrists as to what should be included and excluded. At the Second International Congress of Psychiatry in 1957 the focus was on schizophrenia, and much disagreement was in evidence. The range stretched from people with intractable, incurable, irreversible illness to those who manifested only some autistic thinking.

It is, however, possible to select and specify a section within the range, and we have chosen what we believe to be the symptom complex that most American psychiatrists would accept. The criteria are:

A. *Delusions.* A delusion may be defined as a belief at variance with those beliefs or sentiments accepted in the cultural system to which the individual belongs.[6] An understanding of the beliefs characteristic of a culture is therefore mandatory. In most circumstances the presence of a delusion is presumptive evidence of psychosis, and where there is lack of indication pointing to other psychoses, the most likely possibility is schizophrenia. Further, a common feature is that schizophrenic delusions are directed against cultural sentiments and at the same time are strongly influenced by them.

As is evident, the concept of delusion is primarily a matter of cultural definition, and hence confronts us with the problem of cultural relativity. While there may conceivably be some delusions that would be false in all cultures of the world (for instance, that human beings have wings), it is apparent that an effort to catalogue these would not get us very far. It must be accepted that the content of delusions cannot be the basis of epidemiological comparisons between cultures. It would be a delusion if a man in our society were to believe that semen had wandered up into his head and caused his brains to deteriorate. In parts of India, however, this idea is culturally acceptable, and apparently has considerable history in the East, being known in the Ming Dynasty in China. One is reminded of the belief formerly held in Europe that a woman's womb could move up into her throat and choke her. Delusions can, however, be detected against each culture's network of sentiments for defining reality. This means that as instances of sentiments that are out of keeping with culture, they can be counted in two or more groups that have different cultures.

It remains possible, even probable, that the character of the sentiment system in various cultures may exert a differential influence toward obscuring or revealing delusional behavior. Cultures vary not only as to topics, but also as to the degree of sharpness with which they define credibility. How big a problem this amounts to is something for investigation in particular cultures selected for study.

B. *Schizophrenic thinking.* Like dreaming, schizophrenic thinking is symbolic and wish-fulfilling. There is persistent misinterpretation and preoccupation with inner fantasies, so that the person seems to be out of touch with the world. The concrete and the symbolic are characteristically confused, as in the patient who said and literally meant he was "going up in an airplane to get perspective." Although the schizophrenic himself often makes extensive use of symbols, he has difficulty with other people's symbols and is apt to misunderstand metaphor.

This kind of thinking, so characteristic of schizophrenia, is hard to describe, yet recognizable after one has become acquainted with it. The quality of thought is very different from that shown by the person who is senile, mentally deficient, or slowed up by depression. At the same time, it can be expected to present grave problems for an American or European psychiatrist attempting its detection in a language and a cultural background not his own. For these reasons we do not regard it as a strong criterion, and yet we are disinclined to omit it altogether because of its frequency in cases of schizophrenia. It could, furthermore, turn out in some cultures to be less difficult to detect than we now imagine.

C. *Hallucinations.* Whereas delusions consist in false beliefs, hallucinations consist in false sensory perceptions. Auditory hallucinations—for instance, a voice speaking when nobody is there—are probably the commonest, but parallel disturbances of vision, smell, taste, body feelings, and touch also occur.

Cultural sentiments and definitions present some problems in the distinguishing of this phenomenon. In our own society few hallucinations are sanctioned or "believed in" except by some of the smaller religious sects. Among other societies, however, this may not be the case. Hearing voices and having visions may be an expected part of experience and take place on a basis that has nothing to do with schizophrenia or any other psychiatric disorder. One must distinguish, then, in part on the basis of the cultural acceptability and appropriateness of the hallucination. Duration provides another indicator. Many schizophrenic hallucinations are more or less continuous for years, whereas those that arise purely on a cultural basis are apt to have short duration or occur only from time to time as the situation demands.

So far as cross-cultural comparison is concerned, the remarks made in regard to delusions may be repeated here. It is not the reported voice or vision as such that can be counted and compared cross-culturally but the instances in which the voice or vision is out of keeping with the cultural framework.

D. *Schizophrenic actions.* Schizophrenia is primarily a disorder of thinking, but certain individuals develop related characteristic behaviors that are very striking: withdrawal, gesturing, posturing, or lying in a stuporous state. In time there may be habit deterioration and silly, scattered, superficial talk, with manic features but without the manic's wit. Unusual sexual activity may also occur such as chronic and open exposure and masturbation.

The cross-cultural applicability of this criterion scarcely needs comment. Although exceptional instances and possibilities can be pointed out, behavior of this type is usually recognizable as disordered in all the cultures with which we are familiar.

E. *Inappropriate affect.* This means showing emotion that is unsuitable for a given cultural context or failing to show emotion that is expected. Thus, there may be laughing when sadness or solemnity is called for, or there may be a chronic state of exhibiting little or no outward appearance of emotion. This latter is called "flattened affect," and although it is by no means a necessary part of the schizophrenic syndrome, it is sometimes very marked and arrests attention.

This criterion in general should not give too much difficulty across cultural lines. In India, where for many people the whole goal of life is to downgrade affect, there might be some special problems in distinguishing schizophrenic flattening from other kinds. This is not, however, something to be expected frequently in other cultures; and in any event, since the flattening is only one criterion in a syndrome, it could be evaluated along with others in reaching a conclusion as to whether a schizophrenic complex of symptoms was present or not.

F. *Personal history.* Several characteristics may be noted under this heading. One is that the age of onset is generally from the middle teens to the middle thirties. A first appearance of schizophrenic symptoms after forty is exceptional.

The mode of onset has two common alternative patterns. In one, a normal youth suffers a change of personality over a period of a year or so. Although the particulars of this change vary a good deal, it is usually so striking that everyone around the person takes note of it. "The last year in high school Jim got somehow strange. He was always one of the bunch before, but that year he was different. He kept more to himself, and he seemed to be doing a lot of thinking. He wasn't the same guy at all."

The other mode is one in which a person who has always been a bit rigid, withdrawn, proud, and uncompromising gradually accentuates these characteristics beyond the bounds of normal and then begins to show delusions and other frank manifestations of the disorder.

A third possibility is the sudden appearance of schizophrenia in its full-blown form, perhaps first being manifest in a state of excitement and fear. From clinical experience one would say this is much less common.

There do not appear to be any major and general cultural obstacles to our getting personal history data of this type. There are always chance and situational factors, in our own society and in others, that cause the completeness of history to vary from case to case. This does raise questions of case comparability, but it does not promise to be significantly greater cross-culturally than intraculturally.

Considering the schizophrenic criteria as a whole, and recalling again that they constitute a syndrome, so that one looks for a plurality and evaluates each item in relation to the others, it seems that in most cultures one could detect at the very least the level of impairment that we associate with hospitalization. This is confirmed by the fact that, so far as we know, schizophrenia has been found in every cultural group in which people trained in European psychiatry have worked. The problem lies in the gradation from obvious schizophrenia to conditions that are better described as eccentric or maladjusted. There is also the problem that most if not all cultures provide niches in which persons with some of the milder forms of schizophrenia can fit and in which the symptoms of the disorder are part of a role. Schizophrenic thinking expressed in poetry and painting is at times acceptable as art in our own society. We are not hereby diagnosing any artist as schizophrenic because of his abstract or symbolic style, or because of meanings we derive from psychiatric interpretation of his work. Rather, we take the matter from the opposite side and say that we have known schizophrenic patients who did find a market for their schizophrenic thinking and who did circulate in fashionable bohemian circles without their disorder being at first evident in this subculture. One patient in particular, known to one of us, was an outstanding and successful artist and just as outstandingly schizophrenic. This was eventually obvious to his colleagues when he went to live on top of a pillar like St. Simon Stylites and then became mute.

It has often been suggested that what we call schizophrenia might well be an asset in the role of medicine man or Sadhu. Delusions, hallucinations, posturing, and symbolic utterances of unclear meaning might render the incumbent more rather than less effective. From both clinical and anthropological experience we are inclined to doubt very seriously that this often happens. The healer or priest role has its requirements and regulations, and the unusual behavior that goes with it nearly always has its particular context. The role is, in short, most often a highly integrated node in a social system. The schizophrenic's behavior and thinking are not that well controlled or adaptable, at least not in the kind of patients we commonly see. In fact one of the characteristics of the syndrome is the tendency to wander off all the established pathways of society and to break through its fences, no matter how self-defeating this may appear to be. And even where this countersocial or asocial behavior is not marked, the oddness of the schizophrenic may still be apparent to others of his social group even though he may be performing a role that utilizes some of his symptoms. Thus, one of the seminar members said that in India people will tell you that there are three kinds of Sadhus: the quacks, the real thing, and those who are touched in the head.

We may say again, therefore, that between the grossly evident and the almost normal is a considerable range, and the problem is to hit a similar cutting point for the people in any two cultures to be compared. This does not seem impossible, but it does require working out standards for particular cultures, and at present it is probably not possible for cultures in general.

2. PARANOID STATES

We suggest two criteria taken together as definitive of this condition.

A. *Delusions of persecution and/or grandeur*. The meaning of delusion has already been discussed, and the meaning of "persecution" is obvious. "Grandeur" refers to a role far more splendid, powerful, and important than one's actual role; the person who thinks he is Napoleon is the conventional example.

This criterion, then, involves delusions with a particular kind of content.

B. *Hostility toward others*. This is expressed in a tendency on the part of the subject to interpret the entire world in terms of hostility toward himself. Projection is a part of this interpretation—at least in the simpler sense of the word. That is to say, he reads into the acts of others hostile intentions against himself which are actually his own hostility toward them.*

Paranoid behavior is thought of most often as part of the schizophrenic picture, and yet it occurs widely in other disorders such as brain syndrome and depression. That it occurs alone as a chronic disorder with tremendous logical elaborations on the basis of a few false premises—*paranoia vera*—is a matter

* As is well known, Freud employed a much more complicated definition of projection.

open to question. Many if not most psychiatrists believe that this does not happen, but that people who seem at first to have such a condition sooner or later develop additional symptoms of some disorder, usually schizophrenia. Occasionally they turn out not to be delusional at all but to have justification for their views.

Transient paranoid behavior is probably found from time to time in almost everyone. It seems human nature to blame others for what we do not like but find going on within ourselves. Few things are so painful as self-reproach and few are so relieving as righteous indignation.

With regard to cross-cultural identification, it has to be recognized that societies exist in which hostility, suspicion, and what we would call false beliefs of persecution (e.g., by witches) are exceedingly prevalent. Several familiar questions immediately arise. Are we to regard these sentiments and behaviors as cultural patterns which normal individuals learn through growing up in the society, or do we have instead a clinical paranoid state on a mass scale? And if it is a cultural pattern, how can one ever identify the truly paranoid in such a context?

It is easy to puzzle oneself into a state of paralysis by elaborating further questions along this line. The issue often seems the key obstacle to identification and counting of psychiatric disorders in any culture except our own.

But let us note several things. First, the question comes up in this major form with only one complex of psychiatric symptoms, and not with psychiatric disorder generally. Second, paranoid behavior as a clinical entity is a symptom complex which appears as a component in a number of different syndromes, most commonly schizophrenia. It is also seen transiently in people who are not psychiatrically ill. Third, our definition of a delusion is that it is a false belief *according to the standards of the believer's culture*. That a belief is false according to the standards of some other culture including our own does not therefore make it a delusion. Indeed, one of the features of the clinically observed delusion is its resistance to the conforming pressures of the social group. On the basis of these points, we think that culturally patterned sentiments and behavior reflecting hostility, suspicion, and what persons of our culture would call false beliefs of persecution, are not to be equated with a mass paranoid state in any clinical sense of the word. They can rather be considered as more closely related to a normal capacity for paranoid reaction together with the normal process of culture acquisition. It still remains possible that masses of people in a society could in a short time become hostile and delusional in terms of their own cultural standards. One can visualize this as happening at a time of great stress. Whether or not it should be regarded as normal or abnormal would depend on the results of examining the actual situation and on standards set for dealing with this particular phenomenon. But this is a special case, not one that is general in cross-cultural work. We may conclude, therefore, that the problem of mass paranoid state versus cultural pattern loses some of its formidable character if one breaks it down into more specific parts and is careful about definitions.

Let us return to the question of identifying paranoid symptoms in an individual where the cultural background gives prominence to hostility, suspicion, and beliefs of being persecuted. It is important again to keep in mind that the paranoid symptoms comprise only one of several components in the syndromes we are trying to distinguish. Thus if they were part of the schizophrenic syndrome, it would still be possible in many instances to make an identification through other delusions, hallucinations, schizophrenic thinking, withdrawal, posturing, inappropriate affect, or history of personality change. The problem is further reduced by recognizing that a delusion is such in terms of the culture in which it occurs. The conviction that one is bewitched is not a delusion in a witchcraft culture unless there is something about it that does not fit within the range of the accepted pattern.

It is here, of course, that one begins to get into borderline cases, and competent knowledge regarding the cultural range becomes important. Very often the question is not one of specific items as such, but of appreciation of oddity in how they fit together. This may be illustrated by a conversation one of us had with Dr. T. A. Baasher of the Clinic for Nervous Disorders in Khartoum North, Sudan.

A. Leighton asked Baasher how he would distinguish religious delusion from accepted belief among people coming to his clinic. Baasher replied that he could give no general rules, but he could illustrate it with a case he had seen that involved a murder. Some years ago there had been two religious leaders in the neighborhood of Khartoum who were great rivals. A follower of one of the men began to hear voices telling him to kill his master's rival. It seemed to him that the voices came from a divine source and he set out to execute their command. Since he did not know his intended victim by sight, he wandered from place to place relying on the voices to let him know when he had come upon the man. Several times he saw someone he thought was his target, but the voices said, "No." Eventually one evening he entered a village where a number of men were sitting under a tree talking. One was on a chair, playing with some little sticks. The voices said that this was the man. The religious follower protested that surely not, he was just a poor individual, not a great leader. The voices, however, said, "Don't you see? It's a disguise. Kill." So the follower speared him. Later the follower was arrested for murder and then sent to Baasher for examination.

"Now," said Baasher, "it is not out of keeping with this culture for a man to be extremely devoted to a religious leader, nor is it out of keeping for him to undertake to kill on his master's behalf, and of course he could make a mistake and kill the wrong man, as this disciple did. It is within the cultural range for a religious man to hear voices that tell him to do things, and for him to go and do those things. But the way all these elements fitted together in this case did not make sense. This is especially so since the two religious leaders in question had made up their differences and been friends for over a year prior to the murder.

Item by item, there is nothing that was counter to the culture, but the whole reflected odd thinking, like the Knight's move in chess. I thought he was a paranoid schizophrenic from the story, and examination brought this out."

3. DEPRESSION AND MANIC STATES

The prototype of depression is grief. As a pathological reaction it is characterized by excessiveness and inappropriateness for the situation and for the standards of the culture. Thus it may appear where there is no external cause, where the cause is insufficient, or where the gloom in relation to the cause is excessively prolonged. The sense that it is inexplicable is often very strong. This is perhaps what Shakespeare had in mind when he had Antonio say:

> In sooth I know not why I am so sad;
> It wearies me; you say it wearies you;
> But how I caught it, found it, or came by it,
> What stuff 'tis made of, whereof it is born,
> I am to learn;
> And such a want-wit sadness makes of me,
> That I have much ado to know myself.

Criteria may be stated as: weight loss; sleep disturbance, especially early-morning awakening; constipation; poor appetite; amenorrhea; the subjective feelings of gloom, guilt, poor concentration, and difficulty in thinking; and an objective slowing up of behavior. Throughout the occurrence of such symptoms there is no adequate cause in common-sense terms or by the standards of the culture. Suicidal preoccupations and acts are common. There is often a twenty-four-hour variation, with the worst feelings being in the early morning and improvement occurring toward evening. In some cases negativism and hostility to others as well as to self may be very marked. In a few there are delusions of having committed some unforgivable act or delusions of a somatic type such as having no intestines or blood.

Some depressions are cyclical, so that the patient has a life story of disabling periods with normal performance between, or occasional episodes of manic excitement. Such a history of alternating mania and depression is, or course, indicative of the classic manic-depressive psychosis. This pattern, however, even if classic, is not by any means common.

A number of other subdivisions are also employed in clinical thinking, but we may consider these as too detailed or specialized for the purpose of the present chapter.

The manic state is sometimes not too easy to distinguish from a schizophrenic excitement. Euphoria, humor, and joking are the hallmarks, and like depression the state of excitement may be episodic. Sometimes it is set off by a situation, but then it becomes detached from the situation and goes on and on. Behavior is unconventional and some of the most strict taboos of the society may be broken. The expression of the emotions and of energy takes precedence over convention. Outstandingly there is overactivity. The person is busy all the time, and his busyness is disorganized and distractable like that of a monkey. There is a great deal of playfulness with bursts of anger and hostility if frustrated; and as with the depression there is, as a rule, a lot of difficulty with sleep.

In their full-blown form, both depression and manic states can probably be recognized in any culture. Again, however, protective coloration may be afforded by certain cultural backgrounds. How do you detect depression among people of a generally gloomy culture—as is alleged by some writers to be the situation in India? Or manic states where the culture has a high level of excitement, as is said to be the case in parts of Africa? The problem is the one discussed previously as the borderline case. Culture adds to the difficulty of differentiation, but not necessarily in an overwhelming manner. As with delusions, the standards for "excessively" depressed or elated behavior have to be worked out within each cultural framework. The number of instances, on the other hand, may be open to cross-cultural counting and comparison.

As for the cultures familiar to those participating in the seminar, it was felt that depression and manic conditions probably did occur in all of them. On the other hand, we took note that several clinical studies in Africa reported depression as exceedingly rare and excitement as very common by comparison with Europe and North America.

PSYCHOPHYSIOLOGIC CONDITIONS

These are disorders that are primarily organic in their manifestations and consequences, but in which there are important psychological causes. Clinical studies in Europe and America point to certain symptom complexes as being frequently of this nature. On such a basis we suggest that the following types of illness deserve attention: skin eruptions of the eczematous type, asthma, hay fever, hypertension, hypotension, peptic ulcer, and colitis.

No interferences from cultural factors are to be anticipated in distinguishing these symptoms. The necessary information can be obtained by physical examination and fairly simple questions about personal history.

On the other hand, major difficulties are likely to appear when one tries to establish the role of psychological events as cause. This matter is always difficult, requiring exhaustive investigation in every case, and even then one may not be able to produce strong evidence one way or the other. Cultural differences would surely make the problem worse. Added to this is the possibility that a high morbidity rate of chronic diseases, such as exists in many parts of the world, could well serve to mask those disturbances that have a major psychological component in their etiology. There is also the open question as to which organic syndromes commonly involve psychological factors to a significant degree. Clinical opinion ranges from implicating them in practically all disorders (through such mechanisms as lowering resistance) to a more limited list such as that given above. In cultures other than our own it could well be that a different set of syndromes would have major psychological factors in their origin and perpetuation.

It remains true, however, that despite all these serious difficulties, the manifestations of psychophysiologic disorders are easy to detect cross-culturally. With this one advantage we suggest that a start can be made by counting the syndromes in a sample and seeing whether or not their prevalence, incidence, demographic features, and so on turn out to be the same or contrast markedly from one cultural group to another. With such a procedure, one could go beyond the conservative list of syndromes we have given and note the distribution of all symptoms according to the systems of the body as outlined in the *Manual*. Oriented by knowledge of such comparative distributions, one might then carry out intensive physical and psychological investigation of a selected sample of cases in order to adduce evidence for or against the presence of compelling psychological influences.

PSYCHONEUROSIS

In this section we shall outline two symptom complexes that are clinically common among people of our own culture, and then treat in a more summary fashion several rarer types. Finally we shall discuss cross-cultural application of criteria.

I. ANXIETY REACTION

We begin with the anxiety reaction or state, because anxiety in some form is the chief characteristic of psychoneurosis. Just as depression is like mourning, so anxiety is like fear: it is excessive and has either no object or an inappropriate object. The person so afflicted has the subjective sensation of fear, and at times the outward physiological manifestations, but the feelings are vague and diffuse. Either he does not know why he feels this way, or the causes he alleges appear improbable to others. The discomfort and suffering, on the other hand, are apparent enough.

The criteria proposed are both objective and subjective. Objective criteria may be stated as: fast pulse, rapid respiration, pale skin, sweating, dilated pupils, facial expression of apprehension, poor sleep, and restlessness. Subjective criteria would include: apprehension, worry, fear of dying, palpitations, cold sweats, and nightmares. Since it is rare to see a person in such an acute or severe state of anxiety that the objective criteria are immediately evident, we must usually rely on the patient's story.

2. DEPRESSION

The *Manual*, following the thinking of many psychiatrists, attempts to make a fundamental distinction between psychotic depression and psychoneurotic depression. We must admit, however, that we have not found the points of differentiation sufficiently specific to be workable. The distinctions proposed are too elusive for standardization and the development of reliability in judgment between psychiatrists. As a consequence we suggest that the matter be considered primarily one of degree.

This means that the criteria for identifying psychoneurotic depression are the same as those already outlined for psychotic depression. Applying these in the Stirling County Study [7] yielded one category that contains very few cases, all of which have a history of being severely disturbed, whether episodically or chronically, and another category with many cases, most of which show mild yet exceedingly chronic disturbance.

Both clinical experience and survey work suggest that depression, mixed with anxiety and other symptoms, is a very common type of psychoneurotic disorder. Frequently, especially in the mixed reaction, there is a focusing and overconcern with the functioning of the body, constituting hypochondriacal symptoms.

3. SOME ADDITIONAL TYPES OF PSYCHONEUROSIS

Under this heading the following conditions may be noted. A. *Conversion reactions*. These consist in anesthesias, paralyses, and sensory losses that are recognizable as psychological because the disturbances fail to be consonant with the actual distribution and functioning of nerves.

B. *Dissociative reactions.* Grouped here are the amnesias, fugue states, and multiple personalities.

These conditions appear to be exceedingly rare in the cultures of Europe and America at present, although they may be so dramatic when they do occur as to attract considerable attention and remain long remembered.

C. *Phobias.* People with this condition show unreasonable and incapacitating fears of specific objects or situations, such as elevators, trains, crowds, or open spaces.

D. *Obsessive-compulsive reactions.* Here the trouble is the intrusion of unwanted ideas, or the need to do things repeatedly, despite the feeling that they are foolish.

Referring again to the Stirling County Study, its findings show that psychoneurotic syndromes exclusively of one or another of the six types mentioned above are rare. Although anxiety or depression may dominate the picture, there are often mixtures of symptoms pertinent to the other subcategories. Indeed, the type of psychoneurotic symptom complex most commonly found is one in which the distribution of symptoms is so mixed that it has to be given the label "Other"—that is, as defined by the *Manual*, not specifically in any of the subcategories, although comprising symptoms referable to a plurality of them.

Many studies have indicated that a high proportion of psychophysiologic symptoms are associated with the more purely psychoneurotic. It is unusual to find a case of psychoneurosis unaccompanied by gastrointestinal, cardiovascular, or musculoskeletal difficulties.

To this matter of range and amorphousness in psychoneurotic symptoms must be added still another consideration. Item by item the symptoms comprise feelings and behavior that at one time or another are experienced by almost everyone. This means that the definition of psychoneurosis and the standardization of procedures for its recognition are particularly difficult. A solution has been to define the disorder in theoretical terms rather than in terms of phenomena that can be observed. One such view, for instance, gives emphasis to the dominance of unconscious motivation. This, however, cannot be done in the approach represented here, for reasons given earlier (p. 27).

Our inclination, therefore, is to identify the symptoms, and then estimate the degree to which they produce impairment. These may be considered as two separate steps. That is to say, each individual could be surveyed first to see what, if any, symptoms he shows and how these cluster into patterns. Both number and type of symptoms are relevant to the question of whether a psychoneurosis is present or not. Multiple diffuse symptoms of anxiety could be considered presumptive evidence, but so also could the presence of one clear-cut phobia without any other symptoms at all.

With symptoms identified, the second step would be to judge impairment. Criteria for this are, of course, important in all psychiatric disorders, but in the brain syndromes, mental deficiency, and the psychoses they are implied in the very nature of the symptoms. This is not necessarily so in the case of psychophysiologic and psychoneurotic disorders; it is possible for a person to have many symptoms of the latter character and still function fairly well. We suggest in estimating impairment that attention can be given to four main areas of activity: work, family relationships, community relationships, and recreation. The categories for rating impairment, as proposed in the *Manual*, would appear to be serviceable.

No impairment.
Minimal. Perceptible incapacity, but not exceeding 10 per cent.
Mild. Impairment in social and occupational adjustment, such as 20 to 30 per cent disability.
Moderate. Impairment that seriously but not totally interferes with the patient's ability to carry on his social and vocational adjustment, such as 30 to 50 per cent disability.
Severe. Anything over the preceding.

On such a scale, the division between significant and insignificant impairment can be considered as lying above "minimal" and below "mild." "Moderate" and "severe" could probably mark the line between unhospitalized patients and the majority of those who are hospitalized.

Turning now to the problem of cross-cultural identification, our point of departure is to note again that the psychoneuroses present particular difficulties because of their protean character, the lack of congruence in psychiatric definition, and the large number of marginal cases. To jump directly from this into a study of people in one or more other cultures—particularly an epidemiological study—is to compound confusion. On the other hand, it does seem possible to establish operating definitions and criteria. It cannot be hoped that these will command everybody's support, but it may be possible to make evident just what they are, so that points of agreement and disagreement are clear, as well as the extent and limits of the ground covered by the study. The symptoms and impairment criteria that have been already mentioned in this section are a sketch of operating definitions as these might apply in North America. The question now is: Could they be employed in a cross-cultural study?

The answer sums up what has already been said about other categories of psychiatric disorder. While it is to be expected that attempts to apply criteria in another culture will increase the width of the margins of uncertainty, there is not ground for assuming *a priori* that this renders the problem unmanageable. In the cultures that were used for reference in our seminar there appeared to be no sweeping barriers to the identification of psychoneurotic symptoms and degrees of impairment. The fact remains, of course, that here and there a particular symptom might be difficult to detect.

For instance, anxiety might be hard to distinguish from rational fear under certain circumstances. One of the identifying features of anxiety is its free-floating nature. Genuine fear, however, if great enough may develop a free-floating character, while on the other hand anxiety may condense into a phobia and lose its free-floating quality. In cultures where witches are perceived as a constant threat, very real difficulties may arise in separating psychoneurotic anxiety from rational, culturally determined fear. Obviously, fear of witches should not automatically be labeled a phobia; nor should a preoccupation with witches and witchcraft be seen as an obsession. On the other hand, it is possible to take one's respect for culture too far and assume that fear of witches could not be a phobia. This could lead to finding no phobias in a cultural group in which they were actually present.

What we are saying, in effect, is that the distinction between fear (rational) and anxiety (nonrational) depends on the cultural standards of the group to which the individual belongs. The content will vary more or less from culture to culture, but the principle of relationships remains the same.

The test of whether the object of fear is a legitimate source of concern needs to be qualified. One must consider, too, the person's mode of reaction, which may also be rational or nonrational within the framework provided by the cultural system of sentiments. Poorly controlled handling of emotion may provide a clue as to something psychologically wrong in situations where legitimate witchcraft fear may otherwise be hard to separate from anxiety and phobia.

Although concerned with hostility rather than anxiety, Baasher's story of the religious follower who committed murder (p. 48) illustrates both points we are trying to make. On the one hand there is the detection of oddity or abnormality in the apprehension itself as measured by cultural standards, and then there is the question of further symptom manifestations in the way the emotion is managed or mismanaged.

Finally we should like to suggest that even if anxiety were masked by cultural factors in particular individuals, this would not necessarily prevent our identifying these persons as psychoneurotic. The very protean, or multisymptomatic, character of psychoneurosis argues against this. As was mentioned earlier in connection with schizophrenia, it is unusual to have decision hang on one symptom. If this or that symptom is obscured by a particular context, other elements of the syndrome are apt to be sufficiently in evidence to permit identification. This is true in various situational contexts within our own culture which sometimes obscure one or another aspect of a disorder, and we think it probable that the same will apply in issues of cross-cultural identification.

PERSONALITY DISORDER

Personality disorder refers to a condition that is outwardly similar to psychoneurosis; and in the clinical assessment of cases it is often particularly difficult to decide between the two. In general, personality disorder is conceived as being more diffuse than psychoneurosis, spreading through virtually every aspect of personality. It is also thought to be life-long, beginning at an early age and persisting ever afterward, unmodified by experience. Although there are numerous varieties of this disorder, three of the more common types occurring in our culture may be mentioned for illustration.

A. *General emotional instability*. This means a tendency to fly apart under ordinary tests of life with symptoms of crying, screaming, rage, or general confusion.

B. *Passivity*. A person so afflicted gives in too easily, lets others push him around, and seems to bend without spine to every wind that blows.

C. *Hostility and aggression*. In personality disorder these symptoms are chronic, or frequently provoked by very slight stimulation, and they are extreme in degree.

We shall not discuss here the problem of cross-cultural identification, since we would only be repeating much of what has been said about psychoneurotic and other symptoms. The essential points of concept and method have already been covered.

SOCIOPATHIC DISORDERS

The *Manual* considers sociopathic disorders to be a subgroup under personality disorder, but we find it convenient to list them separately. The reason is that the central criterion of this category is deviance from cultural expectation. The underlying syndrome may be personality disorder, but it may also be mental retardation, psychoneurosis, schizophrenia, and even brain syndrome.

As implied above in the reference to deviance, this group is the most culturally defined of all those reviewed in this chapter. In Western society the category presents major problems because it is so essentially a matter of relationship to norms, and the norms vary enormously from one part of the social system to another. The question may be raised, furthermore, as to whether the behavior represented is a disorder.

The three main divisions of sociopathic disorder are listed below.

1. *Dyssocial.* This represents amoral disregard for the conventions of society.

2. *Antisocial.* Such persons act against other people with robbery and violence.

In the first above there is disregard for the feelings of others in pursuit of one's own hedonistic ends, but there is no deliberate desire to harm. In the second there is direct attack on others, and enjoyment of such acts may be a prime reason for carrying them out.

3. *Addiction.* This commonly means alcohol, but also includes overuse and dependence on a wide variety of drugs.

A feature of all three of these sociopathic patterns, and one that is often used as a confirming criterion, is a curious inability to learn from experience. No matter how costly and self-defeating the behavior proves itself to be, the sociopath appears unable to relinquish it.

The seminar members saw no great difficulty in the identification of sociopaths in other cultures. Most were sure they had encountered just such persons in the course of their field work. The seminar members also felt that in the cultural groups they knew, there was common recognition of the existence of the sociopathic phenomenon. This might be put in terms such as: "Occasionally you find people who are born outlaws; they are against everything and they cannot help it because they are made that way." Or, "There are people who just go their own way regardless, and there is nothing that can be done to change them."

SOME NOTES ON DIAGNOSIS

We have discussed the possibility of identifying symptom patterns and impairment cross-culturally, and we have concluded that if one selects particular cultures instead of trying to deal with cultures in general, he will probably be able to establish operational criteria that will permit the desired comparison at a useful and meaningful level of approximation. We also think that operational steps are facilitated if the detection of symptom patterns and the rating of impairment are used as a primary focus in cross-cultural estimates. At the end of the seminar it was the opinion of most participants, anthropologists and psychiatrists alike, that syndromes as a whole are manageable cross-culturally. When one takes up individual symptoms one by one, there is plenty of opportunity for postulating difficult situations and ground for arguments regarding feasibility, but when one considers the symptoms as components of syndromes, and takes the latter as the unit for counting, the task does not look so difficult. Although problematic cases will undoubtedly occur, we do not expect these to be so numerous as to cause serious statistical difficulty.

When one moves beyond symptoms and impairment to consider full diagnosis, especially with regard to the functional psychoses, the psychoneuroses, and the personality disorders, he must be prepared to meet considerable challenge. There are many subtleties in the diagnostic process that are bound to be affected by cultural differences. A constant awareness of these subtleties is necessary in any work that strives for accuracy and consistency, and it seems appropriate, therefore, to outline a few.

In the psychiatric interview, the patient influences the doctor and the doctor influences the patient; diagnosis is one of the complex resultants of this interaction. The diagnosis depends not only on the symptoms and manifestations of the patient, but also on the doctor's training, familiarity with the patient and his culture, and his attitudes toward the patient, which are in turn influenced by the patient's attitudes toward him. Very often the diagnosis reflects whether he likes or dislikes the patient, and whether he approves or disapproves of him. Unfortunately the hierarchy of values differs from doctor to doctor, from time to time, and place to place. "Sociopathic disorder," for instance, often implies dislike and disapproval. "Depression" is usually more flattering than "schizophrenia," which sometimes simply implies craziness.

The diagnosis may at times be a projection of the physician's personality onto the patient. This is apt to happen in rather obscure cases where the diagnosis is achieved empathetically, that is, by transient trial identification with the patient. Such identification is useful, but one runs the risk of confusing himself with the patient. To employ it skillfully one must have a thorough knowledge not only of the patient and his culture, but also of one's self and of one's own culture.

The psychiatrist who attempts diagnoses in another culture will be influenced by his attitude not only toward his patient but also toward his informants, his interpreters, and his anthropologist colleagues. The diagnosis will also be influenced by the attitudes of the informants and patients toward their own culture, toward Western culture, toward the psychiatrist, and toward mental disease in general.

A diagnosis then is the result of a relationship, whether it be a one-one relationship between psychiatrist and patient, or a more complex one between psychiatrist-interpreter-informant-anthropologist-patient. Spiegel [8] has described his difficulties in establishing relationships and doing interviews with the parents of disturbed children from American-Irish Catholic families of the lower income bracket in the Boston area. He had to learn a new language, a new set of values, and new modes of behavior. One is forcibly struck with the similarities between these difficulties and those found in dealing with psychotic patients. Yet these people were not psychotic, not patients, and not from another culture. These comparable problems of dealing with psychotics and people of other cultures can be described as essentially communication difficulties. The psychiatrist-anthropologist must maintain an orientation in his own culture, in the culture under study, and in the private world of the patient under discussion.

Our interest in culture, however, should not obscure the very important, and possibly common, masking effects that can arise from endemic illness such as tuberculosis. From the discussions at Many Farms one would suspect that the problem is not so much one of disentangling neurotic and psychotic complaints from native superstition and folklore as it is of disentangling such complaints from the organic background and perhaps from the tendency of unlettered peoples to express emotional discomfort in terms of aches and pains.

Notes

1. E. Sapir, "Culture and Personality," in *Selected Writings of Edward Sapir in Language, Culture and Personality*, D. G. Mandelbaum, ed. (Berkeley: University of California Press, 1951).

2. R. P. Knight, "Borderline States," *Bulletin of the Menninger Clinic*, vol. 17 (1953), pp. 1–12.

3. W. McDermott, K. Deuschle, J. Adair, H. Fulmer, and B. Loughlin, "Introducing Modern Medicine in a Navaho Community," *Science*, vol. 131, nos. 3395 and 3396 (January 22–29, 1960), pp. 197–205 and 280–287.

4. J. Thurber, "The Night the Ghost Got In," *My Life and Hard Times* (New York: Harper & Row, 1933).

5. E. Llewellyn-Thomas, "The Prevalence of Psychiatric Symptoms in an Island Fishing Village," *Canadian Mental Association Journal*, vol. 83 (July 1960), pp. 197–204.

6. A. H. Leighton, J. A. Clausen, and R. N. Wilson, eds., *Explorations in Social Psychiatry* (New York: Basic Books, 1957), Editorial Comment to ch. 2 ("Paranoid Patterns" by J. S. Tyhurst), p. 69.

7. D. C. Leighton, J. S. Harding, D. B. Macklin, A. M. Macmillan, and A. H. Leighton, *The Character of Danger: Psychiatric Symptoms in Selected Communities* [Vol. III, The Stirling County Study of Psychiatric Disorder and Sociocultural Environment (New York: Basic Books, 1963)].

8. J. P. Spiegel, "Some Cultural Aspects of Transference and Countertransference," *Individual and Familial Dynamics*, J. H. Masserman, ed. (New York: Grune & Stratton, 1959).

III: Native Conceptions of

Psychiatric Disorder

By Jane M. Murphy and Alexander H. Leighton

EDITORIAL NOTES

An obvious fact about cross-cultural psychiatry is that the knowledge and techniques that have been found useful in our society are not necessarily appropriate for investigating a non-Western group. This chapter attempts to move on from the clinical definitions examined in the last chapter and to delve into problems involved in obtaining the native outlook on such matters. Its orientation entertains the possibility that the indigenous views of another culture might be wholly different from those of Europe and America, or they might be surprisingly the same.

It is theoretically possible, of course, that some cultural groups have no idea of psychiatric disorder at all. This could happen if there were, in fact, no disorders among the members of that society. It could happen if the sociocultural system provided roles that could accommodate as functional members all individuals, equipped with no matter what inadequacies, disturbances, or disorders. Or it could happen if the group chose to ignore disorders—to overlook them if they were there, or to call them "natural" if they could not be overlooked.

It is probably safe, however, to dismiss these possibilities as so unlikely as not to warrant serious attention. There appears to be no culture known today nor at any period in history that exhibits so startling an omission in awareness of human behavior as to lack a concept of mental illness. It would seem equally foolish to expect that any people anywhere consider such physical events as a broken toe or an eclipse of the sun as psychiatric phenomena even though they might figure in the preoccupations or delusions of an individual suffering a psychiatric disorder. Neither does it seem possible that any people would call a man crazy because he thinks of himself as a human being nor that any society, even a druid-worshipping group, could make very good use, as Alfred Kroeber once remarked, of a man who believes himself to be a tree and stands mute in the forest with arms outstretched.

Hence we can assume that there are some bounds to cultural variability. The probability is that within these bounds cultures may differ in the way they conceptualize psychiatric disorder. Some of the patterns we recognize may not be so regarded, as for instance changes with old age or psychoneurotic and psychophysiologic disturbances. The content of psychiatric behavior is likely to vary in some regards. For example, it is inconceivable in view of what is known about cultures that any group would not have standards of crime and sociopathy; but what behavior is considered criminal obviously differs from culture to culture. Among many hunting, gathering, and agricultural groups, an abuse of animals and land is thought of as a far greater offense against the sanctity and viability of the society than beating one's wife or killing an enfeebled old man. It is also certain that the explanatory systems for psychiatric disorder will be different in other cultures.

In approaching cross-cultural studies of psychiatric disorder, we are confronted immediately by a situation that calls for a balance between skepticism and confidence. There is reason for confidence that what we know already is applicable in some ways to all human beings everywhere. The previous chapter indicated that it is not altogether hopeless to attempt identifying disorders, as conceived in clinical psychiatry, among peoples of very different cultural background. Our current methods of discovering and evaluating symptoms also seem to provide starting points. But there is need for skepticism that any analysis limited to these resources alone would be complete. At the very least, important items of content, norms, and specific criteria of deviance might be missed. If we find, as evidence suggests we will, that most cultural groups have a word in their language for "crazy" and if we hold at all to the view suggested in the last chapter that schizophrenia is what people in a particular group call "crazy," then opportunity is at hand for exploring what these people mean by "crazy" and how well it actually does relate to what we define as schizophrenia. Beyond this there is the possibility of picking up information about syndromes such as *látah, koro,* and arctic hysteria which appear to be specific to a given culture, and of gaining illuminating suggestions as to causal relationships.

All of this argues for securing the native viewpoint, or range of viewpoints, and it points to questions that should be recognized concerning the use of data-gathering methods that are predicated on Western psychiatric criteria of disorder. It is commonly accepted, we believe, that the criteria and methods employed thus far in cross-cultural psychiatry have met the requirements of freedom from cultural bias only at certain points and in limited degree. Until the last seven or eight years, most investigations in non-Western areas have been conducted in terms of one or another of the following: hospital admission rates, penal records, vital statistics on homicide and suicide, surveying with the Rorschach test, the T.A.T., the I.Q., or other psychological tests, and observations by itinerant psychiatrists. All of these are in some respects culturebound, although it has long been thought that the Rorschach was less contaminated than most tests; and when the T.A.T. has been used in cross-cultural research it has usually been adapted to show situational stimuli appropriate for the culture being studied. In view of the unknowns that confront cross-cultural psychiatry, however, it seems wiser to begin with a search for criteria of anxiety or intelligence, for example, than to start with a test that presumably but by no means definitely discloses these.

The present chapter is an effort toward the goal of discovering such indigenous criteria of psychiatric disorders. It is exploratory in nature, and the information was gathered mainly by Murphy as a part of a general anthropological investigation with special attention given to health problems in an Eskimo village. The study as a whole has drawn on the observations and assessments made by two psychiatrists and one other anthropologist.

THIS report deals with native conceptualization about psychiatric disorder. In approaching this topic, it is apparent that there exists as background a large literature on the conceptualizing tendencies of non-Western peoples as, for example, Lévy-Bruhl's *Les Fonctions mentales dans les sociétés inférieures*, Franz Boas' *The Mind of Primitive Man*, and Paul Radin's *Primitive Man As Philosopher*.[1] Although much of this literature is now controversial, there is no doubt that the magical philosophies of primitive man have been carefully described and discussed.

In order to illustrate some of the issues involved in the undertaking of this chapter, an example of a similar conceptual problem will be used as an introduction. The example has been suggested by W. H. R. Rivers' report on "The Primitive Conception of Death."[2] Certain liberties have been taken for the sake of conciseness and clarity, but they do not do injustice to what is known generally about non-Western peoples. The example is this:

In Melanesia there is a group of people whose language has two words, "X" and "Y," which, in view of what people say and do, you soon equate with "life" and "death." You draw this conclusion because corpses at the time of burial are called "Y" and are contrasted to healthy, young individuals called "X." If you stay with this group long enough, however, you discover that sometimes people are buried even when they are not dead. You learn that the Melanesians call a person "Y" and bury him if he is very sickly or very old—in other words, they bury people who, according to society, ought to be dead even if they are not. Before long you learn further that the state of "Y-ness" is sometimes thought to be caused by somebody in the group getting angry and casting a spell on the person now designated as "Y." Still further inquiry enhances confusion, because you find that after the person called "Y" has been buried for a while, others now say he isn't "Y" at all but rather "Y^x," which, you gradually discover, means something like eternal-life-after-death.

On taking thought you decide that the Melanesians have a very different conception of death from that given in the medical textbooks and collected clinical judgments of the Western world; and yet you have the uneasy feeling that some aspects of this Melanesian life-and-death business have a decidedly familiar ring and that perhaps your own concepts of analysis are obstructing a nicer division between what is different and what is the same.

As a beginning you ask yourself about the difference between a concept and a word. Following dictionary usage we can agree to call a concept "a mental image of a thing formed by generalization from particulars, an idea of what a thing in general should be." [3] It is impossible to communicate a concept without using words, but it does not necessarily follow that all the concepts held by a group of people will each have a specific label in the language of that group. Nevertheless, in view of the close connection between language and culture, you suspect that this is an important area to explore. Among the Melanesians, you note that what they distinguish by the term "Y," which is somehow related to their conception of death, is the basis of the cultural practice of burying both dead and nearly dead people. The word "Y" is also linked to the cultural beliefs about after-life, as in "Y^x." But the significance of the difference in the Melanesian meaning of "Y" and our meaning of the word "dead" does not altogether convince you that the Melanesians cannot tell a dead man from a live one or that they are unaware of the difference between a state of *rigor mortis* and a state in which the heart beats and breathing goes on, even if these functions are impaired as in a sickly old person.

In an effort to clarify the matter you put yourself in the Melanesian's position and look at some comparable body of thought from one of the Western traditions, as for example the way we distinguish people in our kinship systems. In all likelihood a Melanesian has separate words for *male cousin, female cousin, elder male cousin on the father's side,* and so on, and he would be somewhat befuddled by the compression of all these useful distinguishing words into our blanket English term, *cousin.* He would be correct, we would say, in assuming nevertheless that this evidence does not mean that civilized man is unable to tell men from women cousins or old from young cousins. But he would also be right in noting that our kinship language is important as a reflection of behavioral tendencies. Most English-speaking groups do not have as many rules for distinguishing between people in the cousin category as the Melanesians have.

In addition to the value derived from sorting out the conceptual from the linguistic dimensions of the problem, the Melanesian example indicates that illness and death are attributed to quite different causal mechanisms. At least we note that magical explanations such as the casting of spells account for *part* of the phenomena of illness and death in the Melanesian mind. Magical and nonmagical levels of analysis should be distinguished. Although magical thinking has been given most attention in the literature, there is evidence that no groups of people are entirely ignorant of empirical relationships between cause and effect.

For example, a more thorough investigation of our hypothetical Melanesian group would very probably disclose that while they believe that the burning of effigies kills people and that the soul has an after-life, they also know that eternal life does not exist for physical beings, that old age eventually leads to physical death, and that life may be cut off by such nonmagical acts as the thrust of a knife into a man's heart.

In beginning to explore the interplay between magical and nonmagical concepts of the origin, course, and treatment of diseases, it is possible to refer to a rather impressive literature specifically on the topic of primitive medicine.[4] Although this has bearing mainly for theories and classifications of *physical* disease, there are guidelines for studying *psychiatric* disorders. One of these is the indication given by numerous observers that magical and nonmagical theories have a compatible coexistence insofar as natural causes and processes explain *how* illness and death occur—the nature of these phenomena, in other words—while magical ideas explain *why* it is that a particular person is afflicted. Also, there is no evidence so far that witchcraft activities pertain exclusively to physical illnesses and that some other order of explanation pertains to psychiatric manifestations. As a matter of fact, primitive medicine has been said to represent an uncompromisingly psychosomatic attitude toward both causal explanations and treatment.[5] Various psychosocial experiences such as the perception of ill-will in interpersonal relations and the belief in the potency of "hexing" activities are thought to be the veritable causes of disease. Correspondingly, treatment includes other types of psychosocial experiences such as confession, group pressure, or acting out the belief that the disease has been destroyed or rendered harmless. In view of this fundamentally psychosomatic orientation, one of the first questions to be asked in studying native concepts of mental disorder is whether a distinction is drawn at all between what is physical and what is psychical.

Here again we may find a small but growing literature on

primitive psychiatry and further bits of information scattered throughout numerous ethnographic accounts of non-Western peoples.[6] Most of this material focuses on various kinds of easily observable hysterias and schizophrenias, including the culture-specific syndromes. We can learn, for example, the kinds of behaviors that are called *làtah* or *koro*.[7] Further, we can learn that the Navahos believe incest is specifically responsible for insanity and that the mechanism whereby the mind is affected is thought to be a moth that flutters around in the brain.[8] We learn that among some groups of Eskimos a dog spirit is specifically linked to insanity and that particular kinds of offenses are part of the causal matrix.[9]

There are, however, few systematic analyses of the conceptualizations pertaining to the whole range of disorders recognized in non-Western groups. The purpose of this chapter is to make some progress in that direction. It is not a comprehensive analysis of all the various ways one might approach the problem, nor is any claim made for having achieved generalizations about primitive psychiatry as a whole. Rather, an effort has been made to gauge the parameters of the problem and to present impressions based on the study of a particular non-Western group during a given slice of time.

Site and Relevant Aspects of Eskimo Culture

The questions outlined above were raised during the study of a group of Siberian Eskimos in Sivokak village on St. Lawrence Island in the Bering Sea. The island is situated at a transitional point between the Alaskan, Canadian, and Greenland Eskimo cultures to the east and the Siberian cultures of the Chuckchee, Koryak, and Kamchadal to the west. Until recently the St. Lawrence Eskimos displayed most of the characteristics typical of traditional Eskimo cultures: habitat is usually coastal or island-dwelling; hunting of sea mammals is the main source of food, clothing, and material equipment; wife-exchange is practiced; and religious beliefs center on the shaman as a medico-religious practitioner. The St. Lawrence Eskimos also shared many of the features of traditional Siberian cultures. This affinity was especially noticeable in the form of shamanism practiced on St. Lawrence and among the neighboring Chuckchee.[10]

It is impossible to broach the topic of the psychiatric and medical views of these Eskimos without reference to the beliefs and practices of shamanism. Some background on St. Lawrence shamanizing is therefore imperative.[11] Both men and women shamanize in this group but the most powerful shamans of the past were transvestite homosexuals. St. Lawrence shamans enter the profession on the basis of a "call." The initiation rites are carried out in private but they follow a common pattern. The novitiate goes through a five-day period of isolation, wandering in the cold and subjecting himself to a variety of hardships. During this time the prospective shaman enacts death and resurrection in a performance of breaking the bones of a bird and, presumably, bringing it back to life. It is said that at this time the candidates "go something like crazy"—"out of mind but not crazy." At the end of this period when the initiate begins to feel better and has "straightened up in his mind what was bothering him," he acquires a spirit-familiar who will subsequently assist him in the healing rites.

As a practitioner, the shaman does his curing in a séance. These sessions are usually prefaced by a series of "tricks" of ventriloquism or sleight-of-hand. The room is darkened, and the shaman goes into a seizure; he falls, seemingly unconscious, on the floor, and then he rises as though possessed by his spirit-familiar. In this guise he carries out various rational and magical treatments.

There is a controversial literature on the question whether shamanism itself is psychopathological—whether, that is, it is necessary for a person to be severely disturbed before he can be recruited to this role.[12] The contesting view is that shamanistic behavior is simply theatrical—demonstrating the learned and highly controlled behavior appropriate to a certain role in society.[13] What the St. Lawrence Eskimos think about the normal or abnormal qualities of shamanism as well as their utilization of shaman seizure and homosexuality as points of reference in discussing psychiatric disorder will be taken up later.

It is obvious that shamanism rests on magical beliefs about the causes and cures of disease. The background literature on magical disease concepts must be reviewed briefly in order to give context to the St. Lawrence Eskimo situation. Several useful ways of categorizing such beliefs have been developed, first by Clements in a world survey of available ethnographic literature in 1932,[14] then in a reassessment of his categories by Hallowell in 1935,[15] by Rogers in 1942 and 1944,[16] and finally in a somewhat different approach by Whiting and Child in 1953.[17] Building on earlier work, Rogers in 1944 proposed a topical outline to which the following explanations have been added:

I. Proximate Disease Causes
   A. *Object intrusion:* Sickness is believed to be caused by the intrusion of a physical object into the patient's body.
   B. *Spirit intrusion:* Sickness—especially insanity—is believed to be caused by the intrusion of a spirit into the patient.
   C. *Soul loss:* Sickness is believed to be caused by the loss of the soul—the soul being thought to depart from the body or be stolen by spirits during sleep, sneezing, or fright.
II. Remote Disease Causes
   A. *Black magic:* Sickness is thought to be caused by the sorcery activities of human beings—casting spells, saying evil prayers, burning effigies.
   B. *Dreaming:* Sickness is believed to be caused by an experience in a dream such as the ingesting of an object or the loss of the soul while dreaming.
   C. *Violation of taboo:* Sickness is believed to be caused by a transgression against cultural rules committed by the patient or someone else in his family or group.
   D. *Divine wrath:* Sickness is believed to be caused by the anger of the gods due to some act of omission or commission relevant to the way people are supposed to treat gods.

It is evident from this categorization that proximate and remote causes often work hand-in-hand and that any one disease
may require both kinds of explanations. The curing rites which
emerge from these beliefs involve such varied phenomena as the
magical extraction of an object from the patient's body; exor-
cism of the possessing spirit; the recovery of the lost soul by the
medicine man's supernatural powers; discovery by the medicine
man of the nature of the taboo breach, the eliciting of confession, and the prescribing of acts of expiation; and the medicine man's counteractant sorcery in order to mitigate the force
of the initial black magic.

In classifying the same body of ethnographic literature, Whiting and Child focused on another kind of variation in explanations of illness. Their topical headings are as follows:

1. *Agent:* The illness-producing agent may be a living person with
   supernatural power, a ghost of an ancestor, a human spirit, a god,
   or an animal spirit.
2. *Responsibility:* The patient may be solely responsible for his
   illness, or the responsibility may be entirely in other spheres, with
   other people, etc.
3. *Act:* The illness-producing act may be the breaking of a taboo,
   sacrilege, the failure to perform rituals, etc.
4. *Materials:* The illness-producing materials may be poisons, menstrual blood, spirits, magical weapons, etc.
5. *Means:* The means by which the materials have effect may be
   ingestion, introjection (material being magically taken or thrust
   into the body), removal or loss of the materials, their being used
   in rituals, etc.

Where do the St. Lawrence Eskimos fit into these schema?
Interestingly enough, almost all of these ideas have some cur-
rency in this group although some of the ideas were elaborated
rather differently and some were more prevalent than others. In
his world survey, Clements noted that the "soul loss" idea is
especially common in the Siberian arctic. This dominance was
borne out as well in the St. Lawrence data, but there were also

cases of black magic, taboo violation, divine wrath, and dream experiences.

Spirit intrusion presents a special case. Clements observed that usually the only form of sickness attributed to spirit intrusion is insanity (the utterances of the mad man often being taken as the voice of a resident spirit), although madness may also be explained by soul loss. Clements found that the concept of spirit intrusion was notably absent from Siberian cultures; its absence he believed to be the logical outcome of the high development of the soul-loss idea. It is in the Siberian and Siberian Eskimo groups, however, that spirit possession is the hallmark of shamanism. He explained shamanism, therefore, as an atrophied form of the idea that spirit intrusion causes disease and implied that shamans were sick people. The St. Lawrence Eskimos recognize that spirit possession is a phenomenon of shamanism, but they do not therefore regard shamanism as being equivalent to insanity. Nor did they consider spirit intrusion as relevant to any of the cases of psychiatric disorders recognized and described as such in this study. This fact may well relate to the transitional character of the St. Lawrence culture, since spirit intrusion is better developed as an explanation of mental disorder among the central Eskimo groups. (For example, a schizophrenic Eskimo woman from Southampton Island who believed herself to be host to a fox spirit has been well described by Teicher.[18])

Another aspect of the literature on Eskimo culture relevant to this chapter concerns the culture-specific disorders that have been observed and described, often under the general heading of "arctic hysteria." To the east of St. Lawrence Island—among Greenland, Canadian, and to some extent Alaskan groups—a syndrome called *piblokto* existed.[19] It is impossible to tell how widespread it may have been. Gussow recently collected from historical records evidence on seventeen cases, mainly women, which he summarized as follows: *piblokto* involved episodic and temporary states of excitement with disturbance of consciousness. Some seizures lasted a few minutes; others nearly an hour.

The concomitant behavior included such things as disrobing or tearing off one's clothes, running away, rolling in the snow or jumping into a lake, glossolalia (mimicking animal or bird sounds or jabbering in meaningless neologisms), unusual but harmless acts such as trying to walk on the ceiling, throwing things around, grimacing, mimetic acts, choreiform movements, and coprophagia.[20]

Characteristic psychopathology was also found among the Siberian groups.[21] Especially with women, this appeared to be a "copying mania"—in some places called *amurakh*. It included endless and exhaustive imitative behavior (dancing, running, obscene posturing) which could somehow be "triggered off" by words or gestures known by the rest of the group to produce such an effect. A similar disorder (though not as specifically a female reaction and usually wilder and more paroxysmal) was called *menerik*. This included periods of screaming and dancing which culminated in an epileptoid seizure. This was natively designated as "sickness" when observed in some people, but, as already indicated, this kind of behavior was also a routine and integral part of shamanizing on both sides of the Strait. The differences and similarities between these disorders and what was discussed by St. Lawrence Eskimos will be presented later.

By the time of our investigations of the St. Lawrence culture (1940 and 1954–1955) the island had been in contact with the outside world for nearly a century. For much of that period it was mainly in contact with Russian and American whalers, then with missionaries, with people in the governmental school system, and more recently with members of the United States armed forces. The progressive modernization brought about by these contacts has meant that the 1955 culture of St. Lawrence Island was no longer "primitive" in the classical sense. It was a culture in transition, with a fairly large segment of the population displaying various degrees of bilingual facility. Public shamanism had declined, and there was increased mixing of the ideas of Western and shamanistic medicine. In the process of transition Eskimo views of psychiatric disorder, like everything else, have very probably undergone some modification. These Eskimos exemplify, therefore, what Redfield has described as the mixture of a "great tradition" and a "small tradition." [22]

Questions raised by the influence of contact in the case of the Eskimos have been given considerable attention in the following analysis. The effects of cultural contact add another dimension of complexity and represent a problem of almost insurmountable difficulty, because there are remarkably few isolated non-Western groups left that have not been somewhat influenced by outside contacts. Although a certain amount of reconstruction from early ethnographies is possible, the goals of contemporary research are inevitably plagued by the implications of culture change.

Method

The field work on which this report is based was carried out in the summer of 1940 by Alexander Leighton and Dorothea Leighton and for the year of 1954–1955 by Jane Murphy and Charles Hughes. The data on native viewpoints were part of an epidemiological study of psychiatric disorders in Sivokak village. Of the 495 Eskimos living in the village between 1940 and 1955, 113 were found to have symptoms that A. Leighton identified as falling in the province of psychiatry. The case histories on these 113 Eskimos combine information from various sources. The main source was a series of interviews carried out by Murphy with a bilingual key informant, during which the informant was asked to describe the life and health experiences of each of the Eskimos who formed the base population for the epidemiological study. Since this was the major data-gathering operation from which the analysis of native conceptualization stems, the methodology of this aspect of the research is described in an extended chapter note.[23] Additional sources included comments by other native informants, the available medical records, records of the meetings of the village council (the native governing body), information regarding mainland hospital admissions and federal court actions, life histories of individual Eskimos, comments made by local teachers and public health nurses, and observations recorded in field notes by the two psychiatrists and two anthropologists.[24]

It is obvious that the case materials consist of a welter of information given and recorded in English and derived from both native and Western conceptualization. Also, they include evidence that has varying degrees of reliability and validity. In some cases as many as seven different sources would indicate that one individual had something psychiatrically wrong with him. In other instances the information was fragmentary and far from congruent. (The method used for dealing with this problem of different levels of confidence in an epidemiological study is presented elsewhere.[25])

Having available this collection of data, we could then review the case materials focusing on the comments made by Eskimos. From the specific instances of pathological functioning described by natives we have inferred a general psychiatric orientation and specific psychiatric ideas which, we believe, represent the conceptualizations of this group of Eskimos.

This method is obviously oriented primarily to concepts—in contrast, for example, to the method used by Frake in studying the linguistic categories of physical disease among the Subanun of Mindanao.[26] Our focus on concept does not mean a disregard of language. None of the investigators in this study was able to speak or understand the Eskimo language. Had any one of us achieved proficiency in the language, we would, of course, have been much better equipped to understand more fully the Eskimo's psychiatric concepts. In lieu of this, we tried to make a virtue of a necessity. In order to communicate at all, the Eskimos were forced to explain their ideas through the medium of a limited vocabulary in English. Their knowledge of psychiatric terms used in English was sparse. As will become evident subsequently, they knew several lay terms for psychiatric phenomena, but they knew none of the technical terms such as "depression," "anxiety," "schizophrenia," or "mental deficiency." Their lack of a psychiatrically sophisticated vocabulary in English and our lack of proficiency in the Eskimo language meant that we had to ferret out their psychiatric views uncommitted to the semantic restrictions of either language.

The inability to speak Eskimo did not preclude gathering data about the meaning of particular Eskimo words. Hughes was especially interested in language, and he contributed most of the information that will be presented about the psychiatric concepts that do and those that do not have a label in the Eskimo language. Although this part of the methodology was not exhaustively carried out on St. Lawrence Island, we incorporated greater emphasis on native words in a later study of the Yorubas of Nigeria.[27]

Eskimo Psychiatric Orientation

We are quite certain that the Eskimos referred to in this study do not have a word in their language that directly corresponds to our word "psychiatry." The first question, therefore, is whether they have the *idea* of psychiatry. At no point in the field work was it stated that we were interested in psychiatric disorders, nor was a definition of psychiatry ever offered for them to pick up and elaborate or compare with their own. From the case materials it was possible to determine that they have notions about a variety of behaviors, emotional states, and thinking patterns which they recognize as "something being wrong" and which they clearly distinguish from purely organic disorders. The most succinct statement of this referred to a woman who by several accounts exhibited psychotic behavior. She was the widow of a powerful shaman. After his death she had begun to think that people were trying to kill her through witchcraft. She tried several times to run away in the middle of the winter, and her son would find her wandering on the bank of the lake. This was summarized by the key informant as, "her sickness is getting wild and out of mind, but she might have sickness in her body too." The fact that the body-mind dichotomy was clearly expressed in this statement does not mean the St. Lawrence Eskimos failed to subscribe to the psychosomatic attitude mentioned previously as being characteristic of most primitive groups. Nevertheless, this statement was one indicator among many that the two elements were at times conceived separately.

The next important question is whether or not our subjects recognize the alliance between body and mind. Do they have the idea of psychosomatic interdependencies? If they do conceptualize this interdependence, what criteria can we infer as being employed to mark off what is psychiatric and what not? In reviewing the case materials we observed that the disorders recognized by us as psychiatric were the ones that the Eskimos described as either (1) psychologically expressed, or (2) psychologically derived.

The *psychologically expressed disorders* were those having to do with personality characteristics as reflected in patterns of thought, perception, emotional states, and behavior. These included, for example, what the Eskimos called "out of mind," "not right mind," "ignorant mind," "slow to learn," "bad habits," "too much nervous," "easy to get afraid," and so on. Although all of these phenomena were manifest at the psychological level, the Eskimos had a variety of explanations about what caused them. As indicated in the first example, one type of explanation concerned magic and witchcraft. In these instances a psychological experience is considered to be the causative factor, since witchcraft depends on the psychological readiness to believe in the effectiveness of magic. Surprisingly, this type accounted for relatively few of the cases about which explanation was offered, perhaps because the Eskimos nowadays are somewhat inhibited on this topic. The other types of explanation had more in common with Western psychiatry, but we do not believe they were imported. They appear to have emerged from rational observation of human behavior, and several times they were couched in terms of "this is just what I think myself." There were comments, for example, that indicated some awareness of heredity. The "slow to learn" syndrome was described as "running in that family." A pattern of eccentricity and habitual oddness (which we interpreted as personality disorder) was referred to by the informant as "all those brothers are the same—it's their way." Various kinds of physiological events were also called in to explain psychological manifestations. It seemed to be well understood that states of unconsciousness or delirium might be associated with severe physical illness. A blow on the head was once pointed to as what must have caused a child (who had appeared to be developing normally) to change suddenly in her mind—she talked or sang nonsense incessantly. In addition to the magical, hereditary, and physical explanations, the Eskimos have the notion that life situations may cause psychiatric illnesses. For example, a death in the family might precipitate such an episode. A man who lost a much-beloved daughter went on an unsanctioned shamanizing binge following her death. Like the Eskimo shamans, he claimed that he would bring the dead back to life. He became wild and unrestrainable, carrying out various kinds of quasi-shamanizing activities, until finally a bona fide shaman cured him, and after that nobody "paid any attention to his shaman."

The *psychologically derived disorders*, usually involving physical sensations or mood disturbances, were those which the Eskimos linked to one or another psychological experience. As with the psychologically expressed disorders, even though the Eskimos do not have the technical terms for explaining phenomena as we do, a psychiatric frame of reference could be inferred from the specific case descriptions. For example: an instance of "heart beating too hard" was said to be caused by "too much worrying," one woman was said to faint at the sight of blood and another at being in crowds, a temporary facial paralysis was attributed to "too much brain work," and another conversion reaction producing a temporary inability to walk was said to have been caused because this woman's husband abused her.

It appears from this that the Eskimos in our investigation have a way of identifying and understanding certain kinds of human behavior which can be called a psychiatric orientation. It bears some consonance to Western psychiatric thought, especially as the latter is evidenced in Western lay attitudes. It is markedly divergent in that segment of the conceptual map which involves the particular content of magical theorizing found among Eskimos of this area.

With this background on orientation it is now possible to turn to the specific concepts that constitute the psychiatric thinking of the St. Lawrence Eskimos.

Specific Eskimo Concepts

For purposes of continuity, this section is organized in terms of the major categories of symptom patterns that were discussed in the previous chapter. Taking a topic such as "brain syndrome" or "psychoneurosis," we then review the Eskimo data in order to see what corresponds and what not. It should be emphasized here that we look at these data from a clinical point of view, and our attempt is to construct from multiple cases what in the minds of Eskimos would compare with a clinical *model* of a particular kind of psychiatric entity.

1. BRAIN SYNDROME

One of the commonest brain syndromes is senility. The St. Lawrence people have a word for the condition when "a person's brain no longer controls him, when he is 'out of mind' as in old age." It is impossible to tell from our data whether this is considered an illness or simply one of the natural courses of life. Certainly it was not thought of as an illness for which shaman treatment would be sought. The kinds of aberrant thinking, feeling, and behaving that were noticed by the Eskimos as exemplifying this condition are very similar to what we think of as senility, and consistently these manifestations were related to old age. They included "becoming like a child," "crying a lot," "having to be taken care of," "partly crazy, doesn't know way home, walks to the beach instead, but sometimes is in right mind," "not eating," "picking things up from the ground and eating them," "making odd sounds at night," "trying to kill himself," and so forth.

Regarding other types of brain syndromes there are at least two words in the Eskimo language for convulsions—one of them especially denotes a state of unconsciousness. Unconsciousness was clearly described, as for example in a brain concussion following a hunting accident. Also, a small child, thought by the public health nurse to have a brain tumor or tubercular meningitis—leading ultimately to death—was described by an Eskimo in the following manner. "She was kind of paralyzed, and then she got very sick before she died. She was unconscious, and she was sounding like a little pup, and her face moving in any direction, shaping to this side and that side."

Epilepsy or epileptoid seizures were described several times. In view of the manifest similarities between some aspects of psychopathological seizures and the seizures enacted in shamanism, it seemed to us that this might be an area in which we could find out how the Eskimos conceptualize the differences and similarities, the pathological and the nonpathological, and whether the one might be used to help define the other.

It appeared that our subjects clearly conceived the difference between shamanistic seizure and a variety of kinds of seizures that were defined as illness. The distinguishing characteristic of shaman seizure was possession. The other types of seizures or quasi-seizures, involving "falling down unconscious," ranged from epileptoid seizures to fainting episodes. The Eskimos' distinction between the latter was phrased as the difference between "fits" and "fainting." (Fainting will be discussed with psychoneurotic reactions.)

The kinds of phenomena described as "fits" can, with some

assurance, be equated with what Western psychiatry looks upon as evidence of epilepsy. What occurred in these episodes was "stretching out himself," "foaming coming out of mouth," "shaping or twitching the face," "snoring very loud," "peeing in her bloomers," "when well again, crying because ashamed of pee in bloomers." It seems evident from this that the Eskimos had in mind a certain recognizable syndrome of symptoms which had been observed often enough to become a pattern of illness in their conceptualization.

It was said that "fits" of this nature were caused by the spirit of a fox. For example, the father of a child with "fits" was said to have been hunting one day when he wounded but did not kill a fox. When the fox died, it began to make this trouble for the child. In earlier days, one of the treatments for a child with "fits" was to have him wear as a coat the net then used for catching foxes. We heard reports of children who had recovered from this illness, and there were also adults who had suffered from it all their lives. Apparently the recovery rate (based perhaps on spontaneous remission) was impressive enough for a specific shamanistic treatment to be accepted as effective. Also it is interesting to note that "fits" are the only psychiatric phenomena for which the Eskimos gave such a specific magico-causal explanation.

2. MENTAL DEFICIENCY

From our interviewing it appeared that the St. Lawrence Eskimos do not have a general term for mental deficiency. We suspect therefore that mental deficiency was not conceived as being responsive to shamanistic treatments. Although there was no overall term for the condition, there were many phrases in English used to denote a conception of mental deficiency: "slow to learn," "ignorant mind," and—graphically—"not an eloquent." The behaviors that clustered in this syndrome are as follows: "slow of speech," "looking in some direction, sometimes even without blinking," "very dumb at school; he stayed for years and years in second grade, so he was tall and he just shake his head side to side; and he doesn't hunt; and he couldn't find himself a wife, somebody had to help him," "didn't learn much in school and she has been going too far with most of the boys around here," "never learned to talk until he was five, just sort of grunted, then later he drowned," and "that dull one doesn't talk back to anybody but once she beat up somebody." This pattern was summarized by one informant as, "We call it something like ignorant, a person whose mind is not thinking anything, thick and clumsy, and when told to do a thing, then he do it even if it is harmful, just because he doesn't know anything about it."

As can be seen, there were a number of cases in which mental performance was related to the formal school system which had recently been introduced into the culture. This fact, together with the lack of a specific term, might suggest that the conception of mental deficiency had developed as a response to the testing ground provided in a Western style of education. Certainly it seemed as though school brought these phenomena into bold relief. It is interesting, however, that the same kinds of retarded behaviors were described for certain elderly people who had never been exposed to anything except routine Eskimo culture: "She doesn't know how to fix things at home, and she can't say some of the words in the right way either, Eskimo words"; "He doesn't know much about trapping so he gave it up when he was young and he never hunts, just stays home."

The best evidence that the mental deficiency concept had its origin in the indigenous culture was the fact that people described by the various particulars of this syndrome were traditionally thought to be the handmaidens of sorcerers. It was this kind of person who would be sought out by a black-magic worker and used for errand running. A mentally defective person might be approached by a sorcerer and coerced into collecting nail parings or scraps of hair from the victim against whom evil was to be worked.

3. PSYCHOSIS

There is a specific Eskimo term that can be translated as "crazy" or "insane," and the English word "crazy" was employed with several variations in the case materials—"sort of crazy," "a little bit crazy," "out of mind but not crazy," and so on. Generally the term pointed to patterns of behavior and thought that are indicators of functional psychosis. Sometimes it was used for other syndromes, such as a senile person doing things that were "a little bit crazy"; and a person who appeared in both Eskimo definition and our own observation to have a personality disorder was described as sometimes acting "sort of crazy." (This will be more fully discussed under personality disorder.)

Focusing now on the delusional, hallucinatory, and other states of unreality involving the cognitive dimension of "craziness," we face an area for which our data are spotty. The reason, in part, was that there were relatively few cases of frank psychosis in this small population. In part, too, it was that covert behavior such as delusion is more difficult to observe and describe than overt phenomena such as "fits." However we have concluded from our data that if a St. Lawrence Eskimo goes crazy he is not going to do it in a culturally particularistic way. In other words there did not appear to be a common and specific delusional pattern such as, for example, the *witiko* psychosis with its systematized beliefs and cannibalistic impulses, which has been found among the Northeast Woodland Indians.[28]

Nevertheless the St. Lawrence Eskimos provided us with some insights about their view of certain unusual mental states. One of these conditions was called "thinness." "Thinness" enabled people to "see things which other people don't see," to look into the future, to prophesy, to inspect a world of reality that is normally not observable to other people and thereby to find lost articles. This is considered a highly valuable attribute among Eskimos, and many people cultivated it to the best of their ability. All shamans were "thin," as were also numerous minor diviners ("yawners" as they were called in this culture because divination involved making peculiar gurgling or cracking sounds in the back of the throat). None of the people who were described as "sick in mind" and "crazy" were also called "thin." This is one hint that the Eskimos distinguish between a socially useful and culturally patterned delusion—"thinness"— and the cognitive aberrations of being "crazy."

"Out of mind," on the other hand, is a ubiquitous concept, varying in meaning from unconsciousness and possession to psychotic reactions. When the shaman went into possession, he was said to be "out of mind" but not crazy. Presumably this was a way of saying that the shaman was, for the duration of the séance, not in possession of himself but rather possessed and controlled by his spirit-familiar. As was the case with "thinness," the socially useful aspect of "out-of-mindness," i.e., possession, was not conceived as genuine insanity. What, then, is the stamp of true insanity in the Eskimos' eyes? Within the framework of limited cases, we could not find the one perfect criterion—quite possibly, we suspect, because there simply is no single mark of insanity in the Eskimo view, insanity being conceived instead as the way different elements go together. The psychotic woman mentioned as the first example believed that somebody was trying to kill her through witchcraft. Since witchcraft fear is exceedingly widespread, we could not conclude that a seeming paranoid belief of this nature was a criterion of insanity; the point was, rather, that this belief featured in an illness also involving wildness and running away.

The closest we could come to a specification of a subjective experience designated by the Eskimos as an attribute of "craziness" was the case of a woman who recurrently experienced periods of nervousness, "fits," and being "crazy and out of mind." The report of what she believed had happened to her is as follows. She was married as a teenager to an elderly blind man from the Siberian side. She was greatly mistreated and starved, and she decided that she didn't want to live. She went out in the night during winter, stripped off her clothes, and lay down in the snow so that she would freeze to death. It seemed to her that she went to sleep and then woke up. She saw a lumber house and she went in and found a stove and food, and she ate and got warm. It was like a "white people's" house. She remembered this experience as being similar to a dream. When she woke up she was still in the snow naked and her body had melted the snow clear down to the earth. She did not see the lumber house any more, but her stomach was full. She got up and put on her clothes, and there was nothing wrong with her body; it was not frozen. Then she started to take a journey, and she was led by a light. There was always a light in the sky to show her where to go.

Some of the things this woman believed happened to her are actually the motifs in several folk tales—being led by a light or happening onto a house where food and shelter could be acquired. The difference is that outside of shamanistic possession no other Eskimo to our knowledge said or believed that he had experienced events such as these. The improbability that these experiences were real was enhanced in the Eskimo mind by the oddity of including a "white people's" house rather than the traditional Eskimo house found in Siberia.

As compared to these inner, subjective states of belief and perception, it was apparently much easier for the Eskimos to describe behavioral characteristics associated with "out-of-mindness," as, for instance, running away, hiding in odd places, eating wrong things such as feces, and the manic states of "getting wild"—impulsive, recalcitrant, and sometimes homicidal or suicidal.

Although no specific magical theory was used to account for this order of psychiatric phenomena, it seems abundantly evident that insanity, though variable in its manifestations, is a major anchor point in the Eskimo psychiatric framework.

4. SOCIOPATHIC DISORDERS

A. *Sex deviance.* The Eskimos in this study recognize several kinds of sexual deviance. The concept of homosexuality is especially well formulated, and there are Eskimo words for "womanlike man" and "manlike woman." Homosexuals who became transvestite shamans were thought to be exceptionally powerful, but homosexuality in itself was severely disapproved. There were no transvestites in the population we studied, but one man was a homosexual, and one or two others were said to be "a little bit *anasik*." There was apparently no English word known to the Eskimos for this type of behavior, but "anasik" was described in the following hesitant manner, "Didn't you ever hear in the States . . . ? In the States do they have . . . ? Up here many years ago some men acting like women, and some are pretty worse, they are after young boys too. One died not too long ago—no moustache, baby-skin face, and he keeps sewing all the time. He is a pretty fatty man, but he isn't always a real anasik because later he got a wife."

The St. Lawrence culture recognized wife-exchange between men who had entered into a special kind of brotherhood bond. In addition, the culture was generally permissive regarding occasional nonformalized heterosexual affairs, and divorce could fairly easily be achieved. Nevertheless, the Eskimos appear to have standards of sexual activity that allow them to judge heterosexual excesses of a pathological nature. One of these was voyeurism, described as "he is always showing us funny pictures of naked people or looking into people's windows trying to see girls undressing or sitting on the pot—he's always been that way, it's his habit." Although this pattern involved an artifact brought in from the outside—pictures—the overall behavior was conceived censoriously, and the young man in question was brought before the village fathers for punishment and supervision.

Similar village action was brought to bear in controlling one or two people defined as promiscuous—a girl "going too far with too many boys," or "not controllable by her parents." A young man was sent by the Eskimos to a federal jail because, "among other things, he stays home from hunting and 'forces' all the women, any woman from 16 to 60."

B. *Addiction.* The only intoxicant that could be abused in the recent history of St. Lawrence culture was alcohol. Fly-agaric was used aboriginally on the Siberian side, but there was no mention of it or other local intoxicants by our informants. For many years, however, alcohol was available from American and Russian whalers. In 1878 the St. Lawrence people are reputed to have gone on a rum debauch during the hunting season. Failing to lay in an adequate supply of walrus meat for the winter, the population was decimated by starvation. Later, a self-imposed prohibition against the importation of alcohol was enacted. Throughout the lifetime of most of the Eskimos in our study, alcohol was not easily accessible (this was changing by 1955 when beer could sometimes be obtained privately from soldiers at an installation near the village). This background explains the relative lack of experience with alcohol on the part of the recent population. Nonetheless the concept of overuse or misuse of alcohol was quite clear, on the basis not only of the 1878 debacle, but also of observation of specific individuals. One man who had grown up in the whaling era was known as a "big drunkard," and his sensations during inebriation were described: "He told me he felt as though he were walking two feet above the ground."

C. *Antisocial and dyssocial behavior.* There were numerous acts against the rights of others or against moral prescriptions that the Eskimos considered to be punishable or reprehensible. Some of the individuals who carried out these acts and did not learn from experience or punishment were thought of as quite permanently "bad characters." These acts included stealing, physical violence against others, and repeated swindling. A certain amount of maltreatment of women was not considered to be abnormal—"women used to be pushed low around here"—but even this could be carried too far, as when one man was brought to the village governing body because he beat up his wife "too much." Another kind of sociopathy in the conceptions of these Eskimos is black magic. Although the practice of sorcery and witchcraft, like shamanism, is on the decline, the concept of witching as an antisocial behavior is still viable; for example: "You can't trust that kind of person, he knows songs, is in touch with the devil, and lots of people believe that he killed a man recently with his ways."

5. PERSONALITY DISORDERS

The St. Lawrence language has a term for a person "who knows what he should do but has no sense." By one informant, this was not considered a sickness, nor was it mental deficiency; it meant lack of judgment and often making a nuisance of one's self. As such it seems to parallel rather well our concept of personality disorder. A young man who fitted this pattern was said to be "sort of crazy." For example, "He goes around saying in a false voice, 'I'm the United States of America Legion on this island' "; but all the time he knows, of course, that he is not. The informants said that he is always fooling, and he doesn't take care of himself.

A dimension of personality disorders pertinent to Western psychiatric thinking is the passive-aggressive continuum. It is evident from the comments under sociopathy that aggressive acts were recognized as such in this group. There were other instances, however, when aggression seemed to be thought of as a personality feature even though its expression did not reach the level of intensity that would incline Eskimos to institute severe restrictions and restraints against the person. "Getting mad very easily" was their way of depicting this. A manager of the native store was fired from this post by the village council because "he has got the 'educational' for the job but he gets mad too quick, the same as when he was left in charge of the mission when the missionaries went on leave, it got into a mess with everybody's feelings hurt." This kind of response was noticeable to Eskimos and was easily discussed, partially because it required some kind of action or adjustment on their part. The same was not true of passivity. We have a less definite picture of its conceptualization, especially as to whether it was thought deviant or likely to interfere with normal functioning. There were assessments of people, however, as "very humble," "doesn't talk rough to anybody," "very quiet." It is evident then that Eskimos recognize differences in personality and that some of these differences approximate the aggressive-passive polarization.

6. PSYCHOPHYSIOLOGIC REACTIONS

As indicated earlier, the Eskimos conceive a relationship between psychological events and physiological reactions—"heart beating hard because of too much worry," "headaches due to brain work," and "vomiting but not sick, just throwing up when she hears a bad story." As might be expected, there was no use of words such as "ulcer," "asthma," or "hypertension." To the Eskimos, if they suffered from any of these syndromes, they were described as "belly ache," "trouble breathing," or "headaches." It is not our purpose in this chapter to discuss prevalence, but it is our general impression from the epidemiological investigation that asthma, for example, is uncommon. It may be, therefore, that the Eskimos lack concepts of these more complex psychosomatic reactions because they lack experience with them. It may also be that the heavy burden of tuberculosis and other physical diseases in this population masks the prevalence and reduces the likelihood of conceptualization. (The topic of physiological reactions is the focus of the next chapter.)

7. PSYCHONEUROTIC REACTIONS

The native vocabulary for neurotic traits is quite rich. St. Lawrence Eskimos have a general term for "worrying too much until it makes a person sick," and others for "easy to get afraid"

and "too much nervous, sitting with head down and rocking."
As can be seen, English terms were also used—"nervous,"
"fear," and "worry." The word "anxiety" was never used, but it
appeared that the idea of anxiety was in their minds. We mean
by this that "worry" and "fear" were always qualified as excessive or inappropriate when they were remarked upon as indicators of sickness or malfunction; for example: "You know, he
sometimes worried and afraid too much. 'Alingatuk,' that is
what we call the man who is easy to get afraid when something
happens like bad weather or sickness or out of food. He became
the chairman of this village once, but he was worried too much
that time, he hates to rule the people around here, and so he
refused later on."

There were cases described by Eskimos that correspond to
several of the more specific varieties of psychoneurotic reactions
known to Western psychiatry. One of these was phobic with a
claustrophobic focus: "He has been very sick once, even hates
to stay indoors, always worrying and wants to stay outdoors; he
worrying too much, but I don't know what kind of sickness that
is." Several appeared to be conversion reactions. One of these,
for example, was described as, "She was paralyzed once, can't
walk and can't move around much; she was beaten so bad by her
husband, that was how she became paralyzed, but I guess she
just thought she was sick because later a Coast Guard cutter
doctor ran his fingernail along the sole of her foot; it jumped
and jerked and the doctor told her to try walking a little at a
time and now she is okay."

Some kinds of fainting, as said earlier, were definitely linked in
the Eskimo minds with psychological events. These types of
fainting seemed to be associated with the functioning of the
heart, which served as a premonition that a faint would be experienced: "She is become frightened all of a sudden and get
nervous, heart beating fast," "so nervous she almost collapsed."
These sensations were thought of as "heart attacks," which culminated in a swoon or sometimes in the feeling of choking, and

were concomitants to such experiences as seeing blood, coming near a sick child, or being in a crowd.

Other symptoms of anxiety that the Eskimos meant when they talked of nervousness were trembling, restlessness, and shaking. One case of "nervousness" was actually called "shaking sickness"—this was one feature of the claustrophobic syndrome mentioned above, and the onset of the illness was coincident with the patient's conversion to Christianity. In addition to the equation of "nervous" with "trembling," there was also a meaning that referred to "lack of feeling" in much the same way we would refer to anesthesias: "During that time this side of my face was nervous—no feeling." There were two or three cases in which a reaction focusing on the facial muscles was noted: "Her face getting loose right after marriage—it went loose or something—then she got all right."

8. DEPRESSION

This is not a separate symptom pattern category in the system described in the last chapter because depressive symptoms can feature in several kinds of psychiatric disorders. Since depression is an important psychiatric concept, we wanted to take a special look at the Eskimo view of it.

The concept of suicide has had a long history in the St. Lawrence culture. In the past, ritual suicide was practiced— usually if the person seemed to be suffering an interminable illness, if he thought he could safeguard the life of a sick child by taking his own, or if he were excessively despondent.[29] The pattern of such suicides was highly formalized, and the suicidal act took place in a designated public area. Although we learned of people who had died this way during the memory spans of living Eskimos, no one in our study population had committed ritual suicide.

The idea that a person might contemplate a private suicide in moods of hopelessness or in despair at misfortunes was also recognized, as indicated in the psychotic episode of the woman who tried to freeze herself. Another instance was a crippled girl who, after several unsuccessful love affairs, drank part of a bottle of Clorox in the hope that she would die. She did not die but continued to have periods of depression which she described as involving disinterest in what happened to her; but she said, "If I do die I hope they put a door or window in my coffin so I can reach up and get out of it in case I'm not dead." In addition to this self report of depressive feelings, there were descriptions by Eskimos that they had observed a person to be sad or unhappy even though these emotions did not reach the level of preoccupation with suicidal thoughts. Thus the Eskimo conceptualizations of mood, at least as portrayed through English, indicate that they identify patterns that are closely allied to depression.

9. CONCEPTS FOR SPECIAL PSYCHIATRIC REACTIONS

There were two Eskimo concepts of psychopathology that diverge from the Western psychiatric outline we have been following thus far. One of these is "voodoo" death, a phenomenon observed in a sufficient number of primitive tribes that people in the Western tradition have put a name to it—thanatomania—even though it is rarely seen in our culture.[30] The concept of death through witchcraft activities—psychological death—is well developed on St. Lawrence Island. That it remains viable despite the gradual dwindling of sorcery and shamanism is indicated by the fact that a recent death in the village was explained by numerous Eskimos as being caused by a particular witch and the belief of the deceased that he would die this way. Interestingly enough, the public health nurse in this instance could offer no alternate or more plausible cause of death.

One other kind of psychopathology recognized by the Eskimos differed from what is usual in Western psychiatry. This followed very closely what has been reported as the culture-specific pattern of *piblokto* in the eastern arctic; however, we do not know whether the St. Lawrence language includes a specific term of reference for it. Only one case was reported in this study, and it was described as follows: "I thought at first that she was partly shaman but later on I found out that she does that way once in a while, out of mind a little bit, I think." The patient's episodes were sudden, brief in duration, and not stylized in the manner of shamanism. During these periods of disturbed consciousness she shouted and grimaced. The "out-of-mindness" lasted for only a few minutes.

10. THE CONCEPT OF IMPAIRMENT

The foregoing makes clear that beside these specific concepts of patterns of disorder, the Eskimos have the conceptual equipment for making judgments about *impairment* of functioning produced by psychiatric symptoms and disorders. Many of the cases were partly explained in terms of interference with normal functioning: not hunting, not trapping, not taking care of the house, having to give up a job or leadership role.

Conclusion

This chapter has centered on views of psychopathology found in an Eskimo village. In order to summarize, let us return to the model of a hypothetical culture in Melanesia. This model was used at the beginning of this report to explore ideas about death as a way of illustrating some of the facets involved in cross-cultural comparisons of concepts.

In the Melanesian group, we noted first the differences between their orientations and those of the West. The differences were marked in that they bury not only dead people but also near-to-dead people, that they do not have separate words for dead people and buriable people who are not dead, and that they believe death is caused by the magic of casting spells or burning effigies. The St. Lawrence Eskimos exhibit many of the same kinds of differences regarding psychiatric disorders. We would be struck by the differences in cultural practices were we to see a child wearing a fox-trapping net as a cure for "fits"; or an Eskimo sorcerer picking on a mentally defective person to run his ominous errands; or a psychotic patient being treated by a shaman who, in séance, looks and acts much "crazier" than his patient. Then a study of the Eskimo words on the topic of psychiatric phenomena would disclose the lack of an Eskimo counterpart for some of the general terms, such as mental deficiency and senility, which we consider eminently useful; it would show that many of their designations for psychiatric syndromes are descriptive where ours are diagnostic, and that while some of the patterns of thought, feeling, and behavior which we consider to be psychiatric illnesses they also call "illness," others are looked upon simply as "oddness," "badness," or "unhappiness." In the realm of etiological explanation, differences are also remarkable. Asking Eskimos what they think causes various kinds of psychiatric patterns, we would hear of a patient's father breaking the law of the hunt in wounding but not killing a fox, of an enemy using witchcraft to put a hex on another patient, and of still another patient's soul having been captured by marauding spirits from whom the Eskimo shaman would seek the soul's release.

A longer acquaintance with the St. Lawrence people permits us, however, to discover that in conjunction with these basic differences there are equally basic similarities. In the Melanesian example, further exploration of views about death brought us to the value of distinguishing between the word and the concept. Although the Melanesians have only one word for people they bury—dead or alive—this terminology is not a measure of befuddlement as to who is dead and who is alive. At the conceptual level they distinguish the physical properties of life from death by virtually the same criteria used in the West. In the Eskimo study we found much the same situation. Although their psychiatric vocabulary varied in many respects, our subjects recognized disabilities that correspond to the whole range of major types of disorder identified in psychiatry. Even though their labeled categories were different in terms of omissions and elaborations, they described the symptoms we commonly associate with senility, neurotic reactions, and so on. Since some of the behaviors we think of as psychiatric—seizures and spiritualistic control—figure in shamanistic séances as well as in psychopathology and to some extent the same words were used to describe both types of phenomena, it was of interest to learn that conceptual distinctions are clearly made. In other words, there was no difficulty in differentiating between genuine pathology and socially useful behaviors that bear some resemblance to psychopathology. At this level we can say that the Eskimos share with us many criteria regarding impairment in functioning for telling pathology from nonpathology, just as the Melanesians share common physical indicators of the difference between life and death.

The Melanesian illustration gave further insight into differences and similarities by demonstrating that magical theories about the causes of death coexist with rational theories. These rational theories are similar to ours in several ways—for instance, in the awareness that people die of old age or as a result of physical illness, accidents, and violence. An interplay between magical and natural explanations was also characteristic of the psychiatric orientation of Eskimos in this study. Thus, along with the ideas about soul loss, taboo-breaking, and witchcraft, the Eskimos pointed to further determining influences such as heredity, brain damage through accidents or illness, and personal misfortunes. Their observations of human behavior seem to have led to concepts about body-mind, nature-nurture, disorder-wellbeing that in the gross sense are rather comparable to ours.

From this exercise in studying native concepts of psychiatric disorder we have concluded that there are noteworthy differences between the stream of thought of the St. Lawrence Eskimos and that of psychiatry. There are, however, underlying parallels which strongly suggest that cross-cultural comparisons can reasonably be made.

Notes

1. L. Lévy-Bruhl, *Les Fonctions mentales dans les sociétés inférieures* (Paris: Librairie Felix Alcan, 1922); F. Boas, *The Mind of Primitive Man*, rev. ed. (New York: Macmillan, 1938); and P. Radin, *Primitive Man As Philosopher*, rev. ed. (New York: Dover, 1957).

2. W. H. R. Rivers, "The Primitive Conception of Death," in *Psychology and Ethnology* (New York: Harcourt, Brace & World, 1926), pp. 36–50.

3. *Webster's New Collegiate Dictionary*, 2nd ed. (Springfield, Mass.: G. & C. Merriam Co., 1953), p. 171.

4. For example, "A Bibliography on American Indian Medicine and Health," compiled by William C. Sturtevant for the Smithsonian Institute, Bureau of American Ethnology (mimeographed) contains approximately 400 references.

5. E. H. Ackerknecht, "Psychopathology, Primitive Medicine and Primitive Culture," *Bulletin of the History of Medicine*, vol. 14, no. 1 (1943), pp. 30–67.

6. The most comprehensive study of primitive psychiatry to date is: G. Devereux, *Mohave Ethnopsychiatry and Suicide: The Psychiatric Knowledge and the Psychic Disturbances of an Indian Tribe*, Bulletin 175, Smithsonian Institute, Bureau of American Ethnology (Washington, D.C.: United States Government Printing Office, 1961). A useful bibliography on this topic is: M. I. Teicher, "Comparative Psychiatry: Some References in Ethnopsychiatry," *Revue Internationale d'Ethnopsychologie Normale et Pathologique*, vol. 1, nos. 1 and 2.

7. D. F. Aberle, " 'Arctic Hysteria' and 'Lâtah' in Mongolia," *Transactions of the New York Academy of Sciences*, vol. 14, no. 7 (May 1952), pp. 291–297; see also J. J. Abraham, " 'Lâtah' and 'Amok,' " *The British Medical Journal*, February 24, 1912, pp. 438–439; F. H. G. van Loon, "Amok and Lâtah," *The Journal of Abnormal and Social Psychology*, vol. 21 (Jan.–Mar. 1927), pp. 434–444; P. M. Van Wulfften Palthe, "Psychiatry and Neurology in the Tropics," in *A Clinical Textbook of Tropical Medicine*, C. D. de Langen and A. Lichtenstein, eds. (Amsterdam: G. Kolff, 1936); and P. M. Yap, "The Lâtah Reaction: Its Psychodynamics and Nosological Position," *The Journal of Mental Science*, vol. 98 (Oct. 1952), pp. 515–564.

8. K. Spencer, *Mythology and Values: An Analysis of Navaho Chantway Myths* (Philadelphia: American Folklore Society, 1957), p. 3.

9. E. H. Ackerknecht, *op. cit.*; K. Rasmussen, "Intellectual Culture of the Igulik Eskimos," *Reports of the Fifth Thule Expedition*, Vol. VII, no. 1 (Copenhagen, 1920).

10. W. Bogoras, "Chukchee Mythology," in *Memoirs of the American*

Museum of Natural History, Vol. XII, Pt. I [Publications of the Jesup North Pacific Expedition, Vol. VIII (New York: G. E. Stechert, 1910)].

11. J. M. Murphy, "Psychotherapeutic Aspects of Shamanism on St. Lawrence Island, Alaska," in *Magic, Faith, and Healing: Studies in Primitive Psychiatry Today*, Ari Kiev, ed. (New York: The Free Press of Glencoe, 1964), pp. 53–83.

12. G. Devereux, "Normal and Abnormal: The Key Problem of Psychiatric Anthropology," in *Some Uses of Anthropology: Theoretical and Applied* (Washington, D.C.: The Anthropological Society of Washington, 1956); see also A. L. Kroeber, "Psychosis or Social Sanction," in *The Nature of Culture* (Chicago: University of Chicago Press, 1952), pp. 310–319.

13. E. H. Ackerknecht, *op. cit.*

14. F. E. Clements, "Primitive Concepts of Disease," *University of California Publications in American Archeology and Ethnology*, vol. 32, no. 2 (1932), pp. 185–252.

15. A. I. Hallowell, "Primitive Concepts of Disease," *American Anthropologist*, vol. 37, no. 2 (1935), pp. 365–368.

16. S. L. Rogers, "Primitive Theories of Disease," *Ciba Symposia*, vol. 4, no. 1 (1942), pp. 1190–1201; and "Disease Concepts in North America," *American Anthropologist*, vol. 46, no. 4 (1944), pp. 559–564.

17. J. W. M. Whiting, and I. L. Child, *Child Training and Personality: A Cross-Cultural Study* (New Haven: Yale University Press, 1953), pp. 122–123.

18. M. I. Teicher, "Three Cases of Psychosis Among the Eskimos," *Journal of Mental Science*, vol. 100 (1954), pp. 527–535.

19. E. H. Ackerknecht, "Medicine and Disease Among Eskimos," *Ciba Symposia*, July–August 1948, pp. 916–921; see also A. A. Brill, "Piblokto or Hysteria Among Peary's Eskimos," *The Journal of Nervous and Mental Disease*, vol. 40 (August 1913), pp. 514–520.

20. Z. Gussow, "'Pibloktoq (Hysteria) Among Polar Eskimos: An Ethnopsychiatric Study," in *Psychoanalysis and the Social Sciences*, Muensterberger and Axelrad, eds., Vol. VI (New York: International Universities Press, 1960).

21. M. A. Czaplicka, *Aboriginal Siberia: A Study in Social Anthropology* (Oxford: Clarendon Press, 1914); see also W. Jochelson, "The Koryak," in *Memoirs of the American Museum of Natural History*, Vol. X, Pt. II [Publications of the Jesup North Pacific Expedition, Vol. VI (New York: G. E. Stechert, 1908)]; and S. Novakovsky, "Arctic or Siberian Hysteria as a Reflex of the Geographic Environment," *Ecology*, vol. 5 (April 1924), pp. 113–127.

22. R. Redfield, *Peasant Society and Culture: An Anthropological Approach to Civilization* (Chicago: University of Chicago Press, 1956); see pp. 70–71 for a description of the mixing of disease concepts in Latin

American villages where contact with the Spanish brought knowledge of the humoral pathology of Hippocrates and Galen. See also R. Redfield and M. P. Redfield, "Disease and Its Treatment in Dzitas, Yucatan," *Contributions to American Anthropology and History*, no. 32 (June 1940).

23. The following is an explanation of the concepts and methods employed by Murphy in the key-informant interviewing:

One must take a number of concepts into account when interviewing about psychiatric disorder. An inventory of these ideas includes such terms as: "normal-abnormal," "dominant-deviant," "functional-malfunctional," "natural-unnatural," and "well-sick."

The inventory itself is far from precise, and like the phenomena it purports to catalogue is full of interconnections. It is not immediately obvious which concept or set of concepts is most appropriate for this kind of exploration, nor even which end of the continuum of health to illness offers the best starting point. One way of looking at the matter suggests that in markedly different cultures the initial step should be to construct paradigms of normality and from these to characterize abnormality. Another way suggests that the firmest step is to adhere as closely as possible to our own concepts of disorder and to seek counterparts in native belief.

Decision in this study to work mainly through the apertures of deviance and pathology rather than trying to construct ideas of normality involved a number of considerations. One was that it is doubtful if a person of any cultural background can conceptualize and verbalize normality as well as deviance and pathology. To ask an Eskimo the dimensions of wellness and normalcy is comparable to asking the average man in our society what human nature is. If the question is understood at all, the answer is so axiomatic in the informant's system of thought and feeling that he has difficulty communicating it and is reduced to describing it as "self-evident." "Self-evidence" under such circumstances has a way of being extremely recondite.

The concept of deviance has limitations, too. A deviant mode of thinking, feeling, and behaving is as likely to fall on the superior end of the scale and indicate optimal functioning as it is to indicate malfunctioning. It is usually easier, however, to spot evidences of incapacity and handicap than of exceptional ability. Historically many geniuses have gone unrecognized in their time, but few idiots have, even though the levels and shades of incapacity are extremely difficult to judge without testing and measurement.

Although some understanding of the value and limitations of each of these concepts is essential to the researcher, none is the kind of idea that can readily be explained to a native informant. In this study, psychiatric data were obtained in response to the question: "What sickness has such and such a person had?" or sometimes even more simply: "Tell me about such and such a person." This orientation appeared to help the key informant on two accounts: (1) questions about one person specifically are easier to answer than questions about people in general; and (2) questions about sickness require less generalization than questions about health and normality. Further, the concept of "illness" can be communicated fairly easily, and it can be anticipated that all people have a near equivalent in their own language.

After a conceptual approach has been chosen to guide the interviewing, a number of points about key informant selection and qualification remain to be spelled out in order to make clear both the limitations and the extent of data that can be gathered through this means.

One factor to bear in mind concerns whether special knowledge or common knowledge is sought. For the kind of special knowledge that is of interest in psychiatric epidemiology, an experienced shaman would seem an obvious choice. His knowledge of symptoms and his treatment of a large portion of the population during illness would have given him a fund of directly relevant information. None of the Sivokak shamans, however, was sufficiently bilingual to permit extensive and systematic interviewing in English. Since we were interested in generally held views of disorder, it seemed appropriate to seek someone who could convey common knowledge.

Not all cultures lend themselves to the use of common knowledge as an entré. In some cultures there are areas of knowledge to which only special novitiates have access, and there are cultural segregations that limit the expanse of any one individual's information. In India, for example, the purdah division of life into man's world and woman's world would make a female informant most unlikely as a candidate for an epidemiological study except of women. In Sivokak there are no barriers to a free flow of knowledge about people, and a woman key informant was chosen. The decision to ask her assistance rested on a number of factors such as language skill, willingness, and motivation demonstrated in earlier work. Also intimate health information was more easily conveyed in this culture between two women, investigator and informant.

The interviews were conducted in twenty-four sessions over the five-month period of this aspect of the year's study. They were composed of the informant's comments on a limited number of questions, systematically presented, regarding each individual in the 1940–1954 census. The project was explained as an attempt to find out different kinds of things that had happened to people in the village. The census was described as the means by which we would organize our work. The first question for each person was: "Can you tell me about X?" followed by: "Did he or she marry?" "Who are their children?" "Has X been sick?" "What jobs does he or she do?" "Has he or she been to the mainland?" "How far did he or she go to school?"

The questions were chosen in the hope of getting as full a record as possible of general life experience. It became evident early in the procedure, however, that the questions were not equally appropriate for key-informant interviewing. I soon realized that for a culture where all men are hunters and all women are homemakers, the question about jobs was not giving any new information except about those people who held governmental positions, and those I knew already. Much the same applied to migration. With regard to schooling, I found that the informant could give accurate data about whether a person had or had not finished the eight-grade school on the island and about those few who had gone beyond. But to ask for grade levels was quite unrealistic. Throughout the series I tried to minimize situations that required the self-deprecation of too many responses such as: "I don't know" or "I didn't quite remember that."

After the first two or three sessions the informant had sufficiently internalized the aspects of experience in which I was interested that she usually gave all the information she knew on the basis of my asking simply: "Can you tell me about X now?" It was clear that the questions regarding illness fell on fertile soil, as did also those about marriages and children. For these I consistently pressed to make sure that I had recorded everything she knew, and that I had given her time to remember. For the more expendable questions I was satisfied with what she gave on her own accord.

Key informants have been employed in collecting many different kinds of data such as kinship terms, diet habits, witchcraft, and religion. But to talk of practices is quite a different matter from talking about *people*. The question inevitably comes to mind as to how much information about people is gossip and how much is report of actual events. The opportunity to talk about one's acquaintances may be an open sesame for the expression of personal animosities. On the other hand, if there is no evidence of the informant's personal likes and dislikes, the question of hypocrisy arises. Especially in a psychiatric study this aspect of key-informant interviewing has to be judged in the light of cultural feelings of stigma regarding mental disorder. Can an accusation of mental symptoms stem from malicious intent against a disliked person? Is mental disorder conceived as something to be ashamed of and therefore repressed from information-giving?

The amount of data obtained from the key informant and other native informants suggests that there was little reluctance to communicate psychiatric information. There was certainly less hesitancy to talk about mental illness than about some of the old customs and beliefs.

With the exception of homosexuality no stigma appeared to be attached to it. Where homosexuality was concerned, if it did not take the form of transvestitism, it is as likely that native informants lacked knowledge of it as that they withheld information. It would be hushed up in the in-group as much as to outsiders.

Psychoses and mental deficiency did not appear to be something to hide. Mothers were known to be relatively free with their comments that one or another child had difficulty learning. "Sickness of mind" that reached psychotic dimension was viewed with the same sympathy as were other sicknesses. Likewise psychoneurotic and psychophysiologic symptoms did not seem to be stigmatized by the Eskimos, and it was more a matter of extent of knowledge than of prejudice.

Quite aside from cultural stigma, there are questions about reliability that relate to the internal standards by which a key informant herself judges the accuracy of information. How does she sort items into events versus rumors, facts versus fictions? This is by no means an insignificant problem when the informant has grown up relying on magic to explain many things.

In terms of the broad division between magical "truth" and "truth" in the historical and scientific sense, it seemed to me that the informant's world was starkly dichotomized between the Eskimo truths of her child-hood and the new truths of the white world which she accepted in adulthood. The new criteria did not invalidate past history; they were means of judging current affairs, but they simply did not apply to veri-fication of her past experiences and those of her parents' generation. To her it was absolutely true that people used to die because evil prayers were said against them. "It is a good thing we put away all those old stuffs," she said. Back in those times, people *did* get sick because they broke the law of the hunt and stole someone else's whale; shamans *did* see things and hear things of that other reality. Even in terms of the old beliefs, however, there seemed to be standards of accuracy—what might be called measures of the reliability of magic! Once, in the presence of her sister-in-law, who was secular to both the old and new faiths, the informant recounted a story concerning an entrancing half-woman, half-seal creature who had been seen on an ice floe. Her sister-in-law said that the story was nonsense. The informant insisted: "It's true; *two* people saw her!" Thus, like most Eskimos at mid-century, she believed both Eskimo and "white" at the same time.

I believe that she gave as accurate data as possible from whichever of her two premises was foremost in her mind at the time, and I conceived of it as my job as an anthropologist to decide which premise was operative at any given moment. For example, it was clear that in both of her intellectual worlds she was aware of the difference between rumor and opinion on one hand and events and history on the other. She sensed that I valued her discriminations about the criteria and validity of judgments, and at the end of the study it was possible to divide her information into the categories of what she had actually seen herself; what she had heard from the person in question; what she considered her own opinion ("That's just what I thinks myself"); what she considered rumors, enlightening and unenlightening; what she remembered clearly; what she did not remember; and what she did not recall but thought she could find out, and did find out, from other Eskimos.

Motivation is a complex aspect of this kind of interviewing—both too much and too little being disadvantageous. This informant appeared to be highly motivated, but I do not believe she therefore gave me false impressions based on a preconceived notion of what kind of information would please me. Since our work was never described as a psychiatric study, she never knew fully of this special interest.

In addition to assessing her own standards of accuracy it was also possible to measure the reliability of her data about general health by comparing what she said with the health records. There were only 107 health records available for the population of 495, but in 85 per cent of the overlay cases she correctly designated the symptom system that was described in the record. This obviously does not mean that the nomenclature was the same. It was possible, however, to see that her descriptions, though crude, accurately portrayed a disability of the pulmonary system, the cardiovascular system, or the musculoskeletal system. For example:

Health record of an old man who died in 1942:
"1940: Impetigo contageosa. Lesions about healed. Edema of feet, at times has bloody urine. Urine neg. for protein. Ointment for lesions. 1941: Complaint gastric, vomits dark fluid, pain sometimes, used to drink much whiskey. 1942: Man has jaundice, eyes and entire skin very yellow. Is losing weight rapidly. Has dyspnea, ascites, icterus. Bloody stool and sputum. Died in 1942.

Informant's report of his symptoms:
"During his boyhood when he was a young man he used to be a big drunkard. But he quit when he became older. When he getting older he became unhealthy. Sweating most of the time, always sweating, change his clothing about twice a day, especially in the evening he sweating too much and he doesn't feeling good with his belly too. Later on during his sickness his skin became yellowish. I don't know why it became like that, green or yellow partly, like that all over his skin. And then he died from that, and he had T.B. and he has been vomiting some big chunks of blood, something like that, awful smells too. T.B. that is what he vomits I think. He died in 1944, oh no, 1943. He has been sick and don't feeling good for a long time ago with his urine too. Sometimes he couldn't pass urine so easily I think. It was long before he died that his skin became yellowish too." [Unpublished field notes: J.M.M., 26 June 1955, p. 2.]

In addition to asking about reliability, it is also important to ask how much information one person can give concerning 494 other individuals.

To some extent this depends on the stability of the population, the amount of face-to-face contact between them, and the proximity of living arrangements. Certainly such a method would not be appropriate for a study of urban areas where affiliations are based on class, occupation, or associations that cross-cut residence and where population mobility makes many acquaintanceships temporary and superficial. Where Sivokak village is concerned, the first indication of the usefulness of this technique was the fact that the 494 questions drew no blanks. There was considerable variation in how much the informant knew about each person, but she had something to say about each name.

One of the variations regarding her knowledge of the village population concerned the age of its members. She had less to say about children than about adults. The age group of five years and under received scanty treatment. This made sense, however, for the length of contact with children is less. They have lived so little of their lives that there is not much to note unless they are severely abnormal, do not respond to the shaping processes of culture, or do not survive. As far as the epidemiological evidence of a psychiatric nature is concerned there was no reason to doubt her coverage. She described childhood symptoms that we would call tantrums, mental deficiency, epilepsy, and behavior problems. For other children her descriptions tended to be: "He goes to school. He is beginning to help his father. He is a healthy."

Apparently there were no variations relevant to sex. She knew things of psychiatric interest regarding both men and women. Of the 68 cases she contributed, 38 were women and 30 men. Thus her distribution on the basis of sex was similar to that in the overall total from all sources— 113 cases—which includes 60 women and 53 men.

There were differences in the amount of information (and therefore the likelihood of disclosing the less obvious psychiatric symptoms) that related to kinship ties and proximity. The most detailed account of medical and psychiatric history was of herself, then of her immediate family, and from there the degree of detail went out in waves of diminishing description to the extended family, tribe, and village levels. Detail was also greater for her next-door neighbors and, since she lives in the center of the village, it fanned out to less particular information regarding people who live at the peripheries. Nevertheless her coverage of the population in terms of psychiatric descriptions was sufficiently ample to have made this type of key-informant interviewing useful to a study of native concepts.

24. Grateful acknowledgment is given for the use of field notes gathered by our collaborators, Charles C. Hughes and Dorothea C. Leighton.

25. J. M. Murphy (formerly Hughes), "An Epidemiological Study of Psychopathology in an Eskimo Village" (Ph.D. Dissertation, Cornell University, 1960), pp. 224–231.

26. C. C. Frake, "The Diagnosis of Disease Among the Subanun of Mindanao," *American Anthropologist*, vol. 63, no. 1 (Feb. 1961), pp. 113–132.

27. A. H. Leighton, T. A. Lambo, C. C. Hughes, D. C. Leighton, J. M. Murphy, and D. B. Macklin, *Psychiatric Disorder among the Yoruba: A Report from the Cornell-Aro Mental Health Research Project in the Western Region, Nigeria* (Ithaca, N.Y.: Cornell University Press, 1963).

28. J. M. Cooper, "The Cree Witiko Psychosis," *Primitive Man*, vol. 6 (Jan. 1933), pp. 20–24. See also R. Landes, "The Abnormal Among the Ojibwa," *The Journal of Abnormal and Social Psychology*, vol. 33 (Jan. 1938), pp. 14–33.

29. A. H. Leighton, and C. C. Hughes, "Notes on Eskimo Patterns of Suicide," *Southwestern Journal of Anthropology*, vol. 11, no. 4 (1955), pp. 327–338.

30. W. B. Cannon, "Voodoo Death," *American Anthropologist*, vol. 44, no. 2 (1942), pp. 169–181.

IV: The Use of Psychophysiological Symptoms as Indicators of Disorder among Eskimos

By Jane M. Murphy and Charles C. Hughes

EDITORIAL NOTES

Although interest in "culture-personality" studies declined in the postwar era, serious attention was directed during this period to epidemiological research regarding the distribution of psychiatric symptoms in nonhospitalized populations. It was obvious that one source of guidance for developing methods was a study of previous work with psychological screening tests, particularly as these had emerged during the war. When the Stirling County Study got under way in the fifties, the late Allister Macmillan undertook to examine these screening instruments and to select or construct and standardize a test that would be appropriate for use among adults in rural communities.

The approach found to be most closely allied to the needs of the Stirling Study was that taken by the armed forces in a program of screening for neurotic and related symptoms. Nevertheless the questionnaire had to be remodeled to suit the different situation in which it would be used. Unlike the young males tested for military service, a rural community is not a "captive audience." It comprises, moreover, a broader age range and includes both men and women.

With advance knowledge of the community and in consultation with physicians who knew the area, Macmillan devised a questionnaire which he named the Health Opinion Survey (hereafter called the HOS). For purposes of validation and standardization, the questionnaire was tried out in communities similar to those of Stirling County but at a distance from it.[1] In its original pretesting form, the instrument consisted of seventy-five items dealing broadly with health but with a majority of questions centering on complaints of a psychophysiological nature—that is, queries mainly about physiological sensations such as numbness, fatigue, or weak feelings. Items were taken from the Army's Neuropsychiatric Screening Adjunct with additional questions from other instruments such as the Minnesota Multiphasic Personality Inventory and from suggestions made by local physicians. The questionnaire was administered in private, using mobile trailers fitted out as offices, and the questions were asked by an interviewer. The whole procedure required about twenty minutes, and the questions as well as the presentation of the project were given with as much care as possible to avoid causing anger, suspicion, or embarrassment.

During the stages of standardizing this technique and reducing its size to a manageable number of items for surveying larger populations, two measures of validity were instituted. Responses to the same questionnaire were obtained from local patients, both in-patient and out-patient, who had been diagnosed as neurotic. By means of statistical procedures it was possible to achieve a smaller list of items (twenty questions) and a concomitant scoring system which reached an adequate level of discrimination between the group of known "ill" and another group composed as fully as possible of people who were presumably "well." Another measure as to whether a given pattern of responses indicated the presence or absence of psychiatric disorder was an independent clinical appraisal by a psychiatrist of a subsample of the pretested group.

This work as well as the efforts of others to develop screening instruments has produced series of survey questions for which high frequency of positive responses is *correlated* with what psychiatrists in a clinical context discover to be psychiatric disorder, especially psychoneurosis. The fact that the survey questions tend to concern psychophysiologic sensations rather than, for example, dynamic or interpersonal questions is a matter of empirical demonstration. Correlation is, however, quite a different matter from a clinical definition of psychoneurosis. It should be emphasized that frequent feelings of weakness, upset stomach, and palpitations do not themselves necessarily constitute psychiatric illness.

In the Midtown Study, a rather similar procedure was employed in developing a screening test.[2] Called the Twenty-two Item Screening Score (hereafter referred to as the Twenty-two Item Score), this list of questions also is concerned mainly with psychophysiologic symptoms, and a noteworthy aspect is that there is considerable overlap in the twenty questions selected for Stirling and the twenty-two for Midtown. A study of social status in Mexico, which is the last chapter of this volume, made use of the Midtown screening instrument, while the Stirling HOS is the topic of the present chapter.

On the basis of trying to assess populations of people in Western society, several drawbacks and advantages may be noted regarding instruments such as the HOS. The score on the test when not buttressed by information drawn from other sources tells little or nothing about the type of psychiatric disorder, its duration, or the kind of impairment. The questions also, apparently, register rather poorly some of the more severe reactions such as schizophrenia, mental retardation, and sociopathic behavior. On the other hand, the question lists serve as very good indicators of psychoneurotic and psychophysiologic disturbances—that is, those types of disorder which are prevalent in communities at large. The brevity and rapid scoring make possible the screening of large samples, and the content of the questions is not likely to offend or incline people into giving evasive or misleading answers.

For cross-cultural studies instruments such as the HOS or the Twenty-two Item Score have the further asset that the questions, being mostly concerned with fairly specific sensations, are somewhat resistant to distortion when translated from one language to another. Before assuming, however, that such a screening device can be employed in cross-cultural epidemiology, several questions of feasibility and validity need to be explored in a circumscribed trial situation. It could be, for example, that in cultures other than urban and rural North America these physiological indicators are not highly correlated with anxiety, depression, or other psychoneurotic patterns. In such a case, the questionnaire would fail as a screening instrument.

The present chapter is a report of an exploratory study made in 1954–1955 by two anthropologists, Murphy and Hughes, employing the HOS with a sample of Eskimos from the larger study of psychiatric epidemiology described in the last chapter. Their Eskimo work followed the initial period of the Stirling Study during which they collaborated in using the HOS to gather data about mental health and mental illness in rural Canada. The goal of the trial HOS survey among Eskimos was to scrutinize the test for its usefulness as a method of surveying psychoneurotic symptoms in a non-Western population.[3]

THIS chapter reports a trial experiment in using and analyzing the results of a structured questionnaire for gathering data about mental health in a non-Western culture. For this purpose, a sample of Eskimos from Sivokak village on St. Lawrence Island in the Bering Sea were asked to respond to the Health Opinion Survey questionnaire. A copy of the questionnaire is incorporated in the text, together with some notes concerning its administration. Each question is then reviewed as to its suitability for use in the Eskimo culture. Alternative or additional questions are recommended where knowledge of the culture indicates the possibility of some misunderstanding of the concepts involved, and a quantitative comparison of the Eskimo responses with responses from sample members in the Stirling County Study is presented. In the last section of the chapter, attention is given to methods for scoring the HOS results so that the "illness-wellness" rating provided by each Eskimo's responses can be compared with other evidence on the mental health status of the sample members. The corollary information used in these final comparisons consists of key-informant materials and observational data which have been evaluated by two psychiatrists.

Questionnaire and Preparatory Steps for Its Administration

The Health Opinion Survey questionnaire used in this study is reproduced in Table IV-1. The arrangement of items follows

Table IV-1. Eskimo Health Opinion Survey questionnaire *

Name   Sex   Age   Highest School Grade Completed
1. How has your health been, on the whole?
   1. good   2. medium   3. poor
* 2. Do you have any particular physical or health trouble at present?
   1. no   2. yes
3. What sorts of serious illnesses have you had?
   Illness   *Age*   *How sick were you?*
4. Have you ever had one of the following? (Check any already mentioned in previous question, and omit from mention in this question.)

Illness	Age(s) in years at time(s) of occurrence(s)	How sick were you?	Remarks

---

Eye trouble
Ear trouble
Sinus trouble
Throat trouble

Bronchitis
Pneumonia
Pleurisy
T.B.
Boils & abscesses
Low blood (anemia)
Heart trouble
High blood pressure
Low blood pressure
Stomach trouble
Diabetes
Bowel trouble
Piles
Kidney trouble
Bodily injury
Operations (list)
Rupture (hernia)
Rheumatism
Arthritis
Sciatica
Neuralgia
Tooth trouble
For women: female trouble
Other (specify)

---

5. Have you ever had to go easy on your work because of poor health?
    1. no 2. yes
6. What age were you? For how long did this last?
7. Have you ever had to change your work because of poor health?
    1. no 2. yes
8. What age were you? How long did it last?
* 9. Do your hands ever tremble enough to bother you?
    1. often 2. sometimes 3. never
*10. Are you ever troubled by your hands or feet sweating so that they feel damp and clammy?
    1. often 2. sometimes 3. never
*11. Have you ever felt that you were going to have a nervous breakdown?
    1. often 2. sometimes 3. once or twice 4. never
*12. Have you ever been bothered by your heart beating hard?
    1. often 2. sometimes 3. never
*13. Do you tend to feel tired in the mornings?
    1. often 2. sometimes 3. never
*14. Do you have any trouble in getting to sleep and staying asleep?
    1. often 2. sometimes 3. never

Table IV-1. Eskimo Health Opinion Survey questionnaire (*cont.*)

---

*15. How often are you bothered by having an upset stomach?
    1. nearly all the time   2. pretty often   3. not very much
    4. never

*16. Are you ever bothered by nightmares? (dreams which frighten or upset you?)
    1. many times   2. a few times   3. never

*17. Do your arms or legs go to sleep rather easily?
    1. often   2. sometimes   3. never

*18. Have you ever been troubled by "cold sweats"?
    1. often   2. a few times   3. never

*19. Do you feel that you are bothered by all sorts (different kinds) of ailments in different parts of your body?
    1. often   2. sometimes   3. never

*20. Do you smoke?
    1. a lot   2. some   3. not at all

*21. Are you ever troubled by sick headaches?
    1. often   2. sometimes   3. never

*22. Do you ever have loss of appetite?
    1. often   2. sometimes   3. never

*23. Do you ever have a bad taste in your mouth?
    1. often   2. sometimes   3. never

*24. Does your food ever seem tasteless and hard to swallow?
    1. often   2. sometimes   3. never

*25. Do you feel it is necessary to take vitamin pills for your health?
    1. often   2. sometimes   3. never

*26. Do you depend on patent medicines?
    1. often   2. sometimes   3. never

*27. Do you feel that you are more apt to catch contagious diseases than most people?
    1. yes   2. no   3. undecided

28. How would you say your health was this past year?
    1. excellent   2. good   3. fair   4. poor   5. very poor

29. Do you feel in good spirits?
    1. most of the time   2. sometimes   3. very few times

Now I'd like to ask some questions about the health of your close relatives:

30. How has the health of your mother and father been, on the whole?
    1. excellent   2. medium   3. poor

31. How about your brothers and sisters, how has their health been, on the whole?
    1. excellent   2. medium   3. poor

---

* A portion of the material has been used in earlier studies and is reproduced here by permission of the author's wife, Mrs. Allister M. Mac-

the format employed in the Stirling County Study. The twenty crucial questions are indicated by an asterisk. A few additional questions were asked in both the Stirling and Eskimo studies to provide a rough estimate of the degree to which illness interfered with routine activities and to obtain information on family health history. A further inquiry, not part of the HOS itself, takes the form of a medical checklist.[4]

The HOS was conducted in the last month of a year's visit on St. Lawrence Island. By that time most of the study of social change—the central purpose of the field trip—had been completed, and much had been learned about Eskimo culture and about concepts and prevalence of illness. Thus one of the main preparatory steps for the HOS trial was to formulate *a priori* hunches and reservations about the suitability of each individual question in studying psychiatric disorder in this culture.

For the survey, a census of the population in Sivokak village was prepared from government records compiled by the school teacher. Resident in the village during the survey period and available for the first-hand interviewing were 146 adults over eighteen years of age. A systematic sample of twenty names was drawn by selecting the first appropriately aged person in the census and every subsequent seventh thereafter.[5] Although it was not adjusted for equal representation of men and women, the sampling produced ten male names and ten female names. Five additional questionnaires were obtained from two women and three men. These people had previously given life history data and were included in the HOS survey for supplementation

millan, and the publisher from A. M. Macmillan, "The Health Opinion Survey: Technique for Estimating Prevalence of Psychoneurotic and Related Types of Disorder in Communities," *Psychological Reports*, vol. 3, Monograph Supplement no. 7 (1957), and by permission of the authors and publisher from C. C. Hughes, M.-A. Tremblay, R. N. Rapoport, and A. H. Leighton, *People of Cove and Woodlot: Communities from the Viewpoint of Social Psychiatry* [Vol. II, The Stirling County Study of Psychiatric Disorder and Sociocultural Environment (New York: Basic Books, 1960)].

and cross-checking. Since there is no reason to think that the additional five Eskimos were either especially ill or especially well, the remainder of this chapter focuses on the twenty-five questionnaires in order to reflect as large a number of response patterns as possible. Although the sample is small, it represents 17 per cent of the adult population.

Prior to the survey, we interviewed key informants to find out whether the symptoms and sensations discussed in the HOS questions were known to the Eskimos and whether they could be translated into the Eskimo language. We discovered that all the health items qualified in this minimal way. This does not mean that all items were equally relevant as characteristic expressions of psychiatric disorder in this culture. But whether or not the questions on vitamin pills and patent medicines, for example, applied to the Eskimos in terms of psychiatric malfunctioning, the concepts were understandable to them and could be stated in their language or conveyed by English words that were commonly understood. The questionnaire was administered verbally, either in English to bilingual Eskimos or when necessary in the Eskimo language using experienced interpreters with whom the questions were carefully reviewed before the survey was instigated.

By 1955 the Eskimos in Sivokak village were well accustomed to the procedures of public health programs. People were usually informed of these by the village leaders, who went from house to house telling them to appear at the school or clinic for examinations of one kind or another. Apprehension about tuberculosis, sickness, and death was so vivid and so widespread that cooperation could usually be counted on. Also the Eskimos had previously experienced "home visits" by public health nurses or itinerant doctors who asked many questions. With this as background, there appeared to be a favorable climate for a survey such as the HOS. This was confirmed by the fact that we ran into few problems of rapport.[6] At the end of the survey, we concluded that it was feasible to administer such a questionnaire among Eskimos and that the individual queries were sufficiently meaningful to warrant the further analysis described in the following pages.

Analysis of Twenty Questions

The ideal way to design and standardize an HOS questionnaire for cross-cultural work would be to start with a large list of questions administered in each of several different cultural groups, so that we could be sure the full spectrum of significant psychological reactions and psychophysiological sensations was being tapped. The next step would be to select the questions that most effectively sort the known psychiatrically ill people in these cultures from the known well. The hope would then be to combine the results of the several studies and determine a core set of universally appropriate questions so that cross-cultural comparisons could be made directly from responses to the same questions. This forecasts an extremely long and expensive operation of pretesting, and it presupposes that we know in advance what in reality we are seeking to discover, namely, the ways of identifying psychiatrically ill people in a foreign culture.

Thus for the purposes of gathering data that may illuminate this problem, let us assume at the beginning that certain questions have universal applicability. This is not an unreasonable assumption in view of (1) the common denominators of the human condition such as need for sleep, fatigue after exertion, occasional palpitations as well as other physiological events, and (2) the fact that variations in these functions are probably significant to the psychiatric status of people from widely different cultural origins. For the moment, then, our attitude is experimental. We decided to go ahead and ask the questions that have been found useful in other studies, bearing in mind that culture-specific variations in psychoneurotic and psychophysiological reactions could be reflected by weighting and scoring of the responses. For example, questions about generalized hypochondriacal preoccupations or specific bodily rhythms may be strong indicators in culture A, while sensations of fear may be more important in culture B, even though one would not want to leave out questions of either kind in cross-cultural studies.

It seems worthwhile, therefore, to review the twenty questions in the light of what we know about Eskimos and Eskimo culture and through comparison of the Eskimo response patterns with those of Stirling County residents. Although subsequent sections of this chapter build on the results of this review, the purpose here is mainly to systematize a series of recommendations on how the HOS might be improved in preparing for a large-scale study of Eskimos. It is not intended as a *demonstration* of the relevance or irrelevance of *individual* items from the questionnaire. This is to be especially underscored because there is reason to believe from the Stirling and Midtown Studies that the questions taken separately are not nearly as crucial in indicating disorder as is the totality of responses.

If we start with the question: "What makes a particular Eskimo say 'yes' or 'no' to a given item?" it is obvious that the answer lies in several factors, some of which are more or less idiosyncratic, some related to physical considerations, some to cultural practices and beliefs, some to the wording of the question or the interview situation, and some to psychological phenomena. Because of our interest in cross-cultural comparison, one aspect of the twenty-question review is to ask ourselves, "Does an Eskimo respond in a particular way because he understands by the question the same thing that a resident of Stirling County understands?" The second aspect concerns whether there is a similar psychiatric implication in the questions when asked of Eskimos, that is, do the questions have the same potentiality for either being correlated with or conveying information about emotional upsets. Although we have not operated on the principle that the sensations and feelings queried in the twenty items define psychiatric disorder in either Stirling County or among Eskimos, it is clear that the questions are not an entirely random selection. "Does your food seem tasteless and hard to swallow?" bears a relationship to psychological disturbance in Western culture that would not be true of physical sensations such as experiencing pain when sunburned or frostbitten. Thus we want to look at the questions further to see if it is likely that a psychological dimension will be dominant and the influence of cultural and physical factors minimal.

From this viewpoint, the twenty questions seem to fall into five categories.

1. *Questions centering on views, practices, and patterns of physical illness.*

     2. Present health trouble? *

     27. Susceptible to contagious disease?

     25. Vitamin pills?

     26. Patent medicines?

Attention was immediately drawn to questions relating to physical illness because the Eskimos, like many underdeveloped groups, experience a much greater prevalence of physical disease than do members of our own culture. Further, the history of these Eskimos is typical of that of other arctic inhabitants regarding the introduction of tuberculosis and periodically devastating epidemics of measles and flu, giving evidence that the Eskimos as a group do not yet have immunity to many of the diseases that have less drastic effects in our culture. The possibility of a psychiatric component being related to positive responses about present health trouble or susceptibility to contagious disease might therefore be vitiated. It was our impression, however, that illness was so much a focus of anxieties for the St. Lawrence Eskimos that these questions might be highly correlated with psychological disturbance though not in themselves a direct outcome of such disturbance. Also, the question on susceptibility is appropriately worded: "Do you feel *more*

---

* Although the questions have been rearranged in order, the numbering system has been retained for cross-reference to pp. 112 to 114.

apt to catch contagious diseases than most people?" As such, it seemed an adequate reflector of preoccupation with health.

The questions about need for vitamin pills and patent medicines were the only ones not consistently asked. Such pills and medicines are not part of the existing culture and are not readily available. Thus we asked about them only in situations where understanding was certain. In looking back on our field notes and reviewing the affirmative responses to these questions when they were asked, we found that the acculturated Eskimos seemed to be far more knowledgeable about these matters than we had supposed. The physical isolation of the Island had been largely overcome by trips to the mainland for hospitalization, by National Guard training camps, and by schooling. Mail ordering had also done a great deal to bridge the gap. Western medicine was one of the first and most enduring attractions the white world offered to this physically debilitated population, and "cure-alls" and "wonder drugs" had great significance as objects about which to center, however unrealistically, the hopes and fears concerning the health situation of the Island. Thus, despite our initial misgivings about the four questions involving physical health, fuller knowledge of the Eskimo situation suggested that these items are particularly suitable.

2. *Questions involving food and the gastrointestinal tract where diet habits might be relevant.*

    15. Upset stomach?
    22. Loss of appetite?
    23. Bad taste?
    24. Food tasteless?

A first reaction to the HOS questionnaire when we began to think of it in connection with the Eskimo survey was that, taken as a whole, it seems to emphasize questions involving the gastrointestinal tract. Four out of the twenty items concern some aspect of the alimentary canal—stomach upset, food, taste, and appetite. No other bodily system receives so much attention. Although this focus may be appropriate in Northeast America, it is not necessarily so on St. Lawrence Island. Our reservations, therefore, mainly concern the number of items on this theme and the correspondingly fewer items on other themes that might be more pertinent to the Eskimos. Also, however, there were diet patterns that might influence responses to these questions.

We doubted that "upset stomach" would have much psychiatric significance in the Eskimo population. Gastrointestinal complaints were extremely common as a reflection of generally poor health, mild epidemics of flu, and diet variations. During the times of poor hunting when food was scarce people ate meat that was rotting and which in better times would have been consumed only by the dogs. They did not ordinarily eat "high meat," although as in other Eskimo groups this was sometimes a necessity. The public health nurse for the Island held the view that lean periods were correlated with outbreaks of stomach trouble and attributed this to periodic waves of food poisoning.

Although lean periods were not continuous, food was rarely plentiful. In addition, diet habits were being revolutionized. Many people preferred white man's food to Eskimo food, and some children refused altogether to eat native meat because they found the odor offensive. Although responses about taste and appetite might be somewhat ambiguous in such an underfed population undergoing such change in diet, our skepticism about these questions was somewhat allayed by the fact that outside the HOS situation, Eskimos said they recognize a link between emotional disturbance and at least one of these items—loss of appetite. Of these four questions, then, we have greatest reservations about "upset stomach" and greatest confidence in "loss of appetite."

3. *Questions in which wording might influence response.*

 13. Tired in morning?
 19. Ailments all over?

We did not believe that the "morning tiredness" question would apply to the Eskimos—not because they lack the idea and sensations of tiredness but because they have different sleep habits. People sleep during the daytime and work at night if necessary in view of hunting possibilities. We were consistently impressed by the irregularity of sleep patterns and believed that it was increased by the nearly continuous darkness or continuous light depending on the season of the year. Since the Eskimos do understand fatigue, we would recommend that questions about this sensation be recast in more understandable terms such as, "Do you tend to feel tired a lot?" or "Are you tired even when you wake up?"

The question on ailments is stated: "Do you feel you are bothered by all sorts (different kinds) of ailments in different parts of your body?" This is the most abstract of all the items and requires the greatest generalization from the respondent. We anticipated that questions about specific sensations would be better understood. It was intended that this question elicit responses indicative of hypochondriacal concern and of those psychologically induced organic discomforts that have the distinguishing feature of shifting all around the systems of the body. This intent was probably not conveyed in the complicated wording of the question. Since there are Eskimo words for overconcern with illness and malingering, these phenomena are clearly known to them and would probably have been more profitably explored by two or three more concrete questions.

4. *Questions in which cultural practices might be pertinent.*

    17. Arms or legs asleep?
    20. Smoke?

It seemed to us that the item on "arms and legs going to sleep" would lack psychiatric significance because of a cultural practice of the Eskimos. Customarily they sit on the floor without back support and with their legs extended straight out in front of them. This posture almost invariably produces numbness in people who do not habitually sit that way, and even Eskimos say it becomes uncomfortable and that they frequently have numb feelings. This is one of the few questions that was stated simply

"Do you experience this sensation?" rather than "Are you bothered or troubled by this sensation?" Thus we would recommend a restatement of the question in the latter form in order to reduce the likelihood that a cultural practice will mask the psychophysiological import.

The other question in which cultural practice might predominate is "smoking." In studying a group that does not have tobacco available, this question would obviously be meaningless. As it happens, the St. Lawrence Eskimos, both men and women, have long made use of tobacco in many forms. There were no restraints of propriety to control the use of tobacco except in the presence of missionaries or latterly among those who have adopted the missionary view. Nor were there restraints in 1955 based on medical awareness of the possible ill effects of smoking. Because smoking appeared to be such a common practice, uninhibited by some of the factors that relate to smoking patterns in Stirling County, we would recommend that the question for Eskimos be worded: "Do you feel you smoke too much?"

5. *Questions that do not appear to be distorted by cultural or physical considerations.*

   9. Hands tremble?
   10. Hands or feet sweat?
   11. Nervous breakdown?
   21. Sick headaches?
   14. Trouble sleeping?
   12. Heart beating hard?
   18. Cold sweats?
   16. Nightmares?

The judgment of the adequacy of the "hands tremble" item was supported by descriptions we heard of trembling and shaking as expressions of worry and depression ("shaking sickness" has already been referred to, p. 94). Variations in tendency to perspire were recognized; for instance, one man was described as a "big sweater." We did not hear of this sensation in association with emotional disturbance but neither did we have any evidence that it might not be a psychiatric variable. The phrase "nervous breakdown" was used by some of the acculturated Eskimos, and, as indicated in the last chapter, the concept was approximated by a number of Eskimo words. The phrase "sick headaches" has a colloquial tone that is readily understandable to people in Stirling County. It is doubtful that this was assimilated by the Eskimos, and we presume that their responses refer to ordinary headaches. This did not seem to be a distortion of significance. The question on "trouble sleeping" avoids the difficulties described for "morning tiredness" and seemed to be an adequate way to ask about sleep disturbance.

During the year of investigation we were impressed by the degree to which fear was generated and expressed in the Eskimo group—fear of witchcraft, fear of becoming sick with tuberculosis, fear of going hungry, and fear of the physical dangers of hunting on the ice or being lost in the arctic storms. Much of this was undoubtedly realistic fear, and we realized that the problems of distinguishing between fear and anxiety are somewhat similar to those of differentiating between organic symptoms that stem from physical malfunction and organic complaints that are mainly of psychological derivation. Nonetheless it seemed to us that any symptoms such as palpitations and "cold sweats," which might be a physiological expression of fear, deserved special attention.

We heard many descriptive accounts of people having the sensation of heart pounding. Some were simply the reporting of reactions to "scary" events. We also learned, however, that the Eskimos conceive of this symptom as "psychiatric" in some situations and "normal" in others, that is, they linked it to states of "worrying *too* much" and "*too* easy to get afraid" as well as considering it a normal reaction to psychological trauma. Also the Eskimos look upon palpitations as a premonition of a "faint," and some of them viewed a "faint" as chiefly characterized by the cessation of the heart beat rather than by unconsciousness. A "faint" was, in fact, described as "dying a little bit." As remarked in the last chapter, fainting seemed to be quite frequent among the Eskimos.* Thus, besides noting the appropriateness of the palpitation item, we would recommend further exploration of this area through questions such as, "Do you take weak turns?" "Do you get dizzy or faint often?" and "Do you ever lose consciousness?" [7] Other questions that could be asked as ways of investigating the psychology and physiology of fear would refer to "choking sensations," "hair-raising experiences," and "goose flesh."

We also expected that the item on nightmares might be especially appropriate to a group that practices witchcraft and other forms of spiritualism. During the year there were a number of "scares" which Eskimos elaborated in dreams. For example, two or three people thought they saw a big animal prowling around the village at night. This was so vivid a threat that for several nights young men took turns standing watch to guard the village. Some people had "bad dreams" about this eerie creature. Nor should "voodoo" death be ignored in a group that believes in witchcraft. Among these Eskimos, several deaths were imputed to "voodoo" sorcery, and it would be pertinent to ask about "voodoo" experiences; for example, "Have you ever felt that you were being hexed and might die?"

This concludes the statement of recommendations and conjectures based on knowledge of Eskimo culture. The review can be summarized as an attempt to separate those questions which seem to be equally good indicators for the Eskimos from those questions which might not be. We judged ten questions to be appropriate for the Eskimos in their present form ("present health trouble," "susceptibility to disease," "vitamin pills," "patent medicine," "loss of appetite," "hands tremble," "hands or

---

* Also, as remarked in the last chapter, conversion reactions seemed to be more prevalent than anticipated. Although conversion is not related to the point in hand nor directly relevant to other points in these five categories, we do want to observe that questioning in this area would seem desirable.

feet sweat," "nervous breakdown," "sick headaches," and "trouble sleeping"). Eight questions, we thought, would have different meaning, either being unintelligible because of wording ("tired mornings" and "ailments all over") or referring to behavior and sensations that are especially common for cultural and physical reasons and for which the enhanced or reduced psychiatric implications would have to be established through further work ("smoking," "arms and legs asleep," "upset stomach," "heart beating hard," "cold sweats," and "nightmares"). We were undecided about two questions ("bad taste," and "food tasteless").

The credence of these ideas can now be examined in greater detail by comparing the areas of convergence and divergence in response patterns of the Eskimo sample and two Stirling samples. One of the Stirling groups is a probability sample of 1,003 subjects living in rural communities. The other is a group of ninety-three diagnosed neurotic subjects from in-patient and out-patient services in the general area of Stirling County. The answers from this latter group were those mentioned earlier as having been used in selecting and weighting the HOS scores employed in the Stirling Study.

We know, then, that the two Stirling samples are different: one is a group identified as "symptom-carriers"; the other is a typical community population in which, we can presume, the symptom-carriers are much less concentrated. An assumption made for the twenty-question review as well as for this comparative analysis is that the sample from the Eskimo village is more like that of the Stirling communities than like the population of neurotic patients in terms of the prevalence of ill people. This view rests on the strong unlikelihood that the Eskimo sample would include as great a number of symptom-carriers as a group purposefully defined as neurotic—even though, one could guess, there might be a few more psychiatrically ill people maintained in the Eskimo village owing to the dearth of hospital and clinic services. Figures IV-1 and IV-2 present HOS data on the three populations showing that the Eskimo village sample and the sample of Stirling community respondents are indeed more similar to each other than either is to the sample of neurotic patients.

Figure IV-1 is a diagram of each of the three populations, constructed by scoring the HOS information given by each sample respondent. The scoring system worked out in the Stirling Study has been employed, and it has been assumed that the samples are an adequate reflection of the populations as

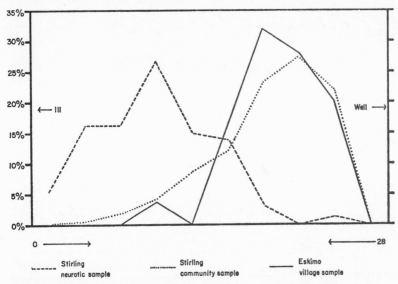

Figure IV-1. Frequency diagram based on raw data of the Stirling weighted scores for three samples. Ordinate = percentage of sample population. Abscissa = Stirling weighted HOS scores. The range is from 0 to 28, low scores meaning illness and high scores "wellness."

wholes. The similarities and differences between the three populations are brought out more coherently by the application of probit analysis as shown in Figure IV-2. This analysis was undertaken in order to examine the consistency of the raw data with the normal distribution of frequencies. By means of this probit technique, it has been possible to project the presumed normal population from the evidence provided in the sample study.[8] This figure appears to verify the similarity of the two

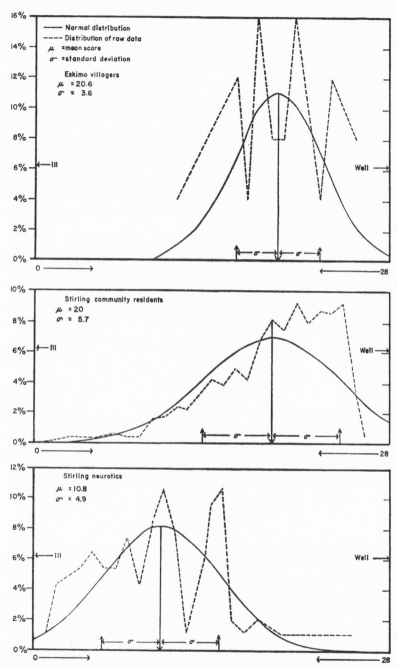

Figure IV-2. Frequency distributions of HOS scores for Eskimo villagers, Stirling community residents, and Stirling neurotics with best-fitting normal curves

community populations and their difference from that of the neurotics.

The next task is to look at the Eskimo and Stirling responses for the individual questions. These materials are given in Figure IV-3. Each lined bar represents two standard deviations around the mean per cent of the Eskimos responding "often," "sometimes," or "never" to each question. The checked bars have the same meaning for the Stirling respondents, and the dotted bars for the neurotics. The use of two standard deviations contributes to the understanding of these data by showing the range in which two-thirds of the responses fall, assuming normal distributions.

Inspection of this chart indicates that there is a characteristic response pattern for the Stirling patients which is different from that of the Stirling community members.* The general paradigm of the patients' response pattern (based on averaging) is for 25 per cent to respond "often," 44 per cent "sometimes," and 31 per cent "never." The paradigm for the community residents is 9 per cent "often," 24 per cent "sometimes," and 67 per cent "never." Because the Eskimo sample is small, the range of 2 standard deviations is considerably broader than the ranges for the Stirling samples. Nevertheless it is immediately apparent that the HOS questions produced a unique distribution of responses among Eskimos. It is theoretically possible that all the Eskimos would have responded "never" to every item, in which case we would have concluded that these questions were probably meaningless and certainly incompetent for differentiating psychiatrically ill Eskimos from those in good mental health. Also the Eskimo pattern is, for some questions, similar to that of the

* Nineteen of the questions provide a trichotomous response pattern; one requires the choice of "yes" or "no." This gives a total of 59 possible comparisons. For the Stirling community residents and the Stirling patients there are only nine instances where the standard deviation ranges overlap. This includes the questions on vitamin pills and patent medicines, which are omitted from Figure IV-3 because not every Eskimo was asked these questions.

Figure IV-3. Comparison of Eskimo and Stirling response patterns*

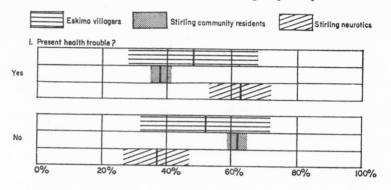

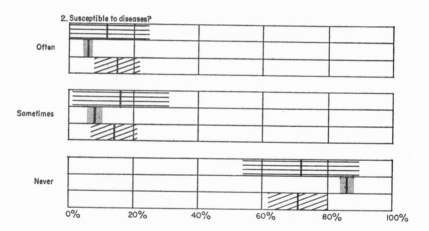

* The diagram for each question is arranged so that the figures at the bottom represent the percentage of the population responding Often, Sometimes, or Never. The bars represent two standard deviations around the mean for the respective population, and the mean for each is indicated by a line through the middle of the bar. The difference in the lengths of the bars is explained by the facts that: (1) the three samples are different in size, and, hence, the range for the smaller sample (the Eskimos) is larger than that for the other two (the Stirling residents and the Stirling neurotics), and (2) where questions drew a particularly large or small number of responses in the Often, Sometimes, or Never category, the range is smaller than if the mean had more nearly approached 50 per cent. It should be further noted that where a question elicited no responses in a given category (and this occurred only for the Eskimos in the Often category for questions 6, 8, 9, 11, and 17, and in the Never category for question 13) the two standard-deviation range for zero, in this instance, is from 0 to 13.7 per cent.

Figure IV-3 (cont.)

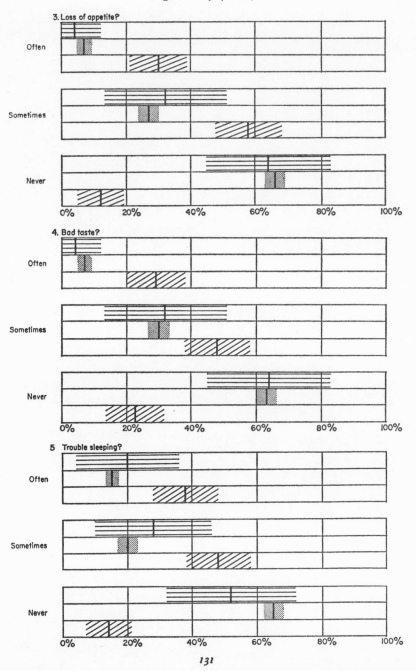

3. Loss of appetite?

Often

Sometimes

Never

0%   20%   40%   60%   80%   100%

4. Bad taste?

Often

Sometimes

Never

0%   20%   40%   60%   80%   100%

5 Trouble sleeping?

Often

Sometimes

Never

0%   20%   40%   60%   80%   100%

Figure IV-3 (cont.)

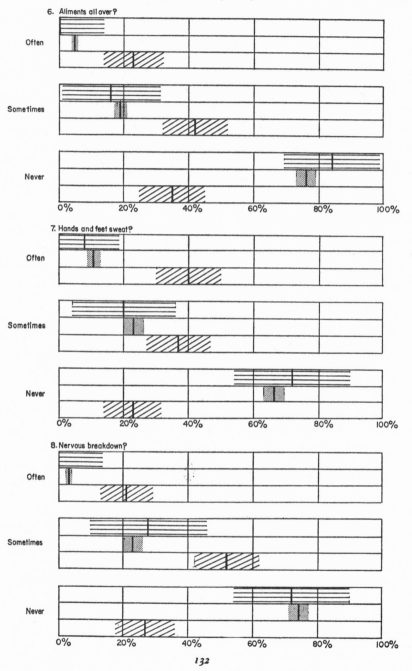

6. Ailments all over?

7. Hands and feet sweat?

8. Nervous breakdown?

Figure IV-3 (cont.)

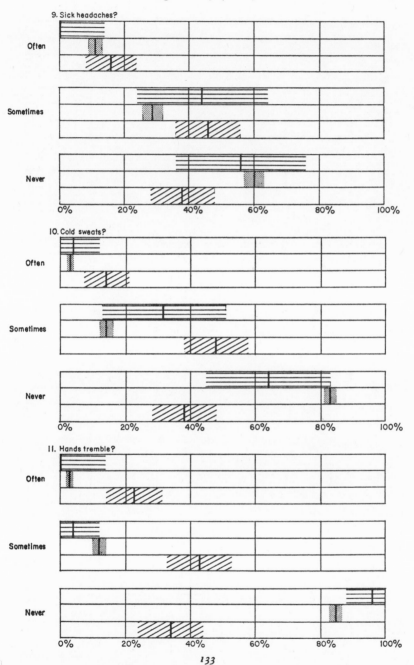

Figure IV-3 (cont.)

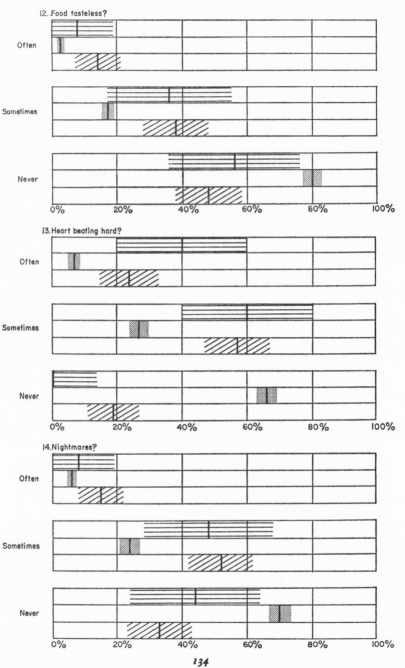

134

Figure IV-3 (cont.)

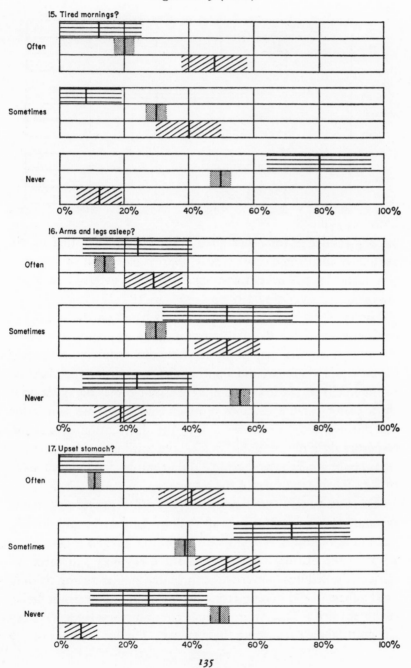

135

Figure IV-3 (cont.)

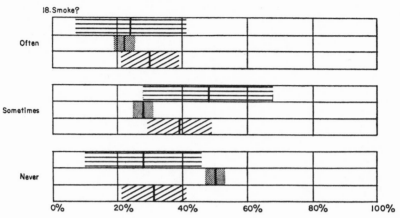

Stirling residents; for other questions it differs from that of the Stirling residents and more nearly approximates that of the neurotics; and for still other questions the Eskimo pattern is ambiguous because it overlaps both.

The interpretation of these patterns is based on the following outline. First, if the distribution of Eskimo responses to a given question resembles that of the community residents in Stirling County and there are no contraindications from the data on Eskimo culture, it can be tentatively assumed that the question is an indicator for the Eskimos in much the same sense as it is for the Stirling people; and second, if the distribution of Eskimo responses does not resemble that of the Stirling residents, attention is redirected to the data on Eskimo culture for suggestions as to the probable meaning of the responses.

The first twelve questions in Figure IV-3 provide the same general kind of response pattern in both the Eskimo and Stirling community samples. (In nine instances the Eskimo ranges comprehend the Stirling ranges on all three responses; in three instances the Eskimo pattern is sufficiently similar to the Stirling and sufficiently different from the neurotics to warrant being included here.) There is no serious contradictory evidence from the cultural data regarding these twelve. The list includes nearly all the recommended items as well as the questions on "bad taste" and "food tasteless," and the query on ailments. We note that the Eskimos have the highest frequency in the "never" category for the item on ailments, suggesting that, as we suspected, this question is difficult to grasp. Nevertheless it follows the Stirling community pattern. The list also includes "cold sweats," which was classified among the fear reactions that might be especially significant among Eskimos.

The only question for which the Eskimo responses do not at all overlap those of Stirling residents concerns palpitations. In this instance the Eskimo pattern is more similar to that of the neurotics. Although somewhat less precise, the same pattern holds for the item on nightmares. The cultural data suggest that heart sensations and bad dreams are areas of considerable importance for our understanding of emotional states of Eskimos. From this evidence and the information that the Eskimo responses for these questions are similar to responses from neurotics, we conclude that these two items are especially good questions to ask Eskimos.

And finally there are four questions ("tired mornings," "arms and legs asleep," "upset stomach," and "smoking") for which the Eskimo responses are, on the whole, different from those of the Stirling residents, though a less perfect divergence is evidenced than is the case with palpitations. It is common for Eskimos to experience these variables "sometimes," and the cultural data suggest that they are probably inappropriate for a psychiatric investigation of the Eskimos.

It can be concluded from this discussion that the HOS instrument could be made more sensitive to Eskimo-specific patterns of psychoneurotic and psychophysiological reactions. Nonetheless the majority of items appear to be useful indicators, and it is worthwhile, therefore, to proceed to the problem of developing a summary score of the HOS responses for each individual Eskimo in the sample. Such a score can then be compared to corollary data on the sample members to yield additional evidence as to whether the HOS is or is not on the right track in spotting cases of psychiatric disorder.

The scoring system designed in the Stirling Study for maximal differentiation between the "ill" and the "well" involves the application of different weights to different items. This system was applied to the Eskimo sample in Figures IV-1 and IV-2 (pp. 127, 128). Since the system was especially apposite to the Stirling samples, there is a built-in bias for the items that are particularly significant in that culture. It is of interest, therefore, to apply an unweighted scoring system to the Eskimo data. This would be a more direct reflection of the Eskimo responses and would serve to index the findings without commitment, at this point, as to which questions are most or least potent. Thus "often" responses were assigned the numerical value of 3, "sometimes," 2, and "never," 1, and a score was compiled for each sample member. By this system high scores register frequent positive responses to the psychophysiological indicators and should, therefore, if our methods are at all accurate, point to poorer mental health than the low scores, which reflect frequent negative responses. As it turned out, the weighted and unweighted scores were highly correlated for the Eskimos. The correlation coefficient is .86 (23 df, $p < .001$).[9] This justifies the employment of either scoring system, but in order to introduce as little speculation as possible we decided to carry out the remainder of analysis using the unweighted scores.

Psychiatric Evaluation of the HOS and Other Materials

It is now possible to consider the relationship of the HOS scores to another method, called a "psychiatric evaluation," which is used to determine the psychiatric functioning of the respondents. In keeping with the procedures of the Stirling Study, this method involves a clinical appraisal of the twenty questions, as well as the medical checklist, the few additional questions on illness interfering with the respondent's work, and certain corollary information. In the Stirling Study the corollary data consisted of comments given by local physicians about each respondent and of hospital records where they pertained. The appraisals were made by psychiatrists, individually at first and then jointly in session, in order to reach agreement that would take account of the clinical judgment of each evaluator. The step-by-step operations involved in this method of evaluation have been published elsewhere and will not be given in detail here.[10] Suffice it for the purposes of this presentation to say that the final results of the psychiatric evaluation can be stated symbolically as a rating of judgment regarding whether the respondent is a "psychiatric case" and the degree to which he is impaired by psychiatric symptoms. The symbols in this rating system are as follows: *A* means "definitely psychiatric," *B* is "probably psychiatric," *C* is "doubtful," and *D* is "probably not psychiatric." The impairment scale reflects judgments about the degree of impairment in total life functioning: "minimal" means up to 10 per cent impairment, "mild" means 20 to 30 per cent impairment, "moderate" means 30 to 50 per cent impairment, and "severe" means 50 per cent or more.

The Eskimo materials were prepared for evaluation in a manner as similar as possible to that employed in the Stirling Study. The full questionnaires comprising responses to the twenty questions, the additional questions, and the medical checklist were reproduced and presented to Alexander H. Leighton and Dorothea C. Leighton who did the evaluations. The identity of each respondent was disguised because both Leightons had been on the island in 1940, and A. Leighton returned in 1955. Thus many of the sample members were known to them.* The comments of the key informant who had assisted in making the

---

* The reason for disguising identity at this stage of the analysis was to insure that the evaluations would be based on comparable information gathered systematically for each Eskimo in the sample and not upon the evaluators' own recollections of these Eskimos.

systematic health survey (described in the last chapter) were included in the protocols presented to the evaluators. These were as close an approximation to the systematic comments from local physicians as we were able to achieve in the Eskimo study.

Since we were interested in the relationship of the HOS scores to the psychiatric evaluations, it was advantageous to convert the psychiatrists' *ABCD* ratings into a numerical value. A statistic found useful for this purpose in the Stirling and Midtown studies is called the "ridit." The ridit, named for the phrase "relative to an identified distribution," is a probability measure with a range from 0.00 to 1.00; the mean for the group investigated being .50.[11] In this system, ridit values that fall above .50 refer to poor mental health relative to the whole Eskimo sample as indicated by the psychiatrists' judgments, and ridits below .50 refer to relatively good mental health. Ridit values were calculated from the Eskimo data, allowing us to translate an *A* rating (high confidence that the individual is a psychiatric case) as the numerical value of .82, *B* as .54, *C* as .26, and *D* as .04 (the last value meaning that the individual is not a psychiatric case). The correlation coefficient of the unweighted HOS scores with the psychiatric *ABCD* ridits is .68 (23 df, $p < .001$).[12]

On several accounts we consider the evaluations a more valid detection of psychiatric disorder than the HOS scores, particularly since (1) the evaluations incorporate, besides the twenty questions, both Western and indigenous materials about psychiatric malfunctioning, and (2) they summarize the impressions of psychiatrists familiar with the St. Lawrence culture and with many Eskimos. The correspondence between the HOS scores and the psychiatric evaluation ridits should not be construed, however, as demonstration of the validity of the HOS. Since the twenty questions contributed to the evaluations, the two measures are not independent and a certain degree of parallelism is to be anticipated. Nonetheless it can be said that when further systematically gathered information about health, personality, and adjustment was added to and evaluated with the HOS responses, the findings were quite consistent with what would have been conveyed about illness and wellness on the basis of the HOS scores alone. A further illustration of this relates to the impairment ratings. Twenty-one of the twenty-five Eskimos were judged to be only minimally impaired; however, the four who were evaluated as mildly impaired had congruently high HOS scores.

A final method of judging the usefulness of the HOS technique was provided in the compilation of materials, other than the key-informant comments, that contributed to the total population study described in the previous chapter.[13] These consist of the public health records, the minutes of the meetings of the village council, comments by other native informants, school teachers, missionaries, and nurses, and the recorded observations of the psychiatrists and anthropologists. None of these sources gave information on each individual in a systematic way, although, when they pertained, the data were often of considerable depth and content. A deficiency of these materials for this HOS assessment is that they were gathered with an eye to discovering the kinds of psychopathology experienced by Eskimos, and there was not a similar effort to note evidence of wellness. Although at this point we still do not have much outside evidence that Eskimos who have low HOS scores or who were evaluated as *D* or *C* are indeed "well," the independent information on *illness* has considerable value as corroboration and in providing further suggestive points.

The full dossiers on each Eskimo were assessed by Alexander H. Leighton. This procedure was patterned on the "psychiatric evaluation" and it produced a new set of ratings. In this second round of evaluations, when the psychiatrist had access to the extraneous case materials, six changes in rating were made. When it was discovered, for example, that one woman was thought by other Eskimos to be mentally deficient, her first evaluation of "*D* with no impairment" was changed to "*B* with mild impairment." Another kind of change related to a re-

Table IV-2. Eskimo HOS scores, psychiatric *ABCD* ratings, and independent evidence of symptom patterns

Case identification	Sex	Age	Unweighted HOS scores	First *ABCD* rating	Symptom patterns	Second *ABCD* rating
a	F	39	39	A mild	Pn +, Pp − Personality disorder *	A mild
b	F	57	39	A mild	Pn +, Pp −	A mild
c	F	34	38	A minimal	Pn −, Pp −	A minimal
d	F	45	37	A mild	Pn +, Pp −	A mild
e	M	76	35	B minimal	Pn −, Pp −	B minimal
f	F	25	35	B minimal	Pn −, Pp −	B minimal
g	M	20	33	B minimal	Pn −, Pp −	B minimal
h	M	55	33	A mild	Pp − Brain-epilepsy *	A mild
i	M	32	33	A minimal	Pn +, Pp −	A minimal
j	F	18	32	C minimal	Pn −, Pp −	C minimal
k	M	56	32	A minimal	Pn +, Pp −	A mild
l	M	32	31	C minimal	Pn −, Pp − Brain-concussion *	A no impairment with concussion
m	F	52	31	A minimal	Pn −, Pp − Brain-epilepsy *	A minimal

n	M	38	C minimal	Pn−, Pp−	C minimal
o	M	17	C minimal	Pn−, Pp−	C minimal
p	F	49	A minimal	Pn−, Pp−	A minimal
q	M	42	C minimal	Pn−	B minimal
				Fainting with loss of consciousness *	
r	F	17	C minimal	Pp−	C minimal
s	F	30	B minimal	Pn+, Pp−	A mild
t	M	40	C minimal	Pn−	C minimal
u	F	70	D no impairment	Pp− Mental deficiency *	B mild
v	M	23	C minimal	Pn−	C minimal
w	M	18	D minimal	Pp−	D minimal
x	F	24	B minimal	Pn+, Pp−	B minimal
y	M	37	C minimal	Pn− Personality disorder *	B minimal

The symbols in the "symptom patterns" column have the following meanings: "Pn" means psychoneurotic, "Pp" means psychophysiologic, "*" means that the evidence of the symptom pattern came *only* from a source *other than* the twenty questions, "+" means that evidence of the symptom pattern came from the twenty questions *as well as* from the independent sources, and "−" means that evidence of the symptom pattern came *solely* from the twenty questions.

estimate of the impairment rating without an alteration of the "caseness" rating. Because of the nature of the extra data, none of the changes was in the direction of increased confidence that the Eskimo in question was psychiatrically well; that is, there were no transfers from an *A* or *B* category to a *C*, for example, or from a mild impairment rating to a minimal. Also, since the absence of additional information could not be taken as an indication of wellness, the *D* rating of "probably not psychiatric" was not used in the re-evaluations. (A case originally evaluated as *D* was, however, retained as such in the second evaluation if no further data were available. This applied in only one instance.) In this final procedure the psychiatrist was given the name of the Eskimo, and he was able to bring to bear his first-hand knowledge of many of the sample members. Owing to the various qualifications indicated about these final assessments, no attempt was made to carry out correlational analysis with the HOS scores. Their usefulness in this chapter is in illustrating a number of points about the symptom patterns indicated and not indicated in the HOS.

Table IV-2 is a summary of much of the material presented in this chapter. It gives the HOS scores, the two psychiatric ratings, and the symptom patterns for each of the twenty-five Eskimos. These data are oriented to the unweighted HOS scores, which are arranged on a continuum with the illness-signifying values at the top and the wellness-signifying scores at the bottom. The column on symptom patterns shows the kinds of symptoms identified by the psychiatrists and the source of evidence for each of the symptom patterns.

Inspecting the information on symptom patterns, we see that the data on personality disorder, brain syndromes, fainting, and mental deficiency were obtained entirely from sources other than the twenty questions, though the two cases of epilepsy were reported in response to the medical checklist. (This is shown in the table by the use of an asterisk.) We are inclined, therefore, to the opinion that the Eskimo experiment agrees with the work in Stirling County in suggesting that the competence of the HOS does not extend to the identification of disorders other than, chiefly, psychoneurotic and psychophysiologic reactions.

The most common symptom patterns are psychoneurotic (Pn) and psychophysiologic (Pp). The fact that such symptoms are registered throughout the scoring scale should not be interpreted against the differentiating ability of the HOS. There is no one in the sample who was evaluated as completely asymptomatic (nor do we consider wellness to be defined as such). Differences in the Pn and Pp patterns involve severity, kind, and amount of symptoms, and these are best measured in the *ABCD* ratings.

Next, it is to be noted that our methods of gathering independent data provided nothing on psychophysiologic symptoms. (This is indicated by the minus signs.) Such symptomatology is not likely to come to the attention of outside informants and observers unless it is severely incapacitating. A face-to-face interview with the subject is probably the best way of gathering such information, and our analysis thus far suggests that the HOS is an adequate and systematic procedure for doing this.

What about psychoneurotic reactions? This is an area of considerable importance because we believe from past experience that the HOS is particularly sensitive to this kind of symptomatology.[14] Because our attitude throughout this chapter has been exploratory, and because our independent evidence is not uniform, we decided to be satisfied if the extraneous data, when available, corroborated our evidence that the four or five individuals at the top of the HOS scale have psychoneurotic symptoms that interfere at least mildly with their functioning and that the four or five individuals at the bottom are mentally healthy in this regard.* (A plus sign indicates that the sources of

---

* This is a more rigorous level of demonstration than it may appear. Since all of these Eskimos are known to the anthropologists and the psychiatrists, it would be possible to use our recollections of them in an

information *other than* the twenty questions gave evidence of the presence of psychoneurotic symptoms.) Thus, three of the four highest HOS-scoring cases were strengthened in the assessment of psychoneurotic symptoms by the outside data. The situation was more equivocal for the low-scoring cases.

The lowest score (23) pertained to a 37-year-old man (Case *y*) who had a long history of being in trouble with his wife and the village council (he was evaluated as emotionally unstable in the larger category of personality disorder), but the key informant said of him, "He hasn't been sick, not very often, he's a healthy." Case *x*, with a score of 26, is a young woman who reported in the medical checklist that she had suffered the sensation of "something moving around in her throat, not an aching, something that felt dry and moved up and down below her Adam's apple." This information was rated by the evaluators as "probably a conversion reaction." The key informant confirmed this disability as well as its cure when the respondent had gone to a mainland hospital for the extraction of all her teeth at the age of 21! This case adds to our view that for the Eskimos the HOS did not adequately explore the problem of various kinds of conversion reactions. The next low scores refer to two young men about whom the key informant said the following:

---

assessment of their gradation from ill to well as indicated by the HOS score. The scores do, in fact, order people pretty much in accord with our impressions of their psychoneurotic characteristics, except for Case *s*—who has the relatively healthy score of 28. (It is the judgment of the investigators that this 30-year-old woman does have psychoneurotic symptoms that have impaired her functioning and that the psychiatric assessment of her as a *B* case is more accurate than the HOS score. Further it is the opinion of the senior author, who interviewed her using the HOS, that this woman was very tense and uneasy about the question-answer interaction and was concerned to create a good, perhaps even a "healthy," impression.) We have not taken the course of using memory because it is not possible, at this point, to be uninfluenced by the HOS scores. Therefore, we have relied entirely on materials put together for the epidemiological study before the HOS scores were known.

Case *w*

He is a healthy boy too now. He hunts lots, bird hunting and seal hunting. He and his brother are saving food for their mother and grandmother now. He isn't sick very much.

Case *v*

I know he went to school up to eighth grade here, finally he sent out to high school. But they found out later on that he got T.B. spot on his lungs, so they sent him outside to the hospital. He came back in 1952 I think after he had gone to the hospital. But he is curing now, but he is still eating pills and the doctors sent him home as he is about to be cured.

The ancillary data for Cases *a*, *b*, and *d* at the ill end of the scale are richer and more convincing, in each case suggesting perduring and generalized psychoneurotic reactions of the anxiety, depressive, and compulsive types. One case of a 45-year-old woman is given as illustration; it was chosen because it is the most concise.

Case *d*

Respondent (R) speaking of herself. R said (through an interpreter) that she always gets an older girl to stay with her overnight if her husband is away hunting or trapping. She has done that ever since she got married. She said she sometimes thinks she hears devils coming and she covers her ears and ducks her head under the covers (J.M.M., 7 April 1955).

Another Eskimo woman (X) discussing the Respondent. X said that she herself is a little bit afraid of going out on the water in a boat, but not as much as R is. When R goes to visit the other village in a big boat with the whole family, she crouches in the bottom of the boat and stays that way all during the journey (J.M.M., 20 April 1955).

R's husband describing his wife in a session with the anthropologist (J.M.M.). One evening J.M.M. was sitting in R's house—R, her husband, and children were present. R put on her parka to go outdoors to get some snow to help stop the nose-bleed which one of the children had developed. She started toward the door, and her husband said to me in English: "Jane, would you go outside with *R?* She is afraid of that 'big dog' that people think is prowling about." I did this, and *R* barely put her foot out of the door and grabbed a handful of snow and was back inside the door in a flash. She doesn't know many English words but she whispered "thank you" to me before we rejoined the group.

Later in the evening *R*'s husband abruptly asked me if I get worried easily. He said that his wife always worries about him. About a month ago he had been out hunting until 5:30 in the evening (which is not very late). *R* became worried and even went to see the old shaman to find out if the boat was in trouble (J.M.M., 14 February 1955).

Anthropologist's observations. All the boats from the village were out hunting late tonight. I was standing with a group of women on the shore about 10:30 P.M. Everyone was a little apprehensive. A small boy came up to the group and spoke to one of the women. This woman turned to me and said in English that *R* had sent the boy as a messenger to say that *R* is worried about her husband and the boats. This woman said that she was going down to *R*'s house to comfort her, and I went along. We found *R* in a great state of excitement. *R* said that she had been shaking and trembling because she is so worried about the boats being gone so long. Soon we got word that the boats were in sight. *R* took my hand and we literally bounded over the snowdrifts to the shore (J.M.M., 20 May 1955).

I think that *R* is the only really compulsive Eskimo I've met—always cleaning her house, always worrying about people tracking mud in, scrubbing the family clothes with Lysol to take the stains out, getting her husband to come with her on a visit to me so that he could translate her question on how it is that white women can keep their houses cleaner than Eskimos. She seems to have trained her children in the same way. Once her youngest child (age 4) had diarrhea. *R* told me that he was just like an adult. He wouldn't lie down and go to sleep because he didn't want to soil his clothes or the bed. So he stayed up, sitting on a piece of cloth (J.M.M., 21 April 1955).

Summary

This chapter has described a questionnaire method, called the HOS, which was given trial in an Eskimo group in order to study the prevalence of certain kinds of psychiatric symptoms in a non-Western culture. The twenty items that constitute the core of the HOS have been reviewed for their suitability as indicators of psychiatric disability among Eskimos. A scoring system was applied to the HOS responses so that the Eskimo sample could be studied in relation to a hypothesized gradation from ill to well. These scores were then analyzed in conjunction with the results of "psychiatric evaluations" of the HOS and other materials. Additional scrutiny of the scores was made in the light of independent materials on mental health and mental illness.

Two questions launched this exploratory study. One was: "Is it feasible and useful to employ a technique such as the HOS in cross-cultural research?" To this we would answer an unequivocal "Yes." The other was: "Does the HOS accurately detect psychiatric disorders among the Eskimos, especially the psychoneurotic and psychophysiologic types?" To this the answer is more circumspect. For the Eskimos, the HOS seems to be more effective in spotting "illness" than in distinguishing "wellness." Nevertheless we may conclude that, although improvements are needed, the technique is generally valid.

Notes

1. A. M. Macmillan, "The Health Opinion Survey: Technique for Estimating Prevalence of Psychoneurotic and Related Types of Disorder in Communities," *Psychological Reports*, vol. 3, Monograph Supplement no. 7 (1957), pp. 325–339. Stirling County is composed of an English and an Acadian French municipality. The standardization study reported by Macmillan was carried out in two neighboring counties which were predominantly English, and the sample included almost no French-Acadians.

2. T. S. Langner, "A Twenty-two Item Screening Score of Psychiatric Symptoms Indicating Impairment," *Journal of Health and Human Behavior*, vol. 3 (Winter 1962).

3. Most cross-cultural epidemiology undertaken to date has relied on

hospital admission rates as a case-finding method. A few studies, however, have approached the problem in a way somewhat similar to what we are considering here. The Cornell Medical Index, composed of 195 items, has been employed as a community screening test among, for example, Kaktovik Eskimos by N. A. Chance ["Conceptual and Methodological Problems in Cross-Cultural Health Research," *American Journal of Public Health,* vol. 52 (1962), pp. 410–417], and among South African Zulu by N. A. Scotch ["A Preliminary Report on the Relation of Sociocultural Factors to Hypertension Among the Zulu," *Annals of the New York Academy of Science,* vol. 84 (1960)].

4. All questions about health (the HOS and the additional queries) as they appear in the Eskimo Health Opinion Survey questionnaire were part of the family life survey used in the Stirling County Study. A copy of the total questionnaire used in the Stirling survey can be found in Appendix C in C. C. Hughes, M.-A. Tremblay, R. N. Rapoport, and A. H. Leighton, *People of Cove and Woodlot: Communities from the Viewpoint of Social Psychiatry* [Vol. II, The Stirling County Study of Psychiatric Disorder and Sociocultural Environment (New York: Basic Books, 1960)]. The health items used in the Eskimo survey appear on pages 509–513.

At the time of the county-wide epidemiological survey conducted in Stirling County, the validation study in neighboring communities mentioned on p. 109 had not been entirely completed. On the basis of analysis in hand, twenty-four items from the pretesting study were selected for inclusion in the "health section" of the larger survey on family and community life. Further validation was possible using data from within Stirling County. The criterion group, composed mainly of psychoneurotics, was expanded by including patients with similar diagnoses from the psychiatric clinic in Stirling County. The twenty questions finally used were demonstrated to discriminate significantly between this criterion "ill group" and a cross section of the heads of households in the communities surveyed in the Stirling Study. It should be noted that twenty questions were discovered as significant in the pretesting study and twenty were also chosen in the Stirling Study. These are not identical lists of questions although the correspondence is nearly complete. All the material presented in this chapter draws on findings from and comparisons to the Stirling Study proper. Further information on these topics is to be found in Chapter 7 and in Appendix E in D. C. Leighton, J. S. Harding, D. B. Macklin, A. M. Macmillan, and A. H. Leighton, *The Character of Danger: Psychiatric Symptoms in Selected Communities* [Vol. III, The Stirling County Study of Psychiatric Disorder and Sociocultural Environment (New York: Basic Books, 1963)].

5. The method of sampling for the twenty names was patterned on one of the surveys conducted in the Stirling County Study. In Bristol, the main town of Stirling County, one of two HOS surveys was carried out

using a 10 per cent systematic sample (*n* of 140) drawn from a census in a way similar to our procedure in the Eskimo study. Criteria of inclusion for the Bristol census were that the individual be eighteen years old or "out of school" and a resident for six months or more in the town.

It was not the goal of the Eskimo survey to provide epidemiological findings for comparison with findings from the Stirling County Study. Nevertheless the Eskimo experiment illustrates a number of problems about cross-cultural sampling and comparisons which will be spelled out here.

Although the sampling methods were similar, analysis after field work indicated that the two populations (Eskimo village and Bristol town)

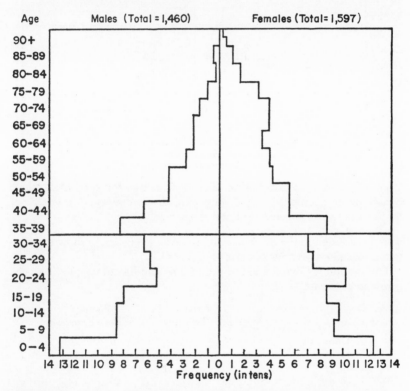

Chart IV-1. Age-sex distribution of the Bristol Ecological Area population (Ninth Census of Canada, 1951). Reproduced by permission of the authors and publisher from C. C. Hughes, M.-A. Tremblay, R. N. Rapoport, and A. H. Leighton, *People of Cove and Woodlot: Communities from the Viewpoint of Social Psychiatry* [Vol. II, The Stirling County Study of Psychiatric Disorder and Sociocultural Environment (New York: Basic Books, 1960)].

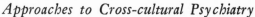

Chart IV-2. Age-sex distribution of Sivokak village for 1955. Dark portions indicate people who died, migrated, or were away in schools or hospitals between January 1954 and August 1955.

were exceedingly different in age and sex characteristics, as shown in the two population pyramids (Charts IV-1 and IV-2).

The age and sex distribution of the Eskimo and Bristol samples is given below in per cents.

Age	Eskimo		Bristol	
	Males	Females	Males	Females
Under 20	20	20	0	0
20–29	20	20	9	20
30–39	20	10	21	34
40–49	20	20	38	15
50–59	20	20	11	20
60–69	0	0	6	7
70 and over	0	10	15	4

Several features of the populations and the samples are to be noted from these charts and figures. It is apparent that the Eskimo population is composed of considerably more young people relative to the proportion of older people than is the case with the Bristol population. Also, for the Eskimos there is a marked absence of people at various points in the decades over thirty-five, which are more fully represented in the Bristol group. It is not surprising, therefore, that the Eskimo sample is composed of more young adults, especially young men, than the Bristol sample. This imbalance in the two samples is compounded by the apparent failure of the Bristol sampling adequately to reflect the actual frequency of individuals between the ages of eighteen and twenty. The total absence of people in this category for the 10 per cent Bristol sample can probably be attributed to the fact that many of them were overlooked in the method used to construct the census for Bristol. The census was prepared by interviewing key informants in a house-by-house survey. The informants were asked to list all the adults in each house, and adults were defined chiefly as "people who are out of school." In the Eskimo study not only was the population composed of more young people than was true of Bristol, but also exact data on the ages of young people were available in the school registries. Every person who qualified on the stricter criterion of birth date was included.

A number of important considerations regarding sampling are inherent in these comparisons. One is the need to be aware of demographic differences, especially as they may be characteristic of Western and non-Western groups. For example, some of the characteristics of the Eskimo population are related to a high birth rate and a high infant mortality rate as well as, at later ages, extraordinarily high morbidity and mortality rates due to tuberculosis. The relative fullness of the age class from twenty to thirty-five in the Eskimo population probably stems from two considerations. This age group is old enough to have become stabilized after attrition from infant mortality and tuberculosis mortality (the rate for the latter at the time of the study being highest for people between eleven and nineteen) and also it is young enough to have profited from recent public health efforts [see C. C. Hughes with the collaboration of J. M. Murphy (formerly Hughes), *An Eskimo Village in the Modern World* (Ithaca, N.Y.: Cornell University Press, 1960), p. 79].

Migration patterns may also influence the demographic profile of a population. Where the Eskimo group was concerned, these factors could be seen to operate selectively in several regards. The darkened portions of the pyramid in Chart IV-2 show the people who were in the village when the schoolteacher made a government census in 1954 but who were not resident in 1955. Out-migration was most common for individuals between the ages of twenty and thirty; otherwise, the sample would have been composed of even more young people. The reasons why young people left the island for the mainland were: schooling, work, hospitalization, or (for the young women) marriage to a white man. For the people older than thirty, the cause of population decrease between 1954 and 1955 was almost exclusively hospitalization and death (two cases).

Comparable emigration data are not available for the Bristol population.

Nevertheless, the gap in the male population for the years from twenty to thirty-five is probably related to the fact that young men do commonly leave the community permanently or temporarily during these years for work, higher education, and military service.

Although these factors are specific to these particular examples of a Western and non-Western group, the problems to which they point are generally pertinent to cross-cultural studies. In many non-Western areas, census materials are inadequate or nonexistent, and such information will have to be obtained as part of the field work. In other words, the special demographic characteristics of the study population will not be known in advance. This situation is one of the arguments for large samples. With sufficient numbers, adjustments for comparing age-specific and sex-specific patterns of responses can be made during analysis.

Another problem that emerges in these population comparisons concerns the definition of adulthood. If the goal is to survey adult populations cross-culturally, some thought needs to be given to the comparability of the cutting points employed to separate adults and nonadults. In the Eskimo study, we were in the unusual position of having precise data on ages for the young people. In retrospect we believe that this, to some extent, obscured the need to combine information on age with the social definition of adulthood. If we had taken the bolder approach of guessing at what was comparable to the Bristol criterion of "being out of school," our knowledge of the culture would have suggested that we focus on an older portion of the population. This does not mean that we could have used school achievement any more effectively than age. In most non-Western groups the educational system, if it exists at all, is not sufficiently standard or compulsory to have the same meaning as in our own society. A qualitative analysis of adulthood in terms of the assumption of responsibilities in various spheres of life such as marriage, subsistence, and community functioning, would suggest that only those people over 25 years be included in the survey. Such a decision would have given a sample more comparable to that of Bristol so far as role and social functions are concerned.

6. Several aspects of structuring the interview setting and developing rapport were brought out in this study and illustrate problems that are common in cross-cultural research. For example, we expected that many of the interviews would be conducted with an interpreter, but as it turned out, all the men except one preferred to be interviewed in English. It was our impression that if some of the men had allowed an interpreter, the interview would have been more satisfactory. Where women were concerned, there seemed to be less sensitivity about using an interpreter. Therefore only one or two women who were fluent in English did not have this assistance.

It may be asked whether there are not serious disadvantages to using interpreters for interviews of the HOS type which concern subjective feelings and subtle psychiatric indicators. Yet in work with Eskimos and many other groups, communication by this means is nearly unavoidable. For most Western researchers the problem of achieving fluency in a non-European language requires an ability that is rare and a linguistic concentration on one group which virtually prohibits a carry-over of personnel in cross-cultural comparative work.

Although numbers of people in non-Western areas are learning one or another European language, a representative sample would likely be composed of some individuals who are monolingual and illiterate, and others who exhibit a range from minimal to excellent fluency in the European language. It seems probable, therefore, that in most cross-cultural studies researchers will reach the conclusion we did, namely that it is more profitable to have an interpreter when needed than to be restricted to communication that is not facile on either side. The presence of an interpreter is so customary in the dealings of the Eskimos with the "white man" that it often does not have the meaning that a third party would in our society. Indeed, for all practical purposes, if we wanted to speak without barriers it would be at least as important to do away with our white skins as to dispense with the interpreters.

Another desideratum for this kind of interview is privacy, which was difficult for us to arrange in the Eskimo situation. It could not be created except by happenstance or by structuring the situation in such an artificial way that gain was immediately counterbalanced. Observation of how activities were actually conducted in Eskimo society led us to believe that privacy was as likely to be traumatizing to them as to be a comfort and an impetus to confidence with us. This seemed to be especially true when it came to using structured techniques and searching out a particular person selected by sampling methods.

The women in the sample were interviewed by Murphy and the men by Hughes. This helped rapport because it fitted with what was most congenial to the Eskimos. In the course of other research we found that Eskimo men were slightly piqued when interviewed by a woman researcher, while Eskimo women were embarrassed to talk at any length alone with a male outsider. We believe that these hesitancies and irritations would have been increased when talking about personal aspects of health.

Field work during the year consisted in participant-observation and in talking with people. We also conducted long series of interviews with some key informants. At the beginning of the year, we had worked out with the village leaders what seemed a fair rate of payment and subsequently used this for all interpreters and interviewers. In planning the HOS we decided to use the rate established for an hour's work.

One problem encountered in the survey was that a male sample member asked in advance how much he would be paid and then decided that he would not give his time except at a higher rate. He was an experienced bargainer for higher prices in the ivory-carving market. He was also something of a deviant, being considerably more antagonistic to the encroaching Western world than was characteristic of most villagers. In a survey of the kinds of symptoms that may in some way reflect the stresses of acculturation, the person who is resistant on these grounds is certainly a type we would not want to see lost from the sample. However in this instance it appeared wiser to make an appropriate substitution than to run the risk of jeopardizing the whole survey by opening it to individual bargaining and the subsequent accusations that might arise about unequal payment.

It seems probable that a survey such as this could be carried out in most non-Western areas without offering financial remuneration although some tangible return for the time given by the participants is an important element of rapport. Except for this one incident, we felt that the payment of a standard fee to all the people who assisted us was a system of mutual advantage which enhanced the quality of collaboration with the Eskimos. In another area, the same might be achieved by gift-giving or by the dispensing of medical treatment and advice.

Another rapport problem was illustrated when the first woman was interviewed. She was very elderly but had been interviewed previously in a series devoted to collecting folk tales. In that context she was willing, cooperative, and appreciative of the money she received. In the HOS her answers were lengthy. More explanatory discussion was carried out in the Eskimo language by the interpreter than was the case with younger respondents. On the other hand only short summaries of these discussions were translated. When the interpreter was pressed to translate everything else that was being said, she answered that she was merely trying to get the ideas across and that there was nothing really to add. This kind of situation is an aspect of using an interpreter—sometimes even the best interpreters—which is familiar to many anthropologists. At the end of the interview when the papers were folded up and put away, we had a casual conversation in which it was translated that the respondent said: "The white woman's questions are very hard to answer!"

Throughout the survey we were aware of the fact that, except in those cases where we had done extensive key-informant interviewing earlier, the respondents themselves structured the situation in ways that apparently hinged on their past experiences with teachers and missionaries and which were difficult to overcome in one sitting. They seemed to view the questions as a cross-examination similar to a school recitation in which one is called on to give "correct" answers. It may be noted in passing that this was also the frame of reference of many respondents in Stirling County and that the interviewers often needed to dissipate the atmosphere of giving a quiz. With the Eskimos we usually introduced the questionnaire by saying that there were no right or wrong answers but that it was purely a matter of what the respondent did or did not feel. This explanation was an important factor in the success of many of the interviews.

An elderly person may indeed find it difficult to remember his health history. It seems unlikely, however, that items about current feelings and sensations are really "hard questions." At the end of the survey, we were fairly sure that the nature of the questions had been understood by most of the respondents and that they were familiar with the concepts of tiredness, trembling, palpitations, and nervous breakdown. It seemed obvious then that the questions themselves were not "hard to answer" but that it was the question-answer situation that was difficult. This pertained especially when a choice was needed as to whether a given sensation was felt "often," "sometimes," or "never" and when mention of an illness had to be amplified in terms of "when it occurred" and "how long it lasted."

This experience underscores the value of trying to find out in advance what interpretation the respondents are likely to make of the interview situation. In many non-Western areas it is probably a unique event, and with careful planning an atmosphere can be created that is devoid of threats and offenses. Among the St. Lawrence Eskimos, for example, it is considered embarrassing to say one's own name. Even though a question about the respondent's name is customary in most surveys in Western society, we avoided asking it among the Eskimos. We knew all the respondents in advance, but had this been otherwise we would have relied on sources of information other than the individual himself to establish identity. In different cultural areas, other kinds of adjustments would probably be necessary to make the question-answer situation an acceptable form of interaction.

Another kind of rapport problem was brought out in an interview with a girl of eighteen. She was shy by nature and far more traditional in her clothes, hairdo, and demeanor than most young women her age. She had spoken to us in English upon occasion but only under the urgency of a message to be delivered or received. The interview was conducted in her home, where previously she had been present on several occasions when her highly articulate father had translated folk tales told by her entirely traditional mother. This family had been very cordial to us, and we anticipated no difficulties in the HOS interview. Several people were in the house at the time, and the interview got under way with no noticeable hardship except that the girl was somewhat monosyllabic. Her father was anxious that she help us properly and once or twice made some further explanation of a question to her in Eskimo. She was the center of attention in their small one-room house. About three-fourths of the way through the interview she suddenly bolted outdoors, to the surprise of everyone—the Eskimos included. There were apologies and explanations on both sides, and we made no attempt to get her to complete the interview; however, by the time of its termination she had responded to the twenty key questions.

This kind of disruption, especially if it is related mainly to personality factors, is likely to happen in a small per cent of cases in all surveys. Nevertheless this particular instance points to a cultural problem as well. One aspect was that by sociocultural definition this girl was not yet an adult. More than that, however, we unwittingly forced her into a role for which she not only lacked experience but which was also diametrically opposed to what was customary for young women in her culture. Traditionally, among this group of Eskimos, fathers and daughters practiced an avoidance pattern, which meant that they rarely exchanged words. Although this pattern is altering, it was still practiced in her family. It seems obvious in retrospect that we had precipitated a reversal of roles which simply put too much strain on her ability to handle the situation. Not only was she in a position of having to talk publicly and directly with her father, but she was also called on to represent the family in a way that was usually left to him. In view of the diversity of role definitions in other non-Western areas, we believe that effort should be made to structure the contact situation as it is exemplified by an interview so that it is appropriate according to age, sex, education, and prestige.

7. Though not among the crucial twenty, items on "weak turns" and "dizziness" followed by probes on loss of consciousness were in the longer lists of questions used in the process of constructing the HOS for the Stirling Study. From what is generally known about hysterical fainting and the "Victorian vapors" in Western society, it seems probable that if the HOS had been developed forty or fifty years earlier these questions might have been included. In a recent article, Abse has put forth evidence for a theory that fainting decreases with increased education, sophistication, and self-awareness [W. Abse, "Hysteria," in *American Handbook of Psychiatry*, S. Arieti, ed. (New York: Basic Books, 1959), pp. 272–291]. The fact that fainting seems to be on the decline in our culture, even in rural areas, and that it appeared as a frequent and significant reaction among the Eskimos at mid-century suggests that this might well be a subject for further cross-cultural research. The accuracy of Abse's interpretation would need more investigation, and the search for causal explanations might be approached from several angles. From what little was known of Eskimo cultures in the early contact period, the psychiatrist, Brill, proposed that their characteristic psychopathology was a hysterical, childlike outburst of impulse expression such as *piblokto* or the copying mania described in the last chapter. He also believed that the Eskimos would *not* display impulse-inhibition in kinds of pathology such as neurotic conversions of the paralytic types or phenomena such as fainting [A. A. Brill, "Piblokto or Hysteria Among

Peary's Eskimos," *Journal of Nervous and Mental Disease,* vol. 40 (1913), pp. 514–520].

8. Probit analysis results in the construction of a graph whose linearity or nonlinearity is the basis for judging the normality or nonnormality of the population distribution. The three graphs in this study were distinctly linear. For further explanation of this technique, see F. J. Moore, *Statistics for Medical Students and Investigators in the Clinical and Biological Sciences* (New York: Blakiston Press, 1951). The tables of probits used are found in *Statistical Tables: For Biological, Agricultural and Medical Research,* by R. Fisher and F. Yates (New York: Hafner, 1963).

9. The fact that the two scoring techniques used in this study yielded closely similar results parallels what was discovered in the Stirling County Study when a simple score was applied to the data on the 1,003 respondents, who also received the weighted scores based on discriminant function analysis. The correlation between the two scores in that study was .88. See D. C. Leighton *et al., op. cit.,* p. 445.

10. For further description of the psychiatric evaluation procedure, see D. C. Leighton *et al., op. cit.,* pp. 45–55, and *Psychiatric Disorder among the Yoruba* by A. H. Leighton, T. A. Lambo, C. C. Hughes, D. C. Leighton, J. M. Murphy, and D. B. Macklin (Ithaca, N.Y.: Cornell University Press, 1963), ch. 5, pp. 83–101.

11. For further details on ridit analysis see I. D. J. Bross, "How to Use Ridit Analysis," *Biometrics,* vol. 14 (1958), pp. 18–38; D. C. Leighton *et al., op. cit.,* pp. 247–249; and T. S. Langner and S. T. Michael, *Life Stress and Mental Health* (New York: The Free Press, 1963), pp. 87–101.

12. The correlation of the *ABCD* ridits with the unweighted HOS scores is better than the correlation of the *ABCD* ridits with the Stirling-weighted HOS scores. For the county sample the coefficient is .57 for the men and .54 for the women (see D. C. Leighton *et al., op. cit.,* p. 208). This finding bolsters our opinion that there is probably a cultural bias reflected in the scoring system worked out for the Stirling County Study and that for the Eskimo Study it was wiser to use the simple scores. Another interesting correlation concerns the relationship between the *ABCD* ridits and a simple score of the fourteen questions (the first fourteen questions given in Figure IV-3, pp. 130–136) that appeared from the item-by-item analysis to be the most appropriate indicators for the Eskimos. The correlation coefficient for the latter is .70 (23 df, $p < .001$). This is by no means a pronounced difference from the correlation for the twenty questions taken as a whole group, which is .68. Nevertheless it suggests that the psychiatrists relied somewhat more heavily on the responses to the fourteen questions than on other responses in making their evaluations.

13. In addition to materials in Chapter III of this volume, see also J. M. Murphy (formerly Hughes), "An Epidemiological Study of Psycho-

pathology in an Eskimo Village" (Ph.D. Dissertation, Cornell University, 1960).

14. The Stirling Study indicates that the HOS works best in detecting a combination of psychoneurotic *and* psychophysiologic symptom patterns rather than either type when it exists without the other. For more discussion of the relationship of HOS scores to symptom patterns, see D. C. Leighton *et al., op. cit.,* pp. 221–225.

V: The Possibility of Using Physiological Indicators for Detecting Psychiatric Disorder

By Edward Llewellyn Thomas

EDITORIAL NOTES

The questions contained in the screening test described in the last chapter seek to have respondents report their subjective feelings and sensations about underlying physiological events. Thus individuals indicate that they do, or do not, feel that they have palpitations, are tired more than they ought to be, go faint at times, or note trouble breathing even when they are not doing strenuous exercise.

The emergence of these kinds of questions as the mainstay in the HOS (and in many other screening devices) is the product of empirical investigation in the development of such tests. For some reason these questions appear to work better than other types in the identification of psychiatric disorders. That is to say, their usefulness is not limited to the specific picture they may give of psychophysiologic disturbances in certain individuals, but rather they correlate with other symptom patterns as determined in clinical investigation by psychiatrists. At the same time it must be recognized that not all forms of psychiatric disorder may be equally well registered by scorings based on these types of questions. Indeed, there is some evidence that psychoneurotic and psychophysiologic symptom patterns show up most readily.[1]

The point is, however, that questions mainly concerned with feelings regarding physiological states may indicate more general psychiatric disturbance. The possibility is raised that underlying such conscious feelings there may be actual disturbance of physiological balance, or that the physiologic patterns of people with psychiatric symptoms may be different from the patterns of those who are not so troubled. An alternative hypothesis is that these psychophysiologic complaints are common ways (perhaps culturally determined ways) of expressing psychological discomfort and have relatively little reference to psychological disturbances as such. Reporting a headache, or feeling sick, or saying that something "gives me a pain" commonly have more symbolic than actual meaning.

Nevertheless, the importance of questions about physiological states suggests that attention be given to the possibility of using physiological tests as an adjunct to other data-gathering operations. On the face of it, the outlook for physiological tests appropriate for epidemiological surveys is not immediately hopeful. It is a type of approach that is high in desirability, but low in feasibility. If tests could be found, however, even if their validity were no higher than that of the screening questions, they would have the enormous advantage of being culture-proof and of avoiding the problems of language variations.

Despite the low level of expectation that one can have at present for physiological testing as a method in epidemiological research, we live in a period of intensive study and rapid advance regarding the physiological aspects of whole-person functioning. In addition to the biochemical research conducted in organic psychiatry, there are new studies of the stresses and strains connected with arctic living, supersonic speeds, and space travel. The question of detectable physiological concomitants of psychiatric disorder may well be one that by its very nature is apt to get its answers—when and if it does—from outside the field of clinical psychiatry. These answers might be picked up as by-products in any one of a large number of physiological and biochemical fields of research.

A further point is that previous attempts to relate physiological tests to psychiatric disorder have generally fastened on one reactive system of the body—galvanic skin resistance, blood pressure, electroencephalogram, and so on. The numerous types of screening devices use questions pertinent not only to one system but rather to a number of systems. It is the total score that makes the difference, and this is based on questions covering musculoskeletal, respiratory, cardiovascular, gastrointestinal, and other aspects of bodily functioning. Thus the possibility is allowed for that multiple patterns of physiologic-sensation disturbance may be associated with psychiatric disorder. Perhaps, then, we may expect better results from physiological tests if we think in terms of not one but rather a battery of tests.

In this situation it has seemed wise to review current literature with the idea of discovering promising areas to watch in the future.

Thomas takes up this review from the vantage point of a medical physiologist engaged in the study of reactions to stress. He gives some orientations regarding the psychophysiology of change and the problems to be expected in assessing physiological factors in people who are undergoing the stress of a rapidly changing cultural environment and in separating the differences in physiological factors that relate to cultural variation from those which may be indicative of one or another kind of psychiatric disorder.

It should be pointed out in advance that his main focus concerns generalizations about what goes on inside people as a result of environmental change. Studies at the level of society and culture have indicated that there are parallel generalizations to be made about the processes of sociocultural change itself, a main one being that no culture is static or entirely stable. There are variations and proportions, but change is both universal and continuous, though it occurs at different rates of speed and in different parts of the whole. In terms of preparing for cross-cultural research, Thomas has found it especially appropriate to talk of the dramatic examples of non-Western groups undergoing extensive, wholesale acculturation. The principles he proposes, nonetheless, apply elsewhere. For our own society, they would have to be explained by somewhat different concepts, such as class and economic mobility, urbanization, and industrialization.

A BASIC hypothesis which has guided this review of physiological indicators concerns what may be called the psychophysiology of change. All living things respond to changes in the world around them by changes in themselves, and all emotional changes are correlated with some physiological change.

The elementary forms of life exist in a strictly physical world and in that sequence of processes we call time. The vital processes consist of physical responses to physical stimuli. Thus their movements are affected by light, temperature, salinity, or gravity, and they may respond to changes in humidity, for example, by such various but immediate physiological responses as encysting or multiplying. Among more complex life forms, a new kind of physical response appears. This is a response to a stimulus that has occurred in the past and that is preserved somehow in the system: the ants store for the winter, and the swallows fly south. Whatever may be the origins of instinct and intuition, they produced a tremendous widening of the stimulus-response relationship.

With the higher vertebrates still another kind of response pattern is evident—a response to a stimulus that is an omen of physical change in the environment rather than the change itself. In this expanded "subjective time" both the conditioned reflex and purposeful behavior are called into play, and omens become further and further removed from the changes they portend. The warning stimulus, then, is like an environmental change in that it can evoke physical responses in the individual. Either the gathering storm clouds or the rain itself causes us to look for shelter, and a sudden clap of thunder may speed the heart or send up the blood pressure just as much as running for cover. Although one stimulus is psychological and the other physical, the response to them is of the same quality.

In all human groups, the stimulus-response mechanisms are vastly more complicated than these illustrations suggest. Man, with all his flexibility of memory, imagination, and foresight, is surrounded by self-made omens, many of which bear such an elaborate relationship to the well-being of the individual that the responses they produce may seem quite unconnected or out of proportion. Human beings have an unusual ability to translate out into the real world thoughts that have arisen in their own minds. When reperceived, these internal impressions may have the same effect as a genuine external stimulus. They may be the beginning of a carefully conceived idea of the structure of the atom, for example, but they also have a wayward tendency to create false omens—the misinterpretation of a creaking stair or the fully developed delusions of paranoid states.

The physiological changes that are continuously occurring in people may be responses to either physical or mental stimuli. It is appropriate to consider whether those due to mental stimuli can be separated from those due to physical stimuli; and, if so, whether their measurement would aid us in discovering the prevalence and following the changes in psychiatric disorders in a community. I have used the phrase "mental stimuli" to clarify in simple terms its difference from "physical stimuli." A more accurate phrase is "the stimuli from a psycho-social-cultural environment," which, though integrally connected with the purely physical environment, can nonetheless be kept distinct conceptually. *If* the physiological changes that attend the stimuli from this psycho-social-cultural environment can be discovered and kept separate from the others—and *if* they can be cor-related, as seems reasonable, with changes in the emotional status of individuals thus stimulated—and *if* changes in emotional status are associated, as also seems reasonable, with at least some kinds of mental disorders—*if* all these conditions can be assumed or satisfied, we may be on the path to finding variables that can be used as objective measurements of psychiatric disorder.

If we view these general propositions in terms of societies ex-posed to rapid and pervasive acculturation, it is evident that individuals will be subjected to both types of environmental stimuli and changes. The whole pattern of life undergoes changes—diet, work, sleep, clothes, shelter, muscular habits, physiological rhythms, as well as family relationships, religion, ideas, and aspirations. All of these forces may generate phys-iological changes. Before considering the possible effects of emotional disturbances in such societies, it is necessary to look at the probable results of the changes in the physical situation. Taking account of these latter is the first step toward devising sufficient control of the innumerable factors to permit isolation of those variables pertinent to our problem.

In such societies, the standard of nutrition will be either im-proving or getting worse. Since nutrition is "adequate" when it allows the individual to function successfully in his own society, there is no absolute standard, and often severe disjunctures occur in a changing society.

Among hunting and gathering peoples, the nutritional cycle of feast and famine may be adaptational, for periodic hunger generates skill and courage; but it can be maladaptive when the group changes to agriculture, and even disastrous if, for exam-ple, they become miners, who work not only as hard or harder but more continuously. Moreover, it is not only a matter of when and how much people eat, but what they either can or choose to produce for food and how they process and prepare it.

Changes in nutrition are reflected in a number of physiological variables such as the vitamin excretion level. But it would be a mistake to assume that such variations are solely physical in origin. The effects of emotion on appetite and gastrointestinal absorption are well known. People brought into resettlement areas, for example, may reduce eating and become emaciated for a time in the same way that some animals will not feed in captivity.

Up to the beginning of this century, contact with Western cultures usually resulted in worsening the sanitary conditions of "primitive" groups by turning them away from customs of sanitation which, though different from ours, were usually effective in keeping most of the people alive and the group as a whole viable. With the introduction of modern public health planning, there have been great improvements. Drainage and antimalarial precautions, for example, have significantly reduced the number of individuals with clinical or subclinical malaria. This means a resulting rise in hemoglobin levels in comparison to the population's former standard. Likewise as the frequency of intestinal parasites goes down, there will be changes in the eosinophil level across the population. Since some work has shown a relationship between eosinophil count and psychiatric disorder, this is a warning that certain indices of emotional and physical stress may be invalidated for use in cross-cultural psychiatry unless secondary control measures can be run or until the new population standards can be constructed. In addition to the problems presented by disrupted nutrition and sanitation, there are also the tremendous variations in endemic diseases and the well-known ravages of introduced diseases, which call in question the tests that have been found acceptable for this kind of research in our own society.

The emotional and psychological stresses that accompany massive social change and cultural disorientation have been documented many times. Perhaps they can best and most briefly be introduced here in terms of imagining ourselves in like circumstances. Imagine that through interstellar communication we are suddenly brought into contact with a civilization as far advanced beyond ours technologically as ours is above that of the Semang or the Hottentots. Within a year this civilization demonstrates to us beyond logical rebuttal that our religion is a myth; that our scientific knowledge, so arduously accumulated, places us at the educational level of a first grader in their sight; that a few devices whose internal workings we cannot understand make obsolete most of our manual and technical skills; and that our scholars turn out to be superstition mongers. They find our economic system ludicrous and our marital habits disgusting. They admire the primitive strength of our art and export all examples of it they can obtain. They give us medicines to cure our diseases, but their views about what causes disease and how the cure works are written in symbols which will take us twenty years to comprehend. They tell us how to become healthier and happier, but what they recommend is repugnant to us.

Suffice it to say that we could expect most of our population to grow more and more distraught as the fundamentals of society disappeared. Hostility and resentment might arise; anxiety, frustration, and suspicion would surely be widespread. Many of the emotional reactions that would be stirred are components of psychiatric disorder, and it seems very probable that the prevalence of psychiatric disorder would increase.

It is important at this point to go further into the beginning hypothesis about the relationship between emotional and physiological changes. We have moved a long way from earlier assumptions that a simple relationship exists between emotion and any one physiological variable. The history of attempts to correlate the psychogalvanic reflex with emotion demonstrates this in its large, confused, and generally unproductive literature. Despite the number of observations which support the view that every emotional change is accompanied by a physiological one, the relationship is essentially complex, and each affects the other through many different mechanisms. Physiological changes may occur before the emotional change and be the cause of it; or the changes may be concomitant, occurring together as a result of some external factor.

Emotional stressors act on the individual through the brain, the central nervous system, and the neuroendocrine system. They can arise outside or inside the individual, but by definition they disturb the person and produce at least a *psychological* response. There is a great variety of emotional stressors, but Engel[2] has divided them into three groups: frustration of drives, threats to the body image, and threats to psychic objects. There is overlapping between these three groups, and an initial stressor in one group may evoke stress situations in the other two. Stress, of whatever variety, is unpleasant to the individual, and he attempts to protect himself through defensive mechanisms which include psychological, physiological, biochemical, and behavioral responses. If an emotional stressor is quickly removed or neutralized and the unpleasantness abated, the psychological response suffices, and the other types of response are hardly noticeable. But if the discomfort continues, the responses may increase, spread, and persist. The persistence of the physiological and biochemical responses may in themselves be stressful to other organic systems in the individual, and the behavioral responses may upset his relationships with the outside world. Thus in body functioning and social relations, as well as at the psychological level, he may begin to demonstrate the effects of mishandled emotion.

These physiological responses to emotion are controlled through the thalamic-reticular portion of the brain stem, which is a coordinating system for the cortical, autonomic, and peripheral nervous systems. The resulting changes are, therefore, widespread and holistic.

The emergency theory of Cannon[3] emphasizes that such emotions prepare the individual for vigorous activity during emergency. To this end the respiratory and circulation rates increase, glycogen is released from the liver, the clotting time of the blood is decreased, the motility of the gut is reduced, thumb sweating starts, and a multitude of other physiological changes make more energy available to the muscles. The general picture is diffuse interference with the resting state, some systems being brought to a high condition of readiness while others are rendered quiescent.

In addition to being diffuse, these responses appear to be nonspecific. Activity seems to be a function of the overall emotional state rather than of a particular type of emotion. For the most part increased emotion produces a high level of activity with enhanced reactions, while decreased emotion, as in apathetic types of depression or sleep, reduces the activity level and the magnitude of the reactions.

With the accumulated background of research and analysis from many workers, there is little question of the fundamental alliance between emotion and physiology. But as Engel has pointed out, the physiology of emotion must in fact go far beyond Cannon's emergency theory, the conditioned reflex physiology of Pavlov, and the general adaptation syndrome of Selye.[4] Current thinking in this field always points out difficulties to be encountered in measuring the diffuse and nonspecific physiological reactions that stem from emotional stress. Thus Rapaport [5] says: "The significance of the physiologic processes present in emotional states is obscured by the fog which conceals all psychosomatic interrelations." These difficulties are compounded when one is trying to design epidemiological measures for whole groups undergoing such stress—this consideration being over and above what was said earlier concerning the actual physical stresses of inadequate nutrition, disease, and so forth.

At the ideal level one might conceive of overcoming the measurement problems in an experimental situation—of measuring every measurable physiological and biochemical variable for each individual of a large group exposed to prolonged emotional stress situations. The study by Pace [6] and his colleagues on infantrymen in combat shows what results can be achieved by this method. But it also demonstrates the great practical difficulties even of dealing with a relatively small group of disciplined men in a limited stress situation. In studying whole societies we cannot, obviously, set up experimental conditions, and we are confined to investigating people under stress only where that stress exists for reasons other than research, using only the restricted number of measurements we can expect people to allow willingly.

Where whole societies are concerned, there is also the problem of constructing norms for each variable appropriate for that group in order to measure change and deviation. An example of this approach to measurement in cross-cultural research is the cephalic index developed by physical anthropologists. Whole groups of people can be called mesocephalic, brachycephalic, or dolichocephalic (these terms expressing the average measure or norm for the group); calipers have been designed on the basis of these standards; and through these instruments two kinds of information can be conveyed—one is the deviation from the group standard exhibited by any single individual, and the other, the variations from one group standard to another.

The analogy between a cephalic index and a psychophysiological index has its limits, however. Techniques of measurement have to be fitted to the phenomena to be measured and *their* peculiarities of change and variation. There is no reason to think that a cephalic index is static because it is structural. It can exhibit change through time in one human group just as much as it exhibits difference between groups. The processes of change, however, are infinitely slower, involving genetic mutation and adaptation, and are pertinent to whole populations rather than individuals. Discovering the causes of these kinds of changes and developing methods for their measurement belong in physical anthropology and genetics. Where psychophysiological changes are concerned we have the remarkable advantage of being able to study them in the life spans of single individuals and groups of individuals living under the emotional stresses we believe to be etiologically significant, though this gain is perhaps overshadowed by the complexities.

The criteria for a particular index are reached by measuring every person in the group, if possible, or by measuring individuals selected by statistical techniques and generalizing to the whole group. In terms of physiological variables, one way of dealing with the problem of standards might be to use a "class serum," which would be composed of pooled specimens from each member of that class, group, or society. Although the "pool" method would need to be used in conjunction with knowledge of individual measurements, the procedure of pooling equal specimens from a large number of subjects would in itself tend to be a self-averaging system, and in a longitudinal study biochemical variables in serial specimens of this pooled material could perhaps be followed in the same manner as serial specimens are followed from one individual. In addition, pooled specimens from similar age and sex groups could also be compared. Pooled specimens taken from the eighteen-year-old male group, for example, at the beginning of the study could be compared with a similar sex-age group at the end of the study.

The pool method would have the further advantage that it might be possible to use only small quantities of specimens from each individual. For blood evaluations it would probably be necessary to take only five drops from the fingertip rather than the larger collections which involve venipunctures. Moreover, the specimens could be measured off by the centimeter, and one part of each sample put into a general pool and another part in a specific sex-age pool.

The most important pooled specimen would probably be blood serum. Pooled urine might also be worthwhile, but the variation in urinary constituents is so great over twenty-four hours that such specimens might be of only limited value. Pooled saliva would be relatively easy to obtain, as would be various mucous secretions.

Physiological Measurements for
Cross-cultural Psychiatry

The continuing success of physiologists and biochemists has given us an extensive list of variables that can be measured. There has also been persistent endeavor to discover physiological changes that indicate emotional stress or provide a clear picture of association with different kinds of psychiatric disorder.

On a number of occasions over the last few years a "breakthrough" appeared imminent, but the research was discredited or reduced in importance by subsequent investigations. The use of ceruloplasmin or adrenochrome levels as indices of schizophrenia are examples of the measurements that seemed promising initially and were later minimized. Much of this confusion arises from the multifactorial complexity of most psychiatric and psychological phenomena and from the history of thought and language which binds us to words and concepts that do not reflect this complexity. Thus the word "schizophrenia" describes a clinical condition which may actually be composed of several fundamentally different conditions. One of the mechanisms that may be involved, as Hoskins [7] showed, is thyroid dysfunction, but this pertains in only a small proportion of the cases classified "schizophrenia." Attempts to correlate schizophrenia with thyroid functioning fail, therefore, except in a selected group of patients.

This multifactorial situation exists also in the field of emotion, but since the physiological responses to emotion are diffuse and nonspecific, it may some day be possible to make a virtue of a necessity. We may find that an integrated measurement of several physiological changes, taken together in sum, has a significance which any one change measurement, taken alone, would lack.

For the present, however, it can be said that a fairly complete survey of the literature has disclosed no widely accepted demonstration of any physiological measurement that bears a strong correlation to emotional strain or to any of the mental disorders (except for those associated with impairment of brain tissue function, such as central nervous system syphilis). Nor has this review suggested any general area in which correlations may be expected to appear as a result of research in the near future. The situation is strikingly like our current preoccupation with the physiological and psychophysiological variables that can be measured and telemetered back from astronauts. Miracles of engineering have provided methods to telemeter a large number of variables from men and animals in space vehicles. But there is still no convincing answer to the question: "Why are we doing all these measurements?" The basic fact that the man or animal is alive and not in gross physiological or psychological imbalance can be established from respiration rate and electrocardiogram. Although many other variables are being measured and telemetered, none at present can be used to indicate the finer changes in which we are especially interested.

The problem shared by astronautical research and cross-cultural psychiatric epidemiology is that decision to use one or another measure rests, to some extent, on practical limitations. From all possible measurements there is at least a clear division between those which are easily made and transmitted, showing gross changes only, and those which are much more complex and expensive but which teeter between being potentially very valuable and entirely valueless.

Conclusion

The main conclusion from this review is that it would be premature at this time to venture into cross-cultural psychiatric studies with physiological tests. It is, of course, possible to suggest a battery that could be managed in the field and that would test multiple aspects of bodily function. Thus one might select the following: resting pulse rate, resting blood pressure, breath holding time, visual acuity, blood serum cholesterol, blood differential leucocyte count, blood eosinophil count, and stain index. It would seem to me, however, that resources would be better invested in working with people of Western culture in places where laboratory resources of considerable magnitude are available. The idea that a *battery* of tests might prove useful is worth exploring. This is particularly so since the study envisioned here, unlike much other work, is not concerned with uncovering physiological causes of psychiatric disorder, but with finding concomitants that might be used as indicators in epidemiological studies. It could best be conducted, in the initial phases, in settings where far more elaborate and controlled laboratory investigations could be carried out than would be possible in the field. Furthermore, the patient group studied should be one that is fully understood from the viewpoint of clinical psychiatry, and it should be matched with controls that have been subjected to parallel investigations in order to ascertain that they are free of psychiatric disorder.

These conclusions are reached after a review of some 201 measurable physiological variables, close examination of 59 relevant tests, and inspection of the selected bibliography given at the end of this chapter.

Notes

1. See "The Health Opinion Survey," ch. 7, in D. C. Leighton, J. S. Harding, D. B. Macklin, A. M. Macmillan, and A. H. Leighton, *The Character of Danger: Psychiatric Symptoms in Selected Communities* [Vol. III, The Stirling County Study of Psychiatric Disorder and Sociocultural Environment (New York: Basic Books, 1963)].

2. G. L. Engel, "A Unified Concept of Health and Disease," *Perspectives in Biology and Medicine*, vol. 3, no. 4 (Summer 1960).

3. W. B. Cannon, *Bodily Changes in Pain, Hunger, Fear and Rage*, 2nd ed. (New York: Appleton-Century-Crofts, 1939).

4. H. Selye, *The Physiology and Pathology of Exposure to Stress* (Montreal: Acta, Inc., 1950).

5. D. Rapaport, *Emotions and Memory* (New York: International Universities Press, 1950).

6. N. Pace, *et al.*, "Physiological Studies on Infantrymen in Combat," Berkeley: *University of California Publications in Physiology*, vol. 10, no. 1 (1956), pp. 1–48.

7. R. G. Hoskins, *The Biology of Schizophrenia* (New York: W. W. Norton, 1946).

Selected Bibliography

Akerfeldt, S., "Oxidation of *N,N*-Dimethyl-*p*-phenylenediamine by Serum from Patients with Mental Disease," *Science*, vol. 125 (Jan. 1957), pp. 117–118.

Altschule, M. D., "Adrenal Function in Some Psychiatric Disorders," Washington: *International Record of Medical and General Practice Clinics*, vol. 166, no. 5 (1953), pp. 190–195.

———, *Bodily Physiology in Mental and Emotional Disorders* (New York: Grune & Stratton, 1953).

Axelrod, L. R., and A. Zaffaroni, "The Extraction of Corticosteroids from Blood and Tissue by Dialysis," *Archives of Biochemistry and Biophysics*, vol. 50 (June 1954), pp. 347–353.

Basowitz, H., *et al.*, "Anxiety and Performance Changes with a Minimal Dose of Epinephrine," *Archives of Neurology and Psychiatry*, vol. 76 (July 1956), pp. 98–105; Correction: vol. 76 (Oct. 1956), p. 419.

Bliss, E. L., *et al.*, "Reaction of the Adrenal Cortex to Emotional Stress," *Psychosomatic Medicine*, vol. 18 (Jan.–Feb. 1956), pp. 56–76.

Bordley, J., C. A. R. Connor, W. F. Hamilton, W. J. Kerr, and C. J. Wiggers, "Recommendations for Human Blood Pressure Determinations by Sphygmomanometers," *Circulation*, vol. 4 (Oct. 1951), pp. 503–509.

Bracewell, R. N., "Communications from Superior Galactic Communities," *Nature*, vol. 186, no. 4726 (May 1960), pp. 670–671.

Brazier, M. A. B., "Physiological Mechanisms Underlying the Electrical Activity of the Brain," *Journal of Neurology and Psychiatry*, vol. 11 (May 1948), pp. 118–133.

Bush, I. E., "Methods of Paper Chromatography of Steroids Applicable to the Study of Steroids in Mammalian Blood and Tissues," *Biochemical Journal*, vol. 50 (Jan. 1952), pp. 370–378.

Caraway, W. T., *Microchemical Methods for Blood Analysis* (Springfield, Ill.: Charles C. Thomas, 1960).

Chapman, L. F., *et al.*, "Highest Integrative Functions in Man During Stress," *Brain and Human Behaviour*, vol. 36, Proceedings of the

Association for Research in Nervous and Mental Disease (Baltimore, Md.: The Williams & Wilkins Co., 1958), pp. 491–534.

CIBA Foundation, *Symposium on the Neurological Basis of Behaviour*, G. E. W. Wolstenholme and C. M. L. Connor, eds. (Boston: Little, Brown, 1958).

Cooper, J. B., "Emotion in Prejudice," *Science*, vol. 130 (August 1959), pp. 314–318.

Davidowitz, J., *et al.*, "An Electromyographic Study of Muscular Tension," *Journal of Psychology*, vol. 40 (1955), pp. 85–94.

Davis, S. W., "Stress in Combat," *Scientific American*, vol. 194, no. 3 (March 1956).

Diagnostic and Statistical Manual of Mental Disorders, by the Committee on Nomenclature and Statistics of the American Psychiatric Association (Washington, D.C.: American Psychiatric Association, 1952).

Diethelm, O., E. J. Doty, and A. T. Milhorat, "Emotions and Adrenergic and Cholinergic Changes in Blood," *Archives of Neurology and Psychiatry*, vol. 54 (August 1945), pp. 110–115.

Dunbar, H. F., *Emotions and Bodily Changes*, 3rd ed. (New York: Columbia University Press, 1947).

Eccles, J. C., *The Neurophysiological Basis of the Mind* (New York: Oxford University Press, 1953).

Eder, H. A., "Determination of Thiocyanate Space," *Methods of Medical Research*, M. B. Visscher, ed., Vol. IV (Chicago: The Year Book Publishers, Inc., 1951), pp. 48–53.

Edozien, J. C., "Biochemical Normals in Nigerians: Urinary 17-Oxosteroids and 17-Oxogenic Steroids," *Lancet*, vol. 1 (Jan. 1960), pp. 258–259.

Elmadjian, F., and G. Pincus, "Adrenal Cortex and Lymphocytopenia of Stress," *Endocrinology*, vol. 37 (July 1945), pp. 47–49.

Engel, L. L., "The Assay of Urinary Neutral 17-Ketosteroids," *Methods of Biochemical Analysis*, David Glick, ed., Vol. I (New York: Interscience Publishers, 1954), p. 479.

Evarts, E. V., "A Discussion of Research Methods as Applied to Physiological Studies of Psychiatric Patients," *Psychiatric Research Reports*, vol. 9 (March 1958), pp. 52–54.

Eysenck, H. J., G. W. Granger, and J. C. Brengelmann, *Perceptual Processes and Mental Illness* (New York: Basic Books, 1957).

Faurbye, A., P. Vestergaard, F. Kobbernagel, and A. Nielsen, "Adrenal Cortical Function in Chronic Schizophrenia (Stress, Adrenaline-test, ACTH-test)," *Acta Endocrinologica,* vol. 8 (1951). pp. 215–246.

Ferguson, R. S., "Some Physiological Responses in Neurotics," *Journal of Nervous and Mental Disease,* vol. 125, no. 2 (April–June 1957), pp. 240–246.

Fink, M., "Quantitative EEG and Human Psychopharmacology," presented at the 118th Annual Meeting, American Psychiatric Association, Toronto, May 1962.

Folch, J., "Biochemical Problems Related to Psychiatric Research," *Psychiatric Research* (Cambridge: Harvard University Press, 1947), pp. 17–37.

Forrer, G. R., "Atropine Toxicity in the Treatment of Mental Disease," *American Journal of Psychiatry,* vol. 108 (August 1951), pp. 107–112.

Fox, H. M., "Psychophysiological Research Methods," *Bulletin of the Johns Hopkins Hospital,* vol. 105, no. 1 (1959), pp. 1–7.

Funkenstein, D. H., M. Greenblatt, and H. C. Solomon, "Norepinephrine-like and Epinephrine-like Substances in Psychotic and Psychoneurotic Patients," *American Journal of Psychiatry,* vol. 108 (March 1952), pp. 652–662.

———, and L. W. Meade, "Nor-epinephrine-like and Epinephrine-like Substances and the Elevation of Blood Pressure during Acute Stress," *Journal of Nervous and Mental Disease,* vol. 119 (May 1954), pp. 380–397.

———, M. Greenblatt, and H. C. Solomon, "Prognostic Tests Indicating the Effectiveness of Treatment," *Association for Research in Nervous and Mental Disease, Proc.* (1951), vol. 31 (1953), pp. 245–266.

———, M. Greenblatt, H. C. Solomon, "Psychophysiological Study of Mentally Ill Patients. I. Status of Peripheral Autonomic Nervous System as Determined by Reaction to Epinephrine and Mecholyl," *American Journal of Psychiatry,* vol. 106 (July 1949), pp. 16–28.

———, M. Greenblatt, S. Root, and H. C. Solomon, "Psychophysiological Study of Mentally Ill Patients. II. Changes in the Reactions to Epinephrine and Mecholyl after Electric Shock Treatment,"

American Journal of Psychiatry, vol. 106 (August 1949), pp. 116–121.

Gantt, W. H., *Physiological Bases of Psychiatry* (Springfield, Ill.: Charles C. Thomas, 1958).

Gellhorn, E., "Clinical Aspects of Psychosurgery: Physiologic Basis of Shock Therapy," *Proceedings of the Royal Society of Medicine*, Supplement 42 (1949), pp. 55–70.

———, *Physiological Foundations of Neurology and Psychiatry* (Minneapolis: University of Minnesota Press, 1953).

———, "Physiological Processes Related to Consciousness and Perception," *Brain*, vol. 77 (Sept. 1954), pp. 401–415.

Gerard, R. W., "The Biological Roots of Psychiatry," *American Journal of Psychiatry*, vol. 112 (August 1955), pp. 81–90.

———, "Metabolism and Function in the Nervous System," *Neurochemistry*, K. A. C. Elliott, I. H. Page, J. H. Quastel, eds. (Springfield, Ill.: Charles C. Thomas, 1955), pp. 458–484.

Goldman, D., "Electroencephalographic Manifestations Associated with Psychotic Illness: Pentothal Activation Technique and Pharmacologic Interrelationships," presented at the 118th Annual Meeting, American Psychiatric Association, Toronto, May 1962.

Goldsmith, H. J., "Physiological Correlates of Psychological Stress with Special Emphasis on Recovery Rate," *Dissertation Abstracts*, vol. 17, no. 12 (1954), pp. 3097–3098.

Goodman, L. S., and A. Gilman, *The Pharmacological Basis of Therapeutics*, 2nd ed. (New York: Macmillan, 1956).

Gotsev, T., *et al.*, *Fiziologicheskii Zhurnal U.S.S.R.*, vol. 42 (1956), pp. 561–565; and *Physiological Abstracts*, vol. 33, no. 5 (Oct. 1959), Abstract 9440.

Granger, G. W., "Personality and Visual Perception: A Review," *Journal of Mental Science*, vol. 99 (Jan. 1953), pp. 8–43.

Grinker, R. R., and J. P. Spiegel, *Men Under Stress* (Philadelphia: Blakiston, 1945).

Grossmann, A., and G. F. Grossmann, "Protein-Bound Iodine by Alkaline Incineration and a Method for Producing a Stable Cerate Color," *Journal of Clinical Endocrinology*, vol. 15 (March 1955), pp. 354–361.

Grundy, S. M., and A. C. Griffin, "Relationship of Periodic Mental Stress to Serum Lipoprotein and Cholesterol Levels," *Journal of* the *American Medical Association*, vol. 171, no. 13 (Nov. 1959), pp. 1794–1796.

Hale, H. B., C. H. Kratochvil, and J. P. Ellis, "Plasma Corticosteroid Levels in Aircrewmen after Long Flights," *Endocrinology and Metabolism*, vol. 18, no. 12 (Dec. 1958), pp. 1440–1443.

Harlow, C. M., and H. Selye, "The Blood Picture in the Alarm Reaction," *Proceedings of the Society for Experimental Biology and Medicine*, vol. 36 (1937), pp. 141–144.

Hebb, D. O., *The Organization of Behavior: A Neurophysiological Theory* (New York: John Wiley & Sons, 1949).

Henderson, D. K., and R. D. Gillespie, *Textbook of Psychiatry*, 9th ed., rev. by D. Henderson and I. R. C. Batchelor (London: Oxford University Press, 1962).

Hildes, J. A., R. Whaley, H. Whaley, and L. Irving, "Old Crow—A Healthy Indian Community," *Canadian Medical Association Journal*, vol. 81 (Nov. 1959), pp. 837–841.

Hill, D., "Theories of the Action of Physical Methods of Treatment in Psychiatry," *British Medical Bulletin*, vol. 6 (1949), pp. 36–43.

Hill, S. R., Jr., *et al.*, "Studies on Adrenocortical and Psychological Response to Stress in Man," *Archives of International Medicine*, vol. 97 (1956), pp. 269–298.

Himwich, H. E., "Thought Processes as Related to Brain Metabolism in Certain Abnormal Conditions," *Journal of Nervous and Mental Disease*, vol. 114 (Nov. 1951), pp. 450–458.

Hinkle, L. E., Jr., and H. Wolff, "Ecologic Investigations of the Relationship between Illness, Life Experiences, and the Social Environment," *Annals of Internal Medicine*, vol. 49, no. 6 (Dec. 1958), pp. 1373–1388.

Hoagland, H., ed., *Hormones, Brain Function and Behaviour* (New York: Academic Press, 1957).

Hoffer, A., H. Osmond, and J. Smythies, "Schizophrenia: New Approach; Result of Year's Research," *Journal of Mental Science*, vol. 100 (Jan. 1954), pp. 29–45.

Kety, S. S., "Biochemical Theories of Schizophrenia," Part I, *Science*, vol. 129 (June 1959), pp. 1528–1532; and Part II, *Science*, vol. 129 (June 1959), pp. 1590–1596.

———, "Blood Flow and Metabolism of the Human Brain in Health and Disease," in *Neurochemistry*, K. A. C. Elliott, I. H. Page, and

J. H. Quastel, eds. (Springfield, Ill.: Charles C. Thomas, 1955), pp. 294–310.

Kolmer, J. A., E. H. Spaulding, and H. W. Robinson, *Approved Laboratory Technic* (New York: Appleton-Century-Crofts, 1951).

Landis, C., and M. M. Bolles, *Textbook of Abnormal Psychology* (New York: Macmillan, 1946).

Laslett, P., *The Physical Basis of Mind* (London: Blackwell, 1950).

Lawson, J. D., "The Free Achilles Reflex in Hypothyroidism and Hyperthyroidism," *New England Journal of Medicine*, vol. 259, no. 16 (1958), pp. 761–764.

———, and A. S. Weissbein, "The Free Achilles Reflex during Treatment of Hyperthyroidism," *American Journal of Medical Sciences*, vol. 238, no. 1 (July 1959), pp. 39–44.

Leighton, A. H., "Mental Illness and Acculturation," *Medicine and Anthropology*, I. Galdston, ed. (New York: International Universities Press, 1959), pp. 108–128.

Luria, A. R., *The Nature of Human Conflicts*, translated from Russian by W. H. Gantt (New York: Liveright, 1932).

Maas, J. W., "A Controlled Psychiatric Study of Military Personnel at Sick Call," *U.S. Armed Forces Medical Journal*, vol. 9, no. 12 (July–Dec. 1958), pp. 1745–1752.

Macmillan, A. M., "The Health Opinion Survey," *Psychological Reports*, vol. 3, Monograph Supplement 7 (1957), pp. 325–339.

Malmo, R. B., and C. Shagass, "Behavioral and Physiologic Changes Under Stress after Operations on the Frontal Lobes," *Archives of Neurology and Psychiatry*, vol. 63 (1950), pp. 113–124.

———, and A. A. Smith, "Forehead Tension and Motor Irregularities in Psychoneurotic Patients Under Stress," *Journal of Personality*, vol. 23 (1955), pp. 391–406.

———, C. Shagass, D. J. Belanger, and A. A. Smith, "Motor Control in Psychiatric Patients Under Experimental Stress," *Journal of Abnormal and Social Psychology*, vol. 46, no. 4 (Oct. 1951), pp. 539–547.

———, and C. Shagass, "Physiologic Studies of Reaction to Stress in Anxiety and Early Schizophrenia," *Psychosomatic Medicine*, vol. II (Jan.–Feb. 1949), pp. 9–24.

———, and C. Shagass, "Physiologic Studies of Symptom Mechanisms in Psychiatric Patients Under Stress," *Psychosomatic Medicine*, vol. II (Jan.–Feb. 1949), pp. 25–29.

——, and C. Shagass, "Studies of Blood Pressure in Psychiatric Patients Under Stress," *Psychosomatic Medicine*, vol. 14 (1952), pp. 82–93.

McCleary, R. A., "The Nature of the Galvanic Skin Response," *Psychological Bulletin*, vol. 47, no. 2 (March 1950), pp. 97–117.

McCulloch, W. S., "Physiological Processes Underlying Psychoneuroses," *Proceedings of the Royal Society of Medicine*, Supplement 42 (1949), pp. 71–84.

McDougall, W., *Outline of Abnormal Psychology* (New York: Charles Scribner's Sons, 1926).

Meduna, L. J., "Physiological Background of the Carbon Dioxide Treatment of the Neuroses," *American Journal of Psychiatry*, vol. 110 (March 1954), pp. 664–667.

Melville, P. H., and A. G. Mezey, "Emotional State and Energy Expenditure," *Lancet* (Feb. 1959), pp. 273–274.

Meyer, A., "The Psychobiological Point of View," in *The Commonsense Psychiatry of Dr. Adolf Meyer*, A. Lieb, ed. (New York: McGraw-Hill, 1948), pp. 590–606.

Morgan, C. T., and E. Stellar, *Physiological Psychology*, 2nd ed. (New York: McGraw-Hill, 1950).

Mowrer, O. H., *et al.*, "Tension Changes during Psychotherapy with Special Reference to Resistance," in *Psychotherapy: Theory and Research*, O. H. Mowrer, ed. (New York: Ronald Press, 1953), pp. 546–640.

Munson, P. L., and F. N. Briggs, "The Mechanism of Stimulation of ACTH Secretion," *Recent Progress in Hormone Research*, Vol. XI (1955), pp. 83–117.

Olds, J., "Neurophysiology of Drive," *Psychiatric Research Reports*, no. 6 (1956), pp. 15–20.

Osmond, H., and J. Smythies, "Schizophrenia: New Approach," *Journal of Mental Science*, vol. 98 (April 1952), pp. 309–315.

Pearson, S., S. Stern, and T. H. McGavack, "A Rapid, Accurate Method for the Determination of Total Cholesterol in Serum," *Analytical Chemistry*, vol. 25 (1953), pp. 813–814.

Persky, H., and H. J. Grosz, "Effect of Anxiety on the Akerfeldt Test," *Science*, vol. 130 (1959), pp. 565–566.

Pincus, G., and H. Hoagland, Part I, "Adrenal Cortical Responses to Stress in Normal Men and in Those with Personality Disorders," *American Journal of Psychiatry*, vol. 106 (1950), pp. 641–650; Part II, "Analysis of the Pituitary Adrenal Mechanism in Man," pp. 651–659.

Price, D., "Preoperative Emotional States and Adrenal Cortical Activity; Studies on Cardiac and Pulmonary Surgery Patients," *Archives of Neurology and Psychiatry*, vol. 77 (1957), pp. 646–656.

Raab, W., and R. J. Humphreys, "Drug Action upon Myocardial Epinephrine-Sympathin Concentration and Heart Rate," *Journal of Pharmacology and Experimental Therapeutics*, vol. 89 (Jan. 1947), pp. 64–76.

Reddy, W. J., D. Jenkins, and G. W. Thorn, "Estimation of 17-hydroxycorticoids in Urine," *Metabolism*, vol. 1 (Nov. 1952), pp. 511–527.

Regan, P. F., and J. Reilly, "Circulating Epinephrine and Norepinephrine in Changing Emotional States," *Journal of Nervous and Mental Disease*, vol. 127 (1958), pp. 12–16.

Reilly, J., and P. F. Regan, "Plasma Catechol Amines in Psychiatric Patients," *Proceedings of the Society for Experimental Biology and Medicine*, vol. 95 (1957), pp. 377–380.

Reymert, M. L., ed., *Feelings and Emotions* (New York: McGraw-Hill, 1950).

Richter, D., and J. Crossland, "Variation in Acetylcholine Content of Brain with Physiological State," *American Journal of Physiology*, vol. 159 (Nov. 1949), pp. 247–255.

Rinaldi, F., and H. E. Himwich, "Alerting Responses in Actions of Atropine and Cholinergic Drugs," *Archives of Neurology and Psychiatry*, vol. 73 (April 1955), pp. 387–395.

Rinkel, M., R. W. Hyde, and H. C. Solomon, "Experimental Psychiatry. A Chemical Concept of Psychosis," *Diseases of the Nervous System*, vol. 15 (Sept. 1954), pp. 259–264; Correction, vol. 15 (Oct. 1954), p. 316.

———, R. W. Hyde, H. C. Solomon, and H. Hoagland, "Experimental Psychiatry. III. Clinical and Physio-chemical Observations in Experimental Psychosis," *American Journal of Psychiatry*, vol. 111 (June 1955), pp. 881–895.

Russek, H. I., "Role of Heredity, Diet, and Emotional Stress in

Coronary Heart Disease," *Journal of the American Medical Association*, vol. 171, no. 5 (Oct. 1959), pp. 503–508.

Saifer, A., and O. F. Kammerer, "Photometric Determination of Total Cholesterol in Plasma or Serum by Modified Liebermann-Burchard Reaction," *Journal of Biological Chemistry*, vol. 164 (Aug. 1946), pp. 657–677.

Schales, O., and S. S. Schales, "Simple and Accurate Method for Determination of Chloride in Biological Fluids," *Journal of Biological Chemistry*, vol. 140 (Sept. 1941), pp. 879–884.

Schenker, V., and A. C. Schenker, "A Tyramine-like Component and Its Responses to Autonomic Stimulation," *Journal of Nervous and Mental Disease*, vol. 128, no. 6 (June 1959), pp. 520–527.

Schlaegel, T. F., Jr., *Psychosomatic Ophthalmology* (Baltimore, Md.: Williams and Wilkins Co., 1957).

Scholander, P. F., and F. J. W. Rought on, "Micro Gasometric Estimation of the Blood Gases. IV. Carbon Dioxide," *Journal of Biological Chemistry*, vol. 148 (June 1943), pp. 573–580.

Selye, H., and Bajusz, "Stress and Cardiac Infarcts," *Angiology*, vol. 10 (Dec. 1959), pp. 412–420.

Shagass, C., "Clinical Significance of the Photomyoclonic Response in Psychiatric Patients," *Electroencephalography and Clinical Neurophysiology Journal*, vol. 6 (Aug. 1954), pp. 445–453.

———, "A Measurable Neurophysiological Factor of Psychiatric Significance," *Electroencephalography and Clinical Neurophysiology Journal*, vol. 9 (Feb. 1957), pp. 101–108.

———, and A. B. Kerenyi, "Neurophysiologic Studies of Personality," *The Journal of Nervous and Mental Disease*, vol. 126, no. 2 (Feb. 1957).

———, "Neurophysiological Studies of Anxiety and Depression," in *Psychiatric Research Reports*, no. 8, American Psychiatric Association (1957), pp. 100–117.

———, and A. L. Jones, "A Neurophysiological Test for Psychiatric Diagnosis: Results in 750 Patients," *The American Journal of Psychiatry*, vol. 114 (May 1958), pp. 1002–1010.

———, "Sedation Threshold, Neurophysiological Tool for Psychosomatic Research," *Psychosomatic Medicine*, vol. 18, no. 5 (Sept.-Oct. 1956).

———, and J. Naiman, "The Sedation Threshold as an Objective

Index of Manifest Anxiety in Psychoneurosis," *Journal of Psychosomatic Research*, vol. 1 (Feb. 1956), pp. 49–57.

———, and A. Kerenyi, "The 'Sleep' Threshold. A Simple Form of the Sedation Threshold for Clinical Use," *Canadian Psychiatric Association Journal*, vol. 3, no. 3 (July 1958), pp. 101–109.

Simpson, S. A., and J. F. Tait, "A Quantitative Method for the Bioassay of the Effect of Adrenal Cortical Steroids on Mineral Metabolism," *Endocrinology*, vol. 50 (Feb. 1952), pp. 150–161.

Singer, E. P., "The Hyperventilation Syndrome in Clinical Medicine," *New York State Journal of Medicine*, vol. 58 (May 1958), pp. 1494–1500.

Slater, E., and P. Slater, "A Heuristic Theory of Neurosis," *Journal of Neurology, Neurosurgery, and Psychiatry*, vol. 7 (Jan.–April 1944), pp. 49–55.

Snydor, K. L., and G. Sayers, "A Technic for Determination of Adrenocorticotrophin in Blood," *Proceedings of the Society for Experimental Biology*, vol. 79 (1952), pp. 432–436.

Sutherland, G. F., "The Salivary Curve: A Psychiatric Thermometer?" *American Journal of Psychiatry*, vol. 116, no. 1 (July 1959), pp. 20–24.

Thurstone, L. L., *A Factorial Study of Perception* (Chicago: University of Chicago Press, 1944).

Voth, A. C., "Individual Differences in the Autokinetic Phenomenon," *Journal of Experimental Psychology*, vol. 29 (1941), pp. 306–322.

Weckowicz, T. E., and R. Hall, "Skin Histamine Test in Schizophrenia," *Journal of Nervous and Mental Disease*, vol. 125, no. 3 (July–Sept. 1957), pp. 452–458.

Weil-Malherbe, H., "The Concentration of Adrenaline in Human Plasma and its Relation to Mental Activity," *Journal of Mental Science*, vol. 101 (Oct. 1955), pp. 733–755.

Wikler, A. W., *The Relation of Psychiatry to Pharmacology* (Baltimore, Md.: Williams & Wilkins Co., 1957).

Wilcott, R. C., "Silverman-Powell Index for Sweating vs. Skin Conductance and the Humidity Index of Surface Moisture," *Journal of Comparative and Physiological Psychology*, vol. 52 (1959), pp. 33–36.

———, "Correlation of Skin Resistance and Potential," *Journal of*

Comparative and Physiological Psychology, vol. 51 (1958), pp. 691–696.

Wolff, H. G., "Life Situations, Emotions and Bodily Disease," *Feelings and Emotions*, M. L. Reymert, ed. (New York: McGraw-Hill, 1950).

Woodbury, D. M., "Effect of Hormones on Brain Excitability and Electrolytes," *Recent Progress in Hormone Research*, vol. 10 (1954), pp. 65–107.

Woolley, D. W., and E. Shaw, "Some Neurophysiological Aspects of Serotonin," *British Medical Journal*, vol. 2 (July 1954), pp. 122–126.

Wortis, J., "Physiological Treatment. A Review of Psychiatric Progress, 1954," *American Journal of Psychiatry*, vol. 111 (Jan. 1955), pp. 515–518.

Ziskind, E., "Isolation Stress in Medical and Mental Illness," *Journal of the American Medical Association*, vol. 168, no. 11 (Nov. 1958), pp. 1427–1431.

VI: Some Criteria of Psychiatric Disorder in Adolescents

By James F. Masterson, Kenneth Tucker,
and Gloria Berk

EDITORIAL NOTES

So far in this book, we have focused chiefly on the problem of identifying psychiatric disorder in adults. We shall turn now to the consideration of young people and children.

Most of the theories regarding cause in psychiatric disorder emphasize infancy and childhood as periods when more or less permanent psychological damage may be produced. Epidemiological work done with adults shows marked variation of prevalence with age: in general the young adult has fewer symptoms, and his chance of acquiring them increases as he grows older. Some research indicates that after age seventy the prevalence of new symptoms may again decline.[1] These correlations indicate the need for extending knowledge below age eighteen or twenty. The importance attached to incidence studies is another reason for surveying groups of all ages. The younger the age group on which longitudinal research can begin, the better are our chances of mapping the important sequences of vulnerability and susceptibility to psychiatric disorder and the environmental processes related to them.

It might be useful at this point to summarize the approaches to basic research that have been treated so far:

1. Prevalence studies among adults in Western society. The bases have been established for work of this type, and a number of projects have been carried out.

2. Prevalence studies among adults in non-Western cultural groups. One of the critical problems here is "cultural relativity," and the necessity for redefinition and transposition of terms in order to make psychiatric surveys in such cultures. Resolution of this problem would provide a basis for cross-cultural comparisons. Some beginnings have been made, but they are scarcely more than that.

3. Prevalence studies among children and adolescents in Western society. The next two chapters are concerned with laying foundations for such studies.

4. Prevalence studies among adolescents and children in non-Western societies. These possibilities are also taken up in the next chapters.

5. Incidence studies that include all age groups in Western society. These, it is thought, will be made possible as a further development from prevalence studies.

6. Incidence studies of all age grades in non-Western groups. Such studies are hardly on the horizon as yet, but progress toward them can be made by the work outlined above. In this final phase the most revealing cross-cultural comparisons will be achieved.

In turning to the problem of identifying psychiatric disorder for epidemiological purposes among adolescents and children, we are at once confronted with the absence of standards and generally accepted criteria for specifying and classifying the phenomena of concern. While adult psychiatry is by no means free of such problems, the situation is much worse with the disorders of young people. One cannot therefore adapt an already existing nomenclature, but must start at a more primitive stage of construction. This means a good deal of preliminary effort within

the framework of Western cultural groups is needed before
cross-cultural comparisons can be achieved.

The present chapter constitutes an exploration into these matters and employs as a point of reference a study of 100 adolescents who attended an out-patient service in New York City.
The system of classification to be described has been devised for
a long-range project in which these cases will be investigated in a
follow-up study to see what alterations or confirmations of
symptoms occur through time. Thus the symptom catalogue was
designed for comparative purposes, each case to be compared
with each other in the study group; each case with itself at a later
date; and ultimately each case as a model by which to compare
the behavior of adolescents in a nonpatient population.

The system is also examined with an eye to its adaptation for
cross-cultural work. In this connection it is necessary to point
out that there is a body of literature, from both the social science
and psychiatric points of view, dealing with the influence of
sociocultural environment on adolescent adjustment.[2] Cultural
variation in the definition and treatment of such phenomena as
age grading is, of course, a key issue in anthropology. Although
it is not our purpose to review the relevant anthropological
literature, it may be said as a matter of impression that much
more attention has been given by anthropologists to cultural
differences in child-rearing practices than to differences in the
adolescent period. A great deal of what has been accumulated
about adolescence consists in descriptive accounts of puberty
rites and other life-cycle events found in different cultures
around the world and reported in the standard ethnographies.
Also available, however, are a number of treatises—largely of a
speculative and theoretical nature—about the relationship between cultural setting and patterns of personality development
and biological maturation. These deal with the question of how
much the compromise between human nature and sociocultural
nature is a matter of human plasticity giving in to the definitions
and prerequisites of culture and how much it is a matter of cul-

ture working with and adapting to the inevitabilities of sex differentiation and a life-arc of birth, growth, prime, decline, and
death.

A dominant though controversial work in the literature is
Margaret Mead's *Coming of Age in Samoa*.[3] This was certainly
the first and to our knowledge the only cross-cultural field investigation to deal solely and directly with the problem of adolescence. It was undertaken at a time when, in the United States,
widespread attention was given to adolescence as an invariable
state, everywhere characterized by storm and conflict. The
study primarily concerned 50 Samoan girls who appeared to
weather through adolescence with no disturbance in the gradual
unfolding of personality and role functioning appropriate for
that culture. This report served a useful purpose in demonstrating that *culture does make a difference,* but this is a point
which would scarcely be ignored nowadays under any circumstances. The controversial aspect is one of relative weight. It
seems clear that not everything is a matter of cultural arrangements nor is it all a matter of the uniformities involved in leaving
childhood and assuming adulthood. We have yet to discover
ways of classifying cultural variations so that full cognizance can
be given to the interplay between these sets of factors.

A rather similar idea, but approached another way, was Ralph
Linton's work on age and sex categories.[4] He observed that age
and sex are basic data which cultures use in the almost infinitely variable elaboration of ceremonies, occupations, and so
on, but that adolescence is not one of the minimal seven differentiations (infant, boy, girl, adult male, adult female, old male, and
old female). This does not mean that adolescence exists in some
cultures and not in others. It merely indicates that it may not be
recognized terminologically or identified by distinctive subcultural patterns of its own such as peer-group associations,
puberty ceremonies, or clearly understood rights and obligations. Adolescence obviously has some distinctive physiological
characteristics which cannot be obliterated by culture, but it is

certainly possible that research might disclose an association between symptom prevalence in this age group and cultural recognition or nonrecognition of adolescence as a stage in the life-cycle.

Linton made explicit his view that in societies where adolescence is linguistically recognized the path for an individual is easier than in those groups where it is not recognized. Although we feel that this should be a guiding thought in designing research, a certain skepticism is also called for. In our own society today, adolescence is certainly talked about—it has ample linguistic recognition. Also our society operates in reference to a number of subcultural institutions for adolescents—peer gangs, guidance programs for occupational choice, and the quasi rites-of-passage of high school commencement and freshman hazing. Yet this recognition does not appear to have lessened the *sturm und drang.*

Cultures may also be sorted regarding life-cycle in terms of Ruth Benedict's propositions about continuities and discontinuities.[5] In some cultures the expectations about a child's development into adulthood shift gradually and are geared to the behavioral capacities of different stages; in others the shift is abrupt. In our society, for example, almost no contribution to family subsistence is expected of a child, and then suddenly it is anticipated that the child will be able to take on this aspect of the adult role without first having been a fledgling. A similar discontinuity exists between the asexuality of prepubescence in our culture and the sexual sophistication expected later.

We do not conceive the points about recognition and continuity to be just other ways of saying Western/non-Western or primitive/civilized. Non-Western, so-called primitive cultures do not universally practice recognition and continuity, and Western civilizations do not universally exhibit discontinuity. There is no doubt, however, that these two factors deserve a place in the classification of sociocultural environment for the purposes of adolescent epidemiology. The framework of sociocultural classification should also touch on such issues as: clear definition of the role of the adolescent as opposed to ambiguity; diversity of occupational alternatives as opposed to a dominant and traditional division of labor; sexual mores, such as virginity being the primary consideration in a desirable wife versus demonstrated fecundity; marriage patterns, such as early, arranged marriages versus delayed self-choice; the work aspects of the adolescent role valued as a responsible contribution to society as opposed to disparagement of the adolescent; balance or imbalance in patterns of work and play; degree of intergenerational conflict; pressures for dependence on family and peer-group conformity as opposed to independence; and, especially in nonliterate cultures, the attitudes toward education and the degree to which it disrupts or threatens the customary way of life. Quite aside from the aspects thought peculiarly significant for adolescents, the catalogue should also refer to the state of the culture as a whole. Is the context for adolescent development stable and integrated, or is all fluid and changing?

THE difficulty in evaluating psychiatric disorder in adolescence is reflected in the sparse literature referring to the problem. A prevalent view in psychiatry seems to be to avoid the issue, to state that one cannot interpret psychopathology or determine diagnosis in adolescence and that, in time, a given symptom may disappear. This dangerous attitude begs the question of diagnosis and may result in overlooking symptoms of a permanent nature which can be identified early and treated before they have a chance to become an integral part of the personality functioning. In an attempt at further understanding of this problem we have undertaken a research project aimed at discovering what kinds of disorder are exhibited by adolescents attending an out-patient service, how these disorders compare with those of a representative group of nonpatient or "normal" adolescents, and what happens to both groups over a five-year period as they pass through adolescence.

By adolescence we mean the period of growth and maturation between childhood and adulthood. The boundaries are, however, extremely difficult to define. Although the emergent functioning of the ovaries and testicles can be taken as the physiological onset, there is no clearly demarked end to the physiological processes of adolescence. Also, the psychological limits cannot be established accurately, for the emotional characteristics of adolescence rarely appear full-blown. Adolescent traits may exist but be masked in a personality which is predominantly childish, or they may appear and then disappear in a transient regression, or they may fluctuate before crystallizing into adolescence. Nonetheless in research it is necessary to establish cutting points by which to select cases, and it is permissible to use chronological age if it is fully recognized as arbitrary and to some extent artificial. Our working definition is the period of time after the twelfth birthday, when puberty will have begun for most adolescents, and up to the nineteenth birthday, when most individuals will have finished high school and be expected subsequently to take a more adult role.

When we consider whether or not psychiatric disorder is present in an adolescent, three questions arise: (1) Is the presenting behavior or symptom evidence of illness? (2) If so, what kind of illness? (3) What does this illness imply regarding treatment and prognosis? In our studies we have observed that these questions are seriously complicated by the influence of the growth process and the personalities of the parents. These two factors have peculiarities unique to adolescence and can confuse what might otherwise be a clear picture.

The phrase "adolescent growth process" as we use it refers to the physical and emotional facets of developmental change. Physical growth has profound influence on the psychological state of the adolescent. The various aspects of physical growth do not occur consistently or together. This creates confusion for the adolescent and also for his parents. For example:

In one year a fourteen-year-old boy grew seven inches to a height of 6′4″ and gained about 30 pounds, weighing 200 pounds. The boy had great difficulty dealing with this new body structure and his parents had even more difficulty remembering that he was still only fourteen.

The other aspect of the adolescent growth process is the ability of the individual to accomplish the "emotional tasks" of adolescence, that is, to change from a dependent child to an independent adult. At the outset his primary relationships are within the family; he does not have a recognized sex role; and he lacks perspective about his standards, his own worth, and his position in relation to others outside the family. As an adult he must function with heterosexual maturity and with realistic acceptance of himself and appraisal of others.

In our own society, the growth process is frequently manifest by heightened intensity of feeling, constant tension between controlling and expressing instincts, shifting of defense mechanisms, and concomitant fluctuations of personality structure. All these aspects make the evaluation of psychopathology difficult. The strength of the instinctual forces and the relative weakness of capacity to deal with them, together with the need for independence and emancipation, produce a type of reaction that is especially characteristic of young people. In our society there is a tendency toward relieving the tensions through acting-out behavior and conflict with authority figures; thus a certain amount of such activity can be considered normal for adolescents.

In a culture where the problems of authority and submission are less acute, it is conceivable that the typical adolescent reaction might be bashfulness or withdrawal. What appears to an outsider as a type of response bordering on psychopathology may in fact be normal to adolescence there (just as acting-out in conflict with authority often is normal among our young people). Only if the pattern were exaggerated or prolonged would it be considered a psychiatric disorder.

Also, the adolescent growth process itself may be so dominant and pervasive that it produces transient symptoms which probably represent temporary excesses rather than an underlying personality disorder. We call this an "adolescent adjustment reaction." The superficial pattern of the symptoms may resemble any of the standard diagnostic categories and thus it must be assessed in terms of several other factors to determine whether it is an adjustment reaction or a more perduring malfunction. If the symptoms are of brief duration and do not reappear, it is reasonable to assume that they are due to the growth process. If the symptoms can be explained in terms of the nature of the growth process there is further reason for attributing them to that source. For example, rebellion may be a way of seeking emancipation, which is one of the tasks of emotional growth and should not, therefore, be called a bona fide disorder. It is also likely to be the adjustment reaction if there has been no past history of symptoms but then a sudden eruption occurs during adolescence. On the other hand, if the symptoms produce substantial impairment in functioning, they can hardly be attributed to the growth process alone.

A second complicating factor is the influence of the personalities of the parents on the adolescent. Often this stage in the child's life places as much stress on the parents as on the adolescent himself. His effort to resolve tensions may stir up similar problems which the parents have only partially solved before. The defenses of the parents against their unconscious strivings may be threatened and anxieties about them aroused. For example:

A mother had a problem in adolescence of untidiness, temper tantrums, rebelliousness, and sexual promiscuity. As the years went by, compulsive defenses developed to handle the underlying problem and the mother became neat, perfectionistic, rigid, and conforming.

However, when her teen-age daughter began to show signs of promiscuity, the mother's compulsive defenses were threatened and she developed considerable anxiety. This appeared to refer to her daughter's behavior, but closer examination showed that it really referred to herself. She was actually so concerned about the threatened release of her own instinctual feelings that she was not able to perceive that her daughter's problems were quite minor compared to her own. She made frantic efforts to control her daughter's behavior in an effort to resolve her own anxiety. The daughter then reacted with rebellion to the mother's inappropriate efforts to control, and the resultant behavior appeared to be more ill than it actually was.

There appears to be a direct ratio between the degree to which parents have resolved the problems of psychological maturation and the degree to which anxiety will be produced in the adolescent as he tries to settle similar problems. As far as our own culture is concerned, we feel the adjustment of the parents has so great an effect upon adolescent psychopathology that one cannot be evaluated without the other. This is particularly true of rebellion, which varies in meaning from being a healthy response to a grossly pathological parent to being the enactment of the unconscious wishes of a parent who stimulates or approves of the rebellious behavior. This consideration may be less crucial, have different content, or involve different people in other sociocultural groups. Elsewhere, for example, the intensity of the parent-child relationship may be disseminated in an extended kinship system, the roles of child and parent may not be so firmly interpenetrated, or authority may be invested in people other than parents.

What has been said about the importance of the growth process and the parent-adolescent relationship is a theoretical approach found useful in dealing with many of the problems presented by adolescents in our clinic. Nonetheless it seems appropriate to mention the limits of its generalizability and where it parallels and where it diverges from other orientations. To begin with, it would be comforting and perhaps illuminating if there were a tidy congruence in the diagnostic problems facing adolescent and geriatric psychiatry. It seems as if we ought to be able to use similar principles of at least biological process in understanding the psychopathological characteristics of both the developmental and involutional periods. Period of life—old age —helps confirm the diagnosis of senile pathology, for example, in a way quite opposite to the confusion introduced by the adolescent growth process. Nor do there appear to be any organic brain syndromes concomitant to abnormalities in physical growth during adolescence like the senile changes that attend the degenerative processes during senescence. Thus, focusing for the moment on the organic side, we may say that the physiological experiences of growing up and growing old do not have the same hazards for the kinds of psychiatric disorders which stem mainly from a malfunction of organic brain process.

On the other hand, talking about the emotional side, there is considerable generality to what has been pointed out as the adjustment problem of dealing with a new life-cycle status, in both going up and coming down the life-arc. On this emotional-adjustment side also, the relevance of the family relationships in which a patient is involved extends far beyond adolescence, although we feel they are especially crucial here. It seems fair to say that the two factors we have isolated for particular attention in dealing with the criteria of adolescent psychopathology are also important in understanding disorders found in any age group, especially if they are of a psychoneurotic, personality, or cognitive nature where social and psychological adjustments are pertinent. There are also considerations, but considerations of a different order, in other types of pathology. Going through adolescence or being in a difficult family situation may certainly complicate life for a young person with, for example, organic brain disease of whatever sort or mental deficiency, but they rarely interfere with the diagnosis.

The discussion so far has elaborated the difficulties involved in accurate evaluation of psychiatric disorder in adolescents. Next we shall present in detail our method for approaching this problem. Essentially, it consists of an attempt to rate the patient's psychiatric state in terms of both symptoms and impairment of functioning.

Concepts of Diagnosis

The concept of "diagnosis" has meaning primarily in terms of differentiating types of psychopathology but also secondarily in terms of etiology, treatment, and prognosis. It is a shorthand way of referring to symptom patterns and at the same time noting the development of symptoms, the patient's history, and his family history. Customarily in medical practice all available information is used in making a diagnosis. Since we hope to develop understanding of the dynamic relationship between types of psychopathology *and* background factors (such as history of illness in other family members, family relationships, treatment of the patient during childhood, his early personality development, or record of organic disease) we shall attempt to specify "diagnostic" groups on the basis of symptoms alone, and then later try to relate these symptom groups to pertinent factors of clinical background. Thus we hope to avoid the error of comparing two entities, one of which was used in the definition of the other.

Another preliminary point must be discussed at this time. There is a prevalent belief that, in adolescents, symptoms may shift from those of a psychoneurotic type to those of a schizophrenic or personality disorder type. Since "neurotic features" and "psychopathic features" may be characteristic of certain adolescent adjustment processes, the possibility exists that adolescents who show this fluid symptomatology are actually schizophrenics who "look like" psychoneurotics or personality disorders. Indeed, if this be true, it may explain the O'Neal and Robins findings in their study of the relation of childhood behavior problems to adult psychiatric status (a thirty-year follow-up of 150 subjects). They found that adult schizophrenics showed much acting-out and had many so-called "neurotic" symptoms as children and adolescents.[6]

In developing a classification for adolescent psychopathology, we were guided by the organization of symptom patterns, outlined primarily for adults, in the 1952 *Diagnostic and Statistical Manual of Mental Disorders*, issued by the American Psychiatric Association (the *APA Manual*). This is especially reflected in the fact that we comprise in our scheme the total range proposed by the APA and encompassed by the broad categories of psychoses, psychoneuroses, psychophysiologic symptoms, brain syndromes, sociopathic behaviors, personality disorders, and mental deficiency.

Analysis of early findings in our study indicated that there are both general similarities and specific differences between adolescent and adult symptom formations. The foci of our categories were the symptoms disclosed in psychiatric examination of our 100 adolescent patients. In order to avoid forcing our observations into a preconceived classification and to encourage a firm alliance between empirical data and the system of categories by which they will be grouped and ordered, we felt that initially the classifications should adhere as closely as possible to the observed symptoms. This required modifying the categories of the *APA Manual* in two ways.

First, in choosing patients for treatment, our department gave little representation, for example, to the categories dealing with hospitalized psychotics, drug addicts, severe acting-out problems, mental deficiency, and organic reactions. In view of this low frequency of cases in certain categories, we have grouped together such disorders as cardiovascular brain disease, toxic brain disease, and mental deficiency under "organic brain pattern." In cross-cultural epidemiology, this category would probably have to be expanded again. Second, several symptom patterns were so heavily represented in our adolescent group that it was felt necessary to give them specific and separate recognition. Thus categories such as "acting-out" and "sex disorder patterns" were added and broadened in meaning in order to highlight types of reactions that are particularly characteristic of adolescents.

We discovered that it was possible to identify symptoms of a great percentage of our adolescent patients by means of fourteen major categories, which are presented below with details of how individual symptoms are catalogued under the main divisions of the system. As an introduction to these symptom lists, the following annotation is an effort to make more precise the correspondence and lack of correspondence between our classification and the *APA Manual*. Our symptom pattern called "thinking disorder" refers to the patterns of psychosis characteristic of adolescents. An adolescent symptom classified here, like those symptoms exhibited by schizophrenic adults, is primarily noted as a disorder of cognitive functioning or orientation. The adolescent categories designated as "anxiety pattern," "conversion and/or dissociation pattern," "phobic pattern," "obsessive-compulsive pattern," "depressive pattern," and "hypochondriacal pattern" deal with the kind of phenomena catalogued in the APA system as psychoneurotic symptoms. Our category of "psychophysiologic pattern" matches the like-named category of the APA. The personality disorders dealt with by the APA system are represented in our scheme by the categories called "hysterical personality disorder pattern," "immature personality disorder pattern," and "compulsive personality disorder pattern." Our categories of "acting-out" and "sexual difficulty" are related to the types of disorder specified by the APA as sociopathic disorders, but we use them in a broader sense, feeling that these symptoms in adolescents are more fluid and appear more frequently in combination with other types of symptoms than is true of adults and that, therefore, they are not entirely congruent with the more stable patterns of sociopathy denoted in the adult classification.

We hope through this approach to make progressively finer

diagnostic differentiations pertaining to adolescents and to shed light on the specific differences between adolescents and adults.

Proposed Classification of Adolescent Psychopathology

Each symptom pattern grouping contains several symptoms which are in one way or another *characteristic* of the entire pattern. If one or more symptoms of a particular grouping were observed, the patient was considered to have that particular symptom pattern. It should be repeated that the symptom pattern groupings are descriptive and *not* diagnostic. Their purpose is to provide a scheme whereby psychopathological data can be analyzed simply and efficiently.

1. *Thinking Disorder Pattern*
   a. Inappropriate affect (giggling; silly behavior; etc.)
   b. Delusions (somatic; paranoid; etc.)
   c. Hallucinations (auditory; visual; etc.)
   d. Bizarre ideation
   e. Bizarre motor behavior (inappropriate gestures; grimacing; etc.)
   f. Mutism
   g. Ideas of reference
   h. Gross confusion of thinking
   i. Disorganization of habits
   j. Thinking disorder (looseness of associations; concreteness; etc.)
2. *Anxiety Pattern*
   a. Generalized anxiety (nervousness) up to panic reaction
   b. Somatic symptoms—autonomic, without organic etiology (dizzy spells; dyspnoea, palpitations; nausea; diarrhea; polyuria)
   c. Nail biting; picking fingers; in general, repetitive motor behavior designed to relieve tension (including "restlessness")

3. *Conversion Pattern and/or Dissociation Pattern*

This grouping includes symptoms of actual organic dysfunction where evidence of organic etiology is lacking.

a. "Anesthesia" symptoms (anosmia; blindness; deafness)
b. "Paralysis" symptoms (paresis; aphonia; monoplegia; hemiplegia)
c. "Dyskinesis" symptoms (tic; tremor; posturing)
d. Automatic behavior; fugue; amnesia
e. Other conversion pattern symptoms

4. *Phobic Pattern*

a. Specific object or situational fear (fear of dirt; fear of closed places; fear of animals; fear of school; etc.)

5. *Obsessive-compulsive Pattern*

a. Obsessive thoughts
b. Repetitive, ritualistic acts (touching; counting; handwashing)
c. Compulsive speech
d. Other compulsions (such as compulsive eating)

6. *Depressive Pattern*

a. Pathologic depression
b. Pathologic self-deprecation
c. Pathologic guilt
d. Suicidal preoccupation
e. Suicide attempt
f. Crying (by history or during interview)
g. Other depressive pattern symptoms

7. *Hypochondriacal Pattern*

a. Somatic complaints without evidence of somatic dysfunction
b. Body overconcern without evidence of somatic dysfunction

8. *Psychophysiologic Pattern*

This grouping includes symptoms of actual somatic dysfunction with organic pathology where psychogenic factors are considered predominant. The following conditions are among many possibilities.

a. Asthma
b. Migraine or tension headaches
c. Colitis
d. Other psychophysiologic pattern symptoms (includes "neurasthenia" or fatigue states)

9. *Hysterical Personality Disorder Pattern*

This grouping is characterized by "persons who are vain and egocentric, who display labile and excitable but shallow affectivity, whose dramatic attention-seeking and histrionic behavior may go to the extremes of lying and even pseudologia phantastica, who are very conscious of sex, sexually provocative, and who are dependently demanding in interpersonal situations." [7]

a. Erotic behavior
b. Dramatic attention-seeking behavior
c. Excessive consciousness of sex or sexually provocative behavior
d. Histrionic behavior
e. Other hysterical personality disorder pattern symptoms

10. *Immature Personality Disorder Pattern*

This grouping includes symptoms characterizing a late or delayed emergence from childhood.

a. Psychological immaturity (as manifested by childish speech, deportment and activities)
b. Enuresis
c. Thumb-sucking
d. History of being easily "picked on"
e. Clinging to parent
f. Choosing friends younger than self
g. Other immature personality disorder pattern symptoms

11. *Compulsive Personality Disorder Pattern*
    a. Overconscientiousness
    b. Overinhibited behavior resulting in greatly restricted, pathological work and play
    c. Other compulsive personality disorder pattern symptoms

12. *Acting-out Pattern*

    This pattern is defined by negative behavioral expressions of emotion.

    a. Juvenile delinquency (destructive antisocial behavior)
    b. Stealing
    c. Temper outbursts
    d. Generally negativistic behavior
    e. Rebellious behavior at school
    f. Physically hostile behavior to parents
    g. Physically hostile behavior to siblings
    h. Overtly hostile behavior—other
    i. Antisocial behavior—other
    j. Pathological lying
    k. Running away from home
    l. Window peeping
    m. Lack of impulse control
    n. Sexual acting-out

13. *Sexual Difficulty Pattern*
    a. Masturbation guilt
    b. Homosexual behavior
    c. Fetishism
    d. Voyeurism
    e. Sexual preoccupations
    f. Sexual deviation—other
    g. Other sexual acting-out (such as promiscuity)

14. *Organic Reaction Pattern and Mental Deficiency*
    a. Psychiatric symptoms derived from brain disease
    b. Mental deficiency

In addition to these fourteen pattern groupings we observed a large number of more generalized and ubiquitous symptoms which, although they do not appear helpful in differentiating symptom patterns, do seem to augment the picture of psychopathology in most patients. These symptoms are the following:

Tension

Concentration difficulty

Tremulousness

Difficulty falling asleep

Nightmares

Obesity

Immaturity by age standards

Poor hygiene

Vanity and egocentricity

Labile affect

Minor physical diseases (colds, headaches, etc.)

Arrogance

Irritability

Demanding in interpersonal situations

Truancy

Low intelligence

Lying

Grand mal epilepsy

Petit mal epilepsy

Poor judgment

Anorexia

Passivity

Blunted affect

Flattened affect

Poor abstractions

Vagueness

Circumstantiality

Blocking

Poor comprehension

Loss of interest in school

Decreased school performance

Decreased social performance

Poor socialization (few friends)

Feelings of inferiority

Withdrawal

Overcompliance

Shyness

Loneliness

Conflict with or about mother or mother surrogate

Conflict with or about father or father surrogate

Unexpressed feelings of hostility

Accident proneness

Apathetic behavior

Evasive, guarded behavior

Denial

Conflict with or about sibling(s) or sibling surrogate(s)

Dating older men

Reading disability

Stuttering

Physical disease or defect (such as hemophilia)

Inarticulateness

Sterile history

Introversion or isolation

Confabulation

Conflict with or about peers

Suspiciousness

Perseveration

Religious conflicts

In evaluating this classification system in terms of preparing for cross-cultural research, we should note several points. Although we can make an adequate beginning by outlining the areas which would need to be covered and specifying the types of symptoms about which questions would need to be asked, it is immediately apparent that whoever used this system would have to be very familiar with the culture and the language of the group studied.

Moreover, the categories at this stage of their development are not composed uniformly of culture-free and culture-bound symptomatology. For example, the items of "truancy," "school performance," and "dating older men" are formulated clearly in terms of institutions and conduct specific to our own society. There might, and yet again there might not, be direct equivalents in another culture. In no place and at no time has life been so simple that it did not require learning; thus counterparts to school performance probably are everywhere available— performance in apprenticeships for adult occupations, for example. We mean that learning is a universal human process and that once we discover what it is that people have to learn in order to be normally productive individuals in their own culture, standards could be constructed from which to estimate "inability to learn." The type of learning obviously varies from one group to another—in our society "school performance" usually means an ability to deal with ideas; in another culture it may mean the ability to make far finer discriminations of sound and smell than we have ever conceived necessary for staying alive or being normally productive. On the other hand, "truancy" could be used only in groups where there is compulsory education, and "dating older men" would not apply in cultures where patterns of friendship and courtship are more formalized and restricted than ours.

Some items would have to be dropped out entirely in adapting this system, some new items would need to be added on the basis of inductive research, and still others would need to be replaced by appropriate substitutes. Gradually, it is to be hoped, the language of psychiatry will become more international and cross-cultural by being increasingly a language of process. Many of the symptoms in this classification are already at such a level. In mind here are "disorganization of habits" and "difficulty sleeping." Habit and sleep are processes. All people have patterns of sleep, dress, eating, and hygiene which, once discovered, are the measure by which to judge "disorganization" and "difficulty." The same can be said about the processes of delusion, hallucination, and depression. They can be defined without reference to specific cultural content, but the job is much more subtle and difficult when, as in these cases, it involves finding the standards by which other cultures operate in terms of what is conceived as appropriate belief or emotion and then of measuring the deviance from common practice which constitutes psychiatric disorder.

Concepts of Impairment

In addition to identifying and classifying symptoms, it is important to make an assessment of the adolescent's functioning and the degree to which it may be impaired owing to the presence of symptoms. An evaluation of impairment is essential for the understanding of adolescent psychopathology, and we anticipate that it will be a valuable tool in separating basic personality disturbances from adolescent growth processes and adjustment reactions. Also, we hope it will assist in establishing standards of functioning appropriate for "normal" adolescents.

Psychiatric impairment is defined in the *Manual* as the "degree to which the individual's total functional capacity is affected by the psychiatric disorder." Unlike diagnosis, which is a qualitative statement, an impairment scale is a quantitative measure of malfunctioning. Impairment indicates nothing about the characteristics of the patient's illness but does tell us that at a given period of time the patient's ability to function normally is diminished to some definable degree.

An impairment scale thus enlarges our concept of illness, for it allows us to specify degrees of illness within diagnostic categories. Impairment can be regarded as a measure not only of the intensity of a patient's illness, but, conversely, also of the strengths and assets within his personality. A patient whose symptoms prevent him from functioning is "sicker" than one who has similar symptoms but who can function adequately. This may sound obvious, but it touches the knotty question of how some individuals are able to convert symptoms into productive effort—"If I didn't have some anxieties, I wouldn't ever accomplish anything." In addition, an assessment of a patient's ability to function frequently indicates whether he is more or less accessible to treatment and influences our estimate of his prognosis. For example, the therapist's treatment procedures, goals, and prognosis for a schizophrenic patient who is minimally impaired differ considerably from those accorded a schizophrenic patient who is severely impaired.

The majority of studies involving impairment have been done as follow-up studies of hospitalized patients. Usually the outcome of illness or the degree of impairment over a span of years have been measured in gross terms. A typical scale is as follows:

A. Functioning without impairment from symptoms at work or in the home.

B. Functioning with minimal impairment from symptoms (for example, up to 50 per cent) at work or at home, or functioning at reduced level without symptoms.

C. Functioning with marked impairment from symptoms (for example, greater than 50 per cent) at work or at home.

D. Unable to function, hospitalized, or suicidal.

It is apparent that finer measurements are needed in studying out-patients, particularly adolescents, who are known to show as wide shifts in functioning as in the appearance and disappearance of symptoms.

In the study "Mothers' Attitudes toward the Social Development of Their Adolescents," Ruth Butler suggested three phases of adolescence—early, middle and late.[8] She noted that adolescents in the early phase appear to have difficulty in organizing social responsibilities and often perform less satisfactorily in school than during the late phase. Focusing on school performance as an area of functioning brought several questions to mind. How significant is impairment of school functioning during the various stages of adolescence in our society? How can this impairment be differentiated from impairment that is a reflection of basic personality disturbance? How does this affect our concepts of adolescent illness, treatment, and prognosis? Besides school functioning, adjustment in other areas and aspects of life seems equally important. Consequently, we devised impairment scales for school adjustment, social adjustment, and family relationships. No attempt is made here to extrapolate from these areas of functioning for purposes of cross-cultural research. Other categories would need to be selected as they pertain to different sociocultural environments. Nonetheless, we feel that these categories could be employed as models for the way in which other categories could be specified and subdivided.

Proposed Scales for Rating Impairment

School Adjustment

A. *Academic functioning*
   1. Doing well
   2. Passing
   3. Passing but not functioning up to capacity
   4. Marginal (i.e., barely passing; not up to grade)
   5. Isolated failures
   6. Multiple failures (including repeated grades)
   7. Not attending school
B. *Deviations from previous characteristics of functioning*
   1. Better
   2. Worse
   3. None

Social Adjustment

A. *Number of friends*
   1. Many friends
   2. Few friends
   3. No friends
B. *Heterosexual activity*
   1. Present
   2. Absent
C. *Age of friends*
   1. Younger
   2. Older
   3. Peers
D. *Intimacy of friends*
   1. Close friend or friends
   2. No close friends
E. *Outside activities* (all activities and interests outside of the home including membership in groups, clubs, and extra-curricular activities)
   1. Outside activities
   2. No outside activities
F. *Deviations from previous characteristics of functioning*
   1. Better
   2. Worse
   3. None

Family Relationships

A, B. *Personality of mother and father*
   1. Positive
   2. Negative
       (a) Overtly pathological
       (b) Aggressive—domineering
       (c) Passive—submissive
   3. Presence or absence of parent
       (a) Present

(b) Absent
    (1) dead
    (2) deserted
    (3) separated
    (4) divorced
    (5) hospitalized
    (6) out of home

C, D. *Attitude and behavior of mother and father to the patient*
1. Accepting
2. Ambivalent—verbalized ambivalence or resentment and observed guilt and/or depression
3. Negative
    (a) Active rejection (domineering, angry, nagging, restricting, demanding)
    (b) Passive rejection (lack of interest, unable to set limits)
    (c) No insight into patient's feelings
    (d) Overindulgent, oversolicitous, overprotective
    (e) Unconsciously stimulating patient

E, F, G. *Patient's attitude toward mother, father, and siblings*
1. Accepting
2. Verbally accepting but negative in behavior
3. Ambivalent
4. Rejecting
5. Overly compliant (patient's positive response to an overtly negative and rejecting parent)

Five impairment scales were designed in order to evaluate functioning in the categories just discussed.

1. SCHOOL PERFORMANCE IMPAIRMENT

In Western culture, school is an area in which the adolescent's capacity to integrate and organize his various strivings is significantly tested. With its requirements for attention, concentration, and self-discipline, school performance is often a sensitive indicator of how well the adolescent functions. Scholastic achievement is our primary index of impairment, behavioral disturbances being indirectly involved insofar as they have affected actual performance in terms of grades or progress:

A. No impairment (students doing passing work of a nature roughly equivalent to their potential as determined by our examination and school report).

B. Mild impairment (adolescents who were "just passing" but clearly not obtaining grades commensurate with their intelligence or capacity; passing subjects on a reduced schedule; failing isolated subjects).

C. Moderate impairment (students who have been left back, could not attend school, or required home instruction).

2. SOCIAL IMPAIRMENT

The ability to form adequate relationships with boys and girls outside the family, to develop interests and hobbies, and to participate in group activities are other important areas of functioning. Adolescents in our culture tend to use identification with a peer group to help in their struggle for emancipation. Frequently, such identification is transitory and precedes the adolescent's readiness to assert his own individuality. The "Social Impairment Scale" is based on the adolescent's relationship with friends and his participation in outside activities as outlined previously. In each of the categories, the adolescent is rated "plus" or "minus." If he had no friends or few friends (only one or two) he was rated "minus." More than two friends was rated "plus." Where the friends were primarily younger than the adolescent (by two or more years) he was rated "minus." Absence of outside social activities was rated "minus." The degree of impairment was then rated according to the following scale:

A. No impairment (no "minuses").

B. Mild impairment (any one or two "minuses").

C. Moderate impairment (any three "minuses").

D. Severe impairment (any four or five "minuses").

3. FAMILY RELATIONSHIP IMPAIRMENT

It is our feeling that disturbances in the family relationship probably have serious repercussions in the growth, development, and functioning of the adolescent in our society and may be directly related to many kinds of psychopathology.

The previous scales attempt to measure a deficit in the patient's own functioning. Family relationship impairment is somewhat different. The element for consideration here is the relationship between the patient and his parents—a bilateral unit—and not just the functioning of either part of the intermeshed whole. Our experience suggests that the level of functioning of the whole unit reflects the individual's functioning within it. If both patient and parents express negative attitudes toward each other, the total relationship is impaired and probably indicates a functional disability on the part of the patient. In our analytic procedure, the relationship is rated good if the parent accepts the patient even though the parent himself may display psychopathology. If the patient's attitude toward his father, for example, is rejecting, as evidenced through rebellious behavior, the relationship is considered at least moderately impaired. When, however, we add that the father's attitude is also one of rejection exemplified in extreme domination, it becomes clear how severely impaired is the total relationship.

The family relationship impairment scale is based only on expressed attitudes and not on the personality characteristics of the principals involved. A separate rating is made for the patient's attitudes toward mother, father, and siblings:

A. No impairment.
    1. Parent accepting.
    2. Patient accepting.
B. Mild impairment.
    1. Either parent or patient is ambivalent and the other is accepting.
    2. Both are ambivalent.

C. Moderate impairment.
  1. Either parent or patient is negative and the other is accepting or ambivalent.
D. Severe impairment.
  1. Both rejecting.

4. "SYMPTOM-INDUCED IMPAIRMENT"

We turn now to factors which are more subjective and therefore harder to evaluate. This impairment scale combines two aspects—objective symptom intensity and subjective symptom distress. These two elements together form a psychopathological impairment rating. For example, one of our adolescents was excessively anxious although he performed adequately in all spheres. Using only the previous impairment ratings, he would be classified as unimpaired. Consequently, a measure of the intensity of the symptom itself (in this case, anxiety) is necessary to obtain a larger perspective of impairment.

Our method of handling the problems involved in establishing a rating for symptom severity is to combine objective evidence of the number, intensity, and duration of symptoms with the psychiatrist's evaluation of the subjective distress as communicated by the patient. From the literature as well as our own experience, we came to the conclusion that comparisons of the severity of one kind of illness with the severity of another kind are qualitatively inappropriate. Despite the contention that, from the dynamic point of view, the differences between psychosis, psychoneurosis, and personality disorder are merely quantitative, their manifestations are so strikingly dissimilar as to make across-the-board comparisons very difficult. For this reason, we rated degrees of severity only within each principal symptom pattern group. For example, we compared one "thinking disorder" adolescent with another "thinking disorder" adolescent, but not with an "anxiety" or "depressive" adolescent. As examples, "severity" and "impairment" are particularized for two symptom pattern categories in the following way:

A. *Thinking disorder pattern.*

1. Mild: a mild tendency to be unrealistic such that the unreality is not focused and perhaps only indirectly detectable. Associated symptoms illustrating this might include: vagueness, extreme suspiciousness, blocking, poor abstractive ability (as determined by psychiatric examination).

2. Moderate: a thought disorder tending to fasten on specific irrational distortions with a decided departure from reality in terms of both perception and behavior. Illustrative associated symptoms: ideas of reference; circumstantiality; inappropriate, personalized abstractions; disorganization of habits.

3. Severe: grossly disturbed ideation, often bizarre and autistic with a breakdown of perception and behavior patterns. Among many others, illustrative associated symptoms include: delusions, hallucinations, bizarre or uncontrolled motor behavior.

B. *Anxiety pattern.*

1. Mild: history of intermittent anxiety or tension or restlessness with or without diminished performance on psychiatric examination.

2. Moderate: either a history of persistent (but not severe) anxiety or evidence of marked anxiety (which must be so stated) on psychiatric examination or both.

3. Severe: persistent, incapacitating conversion or dissociation symptoms.

5. SUBJECTIVE REACTION TO PSYCHOPATHOLOGY

This final impairment scale is based on the adolescent's response to the question: "How much are you upset by your problems?" It is rated in the following manner:

1. Not at all.
2. A little.
3. A great deal.

It is anticipated that these ratings will help differentiate between adolescents with extensive psychopathology who have little or no subjective reaction (and can function well) from those adolescents who may or may not have extensive psychopathology but who are distressed about themselves (and have difficulty functioning). It is our tentative impression that there may be a correlation between degree of subjective reaction to psychopathology and the ability to function.

Summary

In the attempt to develop criteria of psychiatric disorder in adolescence there are many factors specific to this time of life that must be understood. As we have indicated, two of the most important are the nature of the growth process and the relationship of the adolescent with his parents. We have conducted a study that involved examining 100 adolescent out-patients in a metropolitan area of the United States, classifying them according to the degree of impairment shown through their capacity to function at school, in social groups, and in relationship to their parents. It is hoped that by making such objective and specific classifications and then following the patients through their adolescent years, it may be possible to separate the fundamental symptom formations from the transient and superficial ones related primarily to the adolescent phase of development. In addition, we have reviewed our approach and procedures in the light of feasibility for cross-cultural research, and we believe that this effort carried out in our own society could serve as a model for other research, whereby it would be possible to add the comparative dimension of how a universal period of life may have different psychopathological characteristics in different cultural groups.

Notes

1. D. C. Leighton, J. S. Harding, D. B. Macklin, A. M. Macmillan, and A. H. Leighton, *The Character of Danger: Psychiatric Symptoms in*

Selected Communities [Vol. III, The Stirling County Study of Psychiatric Disorder and Sociocultural Environment (New York: Basic Books, 1963)]; L. Srole, T. S. Langner, S. T. Michael, M. K. Opler, and T. A. C. Rennie, *Mental Health in the Metropolis: The Midtown Manhattan Study* [Vol. I, Thomas A. C. Rennie Series in Social Psychiatry (New York: McGraw-Hill Book Company, 1962)].

2. For examples see: S. Lorand, and H. I. Schneer, eds., *Adolescents— Psychoanalytic Approach to Problems and Therapy* (New York: Paul B. Hoeber, Inc., 1961); D. P. Ausubel, *Theory and Problems of Adolescent Development* (New York: Grune & Stratton, Inc., 1959); B. H. Balser, *Psychotherapy of the Adolescent* (New York: International Universities Press, Inc., 1957), chs. 1 and 8; E. Beaglehole, and P. Beaglehole, "Personality Formation in Pukapukan Children," in *Language, Culture and Personality: Essays in Memory of Edward Sapir*, L. Spier, A. I. Hallowell, and S. S. Newman, eds. (Salt Lake City: University of Utah Press, 1960); S. Berman, "Psychotherapeutic Techniques with Adolescents," *American Journal of Orthopsychiatry*, vol. 24 (April 1945), pp. 238–245; A. Gesell, and others, *Youth: The Years from Ten to Sixteen* (New York: Harper & Row, 1956); S. Glueck, and E. Glueck, *Juvenile Delinquents Grown Up* (New York: Commonwealth Fund, 1940); R. J. Havighurst, and H. Taba, *Adolescent Character and Personality* [in collaboration with the Committee on Human Development, the City of Chicago—Andrew W. Brown and others (New York: John Wiley & Sons, Inc., 1949)]; L. Josselyn, "The Ego in Adolescence," *American Journal of Orthopsychiatry*, vol. 24 (April 1944), pp. 223–227; A. B. Landolt, "Follow-up Studies on Circular Manic-Depressive Reactions Occurring in the Young," *Bulletin of the New York Academy of Medicine*, vol. 65 (1957), p. 33; J. F. Masterson, "Prognosis in Adolescent Disorders," *American Journal of Psychiatry*, vol. 114 (June 1958), p. 12; J. F. Masterson, "Prognosis in Adolescent Disorders: Schizophrenia," *Journal of Nervous and Mental Diseases*, vol. 124 (Sept. 1956), p. 3; M. Mead, "Adolescence in Primitive and in Modern Society," *Readings in Social Psychology*, T. M. Newcomb and E. L. Hartley, eds. (New York: Holt, 1947), pp. 6–14; T. Parsons, "Age and Sex in the Social Structure of the U.S.," *Personality in Nature, Society and Culture*, C. Kluckhohn, H. A. Murray, and D. M. Schneider, eds. (New York: Knopf, 1949); *Sources of Information on Behavioral Problems of Adolescence*, compiled by the Committee of Academic Education, American Psychiatric Association, with the professional assistance of Professor Vaclav Mostecky and his staff; J. W. M. Whiting, *Becoming a Kwoma* (New Haven: Yale University Press, 1941).

3. M. Mead, *Coming of Age in Samoa* (New York: Morrow, 1935).

4. R. Linton, "Age and Sex Categories," *American Sociological Review*, vol. 7, no. 5 (Oct. 1942), pp. 589 ff.; R. Linton, *The Study of Man* (New York: Appleton-Century-Crofts, Inc., 1936), pp. 118–119.

5. R. Benedict, "Continuities and Discontinuities in Cultural Conditioning," *A Study of Interpersonal Relations*, P. Mullahy, ed. (New York: Hermitage Press, Inc., 1949).

6. P. O'Neal, and L. Robins, "The Relation of Childhood Behavior Problems to Adult Psychiatric Status: A 30-Year Follow-up Study of 150 Subjects," *American Journal of Psychiatry*, vol. 114, no. 11 (May 1958), p. 961; P. O'Neal, and L. Robins, "Childhood Pattern Predictive of Adult Schizophrenia: A 30-Year Follow-up Study," *American Journal of Psychiatry*, vol. 115, no. 5 (Nov. 1958).

7. P. Chodoff, and H. Lyons, "Hysteria, the Hysterical Personality and 'Hysterical' Conversion," *American Journal of Psychiatry*, vol. 114, no. 8, (Feb. 1958), pp. 734–740.

8. R. M. Butler, "Mothers' Attitudes Toward the Social Development of Their Adolescents," Part I, *Social Casework*, vol. 37 (1956), pp. 219–226, and Part II, pp. 280–288.

VII: Criteria of Psychiatric Disorder in Children

By Albert C. Sherwin and Marie-Louise Schoelly

EDITORIAL NOTES

This chapter, like its predecessor, is concerned with building a platform, rather than taking off from one already established. Indeed, the field of child psychiatry is even less ready for epidemiological studies than is the field of adolescent psychiatry. This is not to imply, of course, that childhood has been ignored by psychiatry. On the contrary, during the last half-century of development in psychopathological theory it has come to have a central position. But the consideration of childhood in theoretical terms is not quite the same thing as direct investigation of individual human beings at the time they are living through its periods and phases. In the main, childhood psychology has been inferred from the free associations and dreams of adults, and is conceived as a time of antecedents to later, more obvious, consequences. Among the antecedents, attention has been particularly directed at child-rearing practices as having potentials for good and bad adjustment in later life. Without questioning the value of this approach it may be pointed out that it is clearly different from the subject matter of the present chapter.

Sherwin and Schoelly are concerned with children under the age of twelve rather than with childhood as such. They deal with manifest disturbances of behavior and feelings of children, rather than with causes of later difficulties that emerge only after the children have grown up. Their report is based on clinical experience in an out-patient department and looks toward the problem of establishing criteria that might be used in epidemiological studies. As in the previous chapter, the first issue of concern is the development of criteria that are appropriate within the framework of Western culture, although cross-cultural possibilities are kept in mind.

Communication is always a paramount problem in psychiatric studies, but it is particularly so where children are the focus. They begin with exceedingly limited capacity to communicate and progressively develop it throughout the childhood period. This fact alone makes for particular difficulties in identifying suitable criteria by which to judge the presence or absence of psychiatric disorder, and in obtaining the necessary information after criteria have been selected. A means of dealing with this, the one chosen by the authors, is to interview the mother as the person most closely associated with the child, and so best able to observe and communicate. This course has been taken in a number of studies including those dealing with child-training practices in non-Western cultures.[1]

Such an approach, however, raises formidable questions as to just what kind of information is being obtained. A mother's view of her child is not commonly thought of as outstandingly objective; moreover, undetected situations will occur in which the mother's report is more colored by her own psychiatric symptoms than by the realities of the child's behavior. The main alternatives to this approach appear to be two: testing procedures and prolonged direct observation of the child. The first of these is open, at the present stage of knowledge, to as many questions and uncertainties as is analysis based on mother interviews. While there exist trustworthy tests for several specific types of performance including a number of aspects of intelligence, there are no tests that can be relied upon to detect all, or even most, types of psychiatric disorder. Prolonged observation (including intermittent multiple observations) is probably the most valid approach available, but it is so costly and so difficult to arrange as to be impracticable in epidemiological research. The authors therefore turn to the mother as the source of information, but also include some limited observation and interviewing of the child.

Several points can be made regarding the specific cross-cultural considerations of this chapter. Although it is precisely in the area of cultural differences in child-rearing practices that, up until the last few years, psychiatry and anthropology have most firmly joined hands, this work has been almost entirely concerned with theoretical implications.[2] In "culture and personality studies" the predominant framework has been psychoanalytic. With the structure which this offers for the organization of data about child experiences, psychoanalytic theory was a way to analyze cultural practices and hopefully to account for the variability of personality associated with being Japanese, Russian, Irish, or Italian.[3] It appeared, also, that these variabilities of personality could be described by psychiatric terminology —an obsessive personality type being characteristic of one group, a hysterical type of another, anxiety of another, and so on—often with the idea that these personality summaries would help illuminate other cultural and historical facts such as religion, philosophy, and national policies.

That there *are* different cultural patterns of handling children is, of course, evident. Some peoples swaddle their infants, some diaper them, some do neither. Some groups uniformly breast-feed, or wet-nurse, or bottle-feed their babies. Some groups lavish attention on little children, others are harsh and reserved; some encourage independence and individual achievement, others seem to let the child's personality unfold without much direction or even attention. These differences can be interpreted to mean that the adults of such and such a group ought to be prone to be neurotic or nonneurotic or to display some particular aspect of neurosis. In the Kardiner and Linton studies, which were a pioneering effort, hypotheses of this nature were investigated using Rorschach tests as the main evidence for the psychiatric characteristics of adults in various cultural settings.[4] Although work of this type has had a stimulating influence on cross-cultural psychiatry, better methods are needed either to refute or substantiate such theoretical formulations.

Since this early work, comparative studies of child-rearing practices have become much more numerous and have been formulated in several different directions so that there is now a large literature on the practices of dealing with children, but still very little on the cross-cultural study of psychiatric disorders in children.

In many non-Western societies, there loom several noteworthy complicating factors that require attention in planning epidemiological research on children. One is the high birth rate and correspondingly high infant mortality rate. The population of children in such areas has, in other words, demographic features which are specific to the fact of their being children. The turnover is much more rapid than in the adult segments, and with this high mortality goes high morbidity. Consequently it is likely that the battery of case-finding methods for children would need to be especially geared both for detecting organically based psychiatric disorders and for distinguishing between organic and psychological disturbances. A further point is that in some cultures the children who exhibit certain psychiatric disorders face quite different problems of survival than do children in Western culture. In several of the so-called primitive societies infanticide has been practiced in the past and may still be done surreptitiously with regard to severely handicapped children. But even where there is no deliberate killing, there are still problems of survival under certain living conditions. In the Eskimo study discussed in Chapters III and IV, the exploratory excursion into the prevalence of symptoms among children disclosed mainly the behavior characteristics of mental deficiency and brain syndrome, and further that most of the children exhibiting these patterns died before reaching adulthood.

These aspects of morbidity and mortality draw attention to two points in cross-cultural psychiatric epidemiology: children constitute a distinctive demographic segment confronting study efforts with particular problems of major proportions; and the understanding of the epidemiology of children (including mortality characteristics) is essential to the understanding of cause in many psychiatric disorders among adults.

IT is appropriate to begin this presentation with a brief discussion of the problem of criteria. It has already been noted that prevalence studies have generally excluded children. In part this omission stems from the difficulty of establishing impairment criteria for children who, by nature, are constantly changing and growing. Various behavioristic manifestations, such as thumb-sucking or temper tantrums, constitute normal phenomena at one age, become mildly pathologic at another, and assume an even more serious significance at a more advanced age.

Other difficulties about criteria involve the present state of knowledge concerning childhood psychopathology. A brief review of this will serve as introduction to the description of our prevalence research with children. General clinical experience in Western society suggests that the child with a psychiatric disorder primarily exhibits disturbances in activity and behavior. Often there are associated manifestations of anxiety, but these are most clearly discerned in behavioral phenomena such as restlessness, nightmares, night terrors, or compulsive activity. Even the thinking disturbances of psychoses in children are mainly evidenced in bizarre behavior; and intellectual defects are often detectable only through primitive and retrogressive characteristics in play and other activities. Thus, the psychiatrically impaired child can be spotted by the overt nature of his psychopathology. In this one regard, then, the task of epidemiology is made easier for children than for adults. But it does not mean that children suffer solely from acting-out disorders. Rather it means that during childhood, psychopathology asserts itself more clearly in action than in words.

With the possible exception of true paranoid reactions (delusions are exceedingly rare in children) most of the diagnostic entities encountered in adult psychiatry have counterparts in child psychiatry. As with adults, neurotic disorders are characterized by excessive anxiety (manifest in children as indicated above, for example, by restlessness, nightmares, frightened behavior, and inattentiveness) or by symptomatology that can be interpreted as defense against anxiety. Of the latter, phobic and psychophysiologic symptoms are common among children. Compulsions are more frequent than obsessions, again indicating the predilection for behavioral manifestations. Depressive reactions occur but are very rare indeed. Thinking disorders, represented by autistic, schizophrenic, or schizophrenic-like disturbances as well as acute and chronic organic psychoses, are probably more prevalent among children than they were once thought to be. Situational reactions analogous to reactive states of adulthood may also be observed.

Retardation and mental deficiency are obviously manifest during childhood and are almost always associated with disturbances of conduct. The same applies to the epileptic child. He may display other kinds of psychiatric symptoms secondary to the reaction to the epileptic condition or he may give vent to explosive activities which can reach dangerous proportions. Finally, the so-called "primary behavior disorder," which is similar in some overt characteristics to personality disorder in adults, is frequently encountered among children.

Thus the diagnostic concepts of adult psychiatry are useful as points of reference in developing criteria for children. Yet they fall short of the exactness necessary for case-counting purposes. Some efforts have been made to construct distinct systems of classification for childhood disorders. The American Psychiatric Association provides a special classification on children, but their categories are broad and tentative in character.[5] By contrast Kanner's classification is complete but unwieldy in detail.[6] The concepts of diagnosis and treatment generally employed by child psychiatrists in the United States lean heavily toward neurotic patterns, as though these types of syndromes were especially characteristic or most prevalent where children are concerned. If this were actually the case, the APA categories would be considered more adequate for our purposes. Even if the concept of neurotic patterns were broadened to include all behavior disorders in which a significant measure of overt anxiety is also manifest, there are many signs from our clinical experiences as well as those of others suggesting that "primary behavior disorders" characterized by limited neurotic mechanisms are more common in our culture as well as more serious than the straightforward anxiety responses. But to apply to these disorders the diagnostic view of adult personality disorders also seems inadmissible in the light of the variety and special dimensions of such disorders in children.

Evaluation and diagnosis of children brought to a psychiatric clinic are customarily based upon three sets of data. The first concerns present symptomatology and the developmental history of the child. The second is based upon exploration of the parent-child relationship. The third emerges from examination of the child, often using psychological testing of a projective nature from which interpretations of areas of conflicts are made. Such interpretations become part of the diagnostic formulation and influence subsequent treatment. They frequently focus upon those conflicts which are thought to be intimately connected with the child-parent relationship in terms of Freudian dynamics.

Until recently, most child guidance clinics have been quite specific in insisting upon psychoanalytically oriented treatment and diagnostic procedures. These involve intensive casework with one or both parents as well as prolonged treatment of the child. Such methods, requiring a team approach (psychiatrist, psychologist, and caseworker), are eminently suitable for neurotic children but are far less effective with children displaying primary behavior disorders. Patients are often selected so as to rule out those cases where anxiety is not a prominent feature or where participation of the family is not anticipated. Thus cases of primary behavior disorders are ignored or rejected as untreatable despite the inherent danger which they represent to the community.

The criteria applied in the average child guidance clinic are not entirely adequate, therefore, to the problem of establishing criteria for psychiatric impairment as it occurs in the total community. This is related not only to the limited experience of clinicians with these conditions but also to the fact that clinical criteria bear little relation to the social factors of child-community or family-community contacts. Up to the present child psychiatry has focused—or perhaps riveted—its attention upon the parent-child relationship and upon intrafamilial pathology almost as if the family could be treated and understood without reference to the community. Inasmuch as the severely impaired child—at least when he reaches school age—does not restrict his behavior deviations to the home setting, community pressures and expectations need to be considered. Bearing in mind that abnormal behavior deviates in the direction of passivity or of aggressivity, it seems probable that a yardstick for measuring degrees of deviation in one direction or the other as well as degrees of impairment is to be found in the community expectations of a child at any particular age.

For example, in our society the community accepts temper tantrums in a three-year-old but rejects them in an eight-year-old. A two-year-old is not expected to be quiet on a train whereas a noisy nine-year-old under such circumstances causes general annoyance and criticism. A certain amount of rough-housing is tolerated in an eight-year-old boy, but stealing, playing hookey, or destroying property are unacceptable. The community standards are established by key figures such as doctors, educators, ministers, and other leaders as well as by parents in general. A child is often referred to a psychiatric clinic because, for his age, his behavior in social institutions is out of keeping with these standards. Even when a mother brings a child because of her own concern about the youngster's behavior, such worry is often related to observations that friends or relatives have made about the child.

In modern urban situations both parents and children belong to more than one community, and sometimes the standards of these different communities conflict with each other. For example, the average adult belongs to a particular socioeconomic group and often to a certain religious group and is also a member of a local community as well as a national community. Thus, our approach to community expectations has much in common with the social science concept of "reference group" and, at a more general level, with that of cultural expectations.[7] Although we have looked to community expectations in our attempt to develop research criteria for urban children in this society, the parallel to different cultural expectations about childhood behavior is clear. In a cross-cultural study the content of these expectations would need to be identified by interviewing key informants. Some expectations about child development, such as walking, learning to talk, and toilet training, are undoubtedly universal, although the expected age of achievement may vary from one group to another. Other expectations, such as learning particular skills or particular types of interpersonal relations, are presumably specific to different groups.

In our society a child's most immediate community is the school. As he grows older, he, like his parents, may belong to several communities and may have to deal not only with differences between their standards but also with the differences between them and those of his parents. His friends may be permitted to do things that he is not allowed to do, so that he experiences difficulty in being accepted. In adolescence he may be torn between adhering to the official school-community or to a gang that grows up in the neighborhood, both of which may have standards at variance with those of his parents. The child who is a member of a minority group is of special interest. His parents' expectations may be consistent with those of the minority group but in conflict with those of the community at large.

With these considerations in mind, it has appeared to us that for children above the age of three, the most plausible way of arriving at criteria for psychiatric impairment would be to evaluate their functioning in terms of the community expectations of the average child at different ages. Although it is obvious that community research needs to be developed in order to plot these variable expectations in more precise terms, for the purposes of presenting our method we have established our standards with the idea of community in mind and with content suggested by our clinical experiences and general observations.

Research Methods—Gathering Data

Based on these theoretical concepts, a method has been designed for determining psychiatric impairment of children in our culture. It calls for the administration of a questionnaire to one parent by a skilled interviewer as well as a brief examination of the child by a psychiatrist. The reliability and validity of such a method have been studied by Lapouse and Monk.[8] They reinterviewed mothers and compared these data with information obtained earlier from mothers and their children. Although this study encountered expected difficulties and presented some discouraging elements, it did not rule out the efficacy of such a method.

Parents of over fifty children already known to our clinic were interviewed with an initial form of the questionnaire. Results were checked against clinical findings, and attempts were made to rate the data in terms of impairment. Weaknesses of the questionnaire were thereafter modified and a new instrument developed which was once again tested using over fifty clinic cases. The questions concern the general areas of a child's functioning (home, school, and social relations), and further items are asked in order to obtain demographic data and social attitudes of parents. The questions about psychopathology have been coded in accordance with the nature of symptoms (A = anxiety; B = behavior symptoms). Such coding has been found helpful, since the impairment ratings are determined in reference to areas in which malfunctioning occurs as well as to nature of symptoms.

In rating psychiatric impairment in a child, questionnaire information has been employed in two different ways. The first of these considers the child's performance in the important areas of his life as well as those aspects of his functioning which transcend or apply generally to all areas. The other evaluates impairment in terms of the nature and intensity of various kinds of symptomatology such as anxiety or disturbances in conduct, habit, mood, or thinking. The latter method is the one most often used by the clinical psychiatrist in making a judgment about the severity and type of illness under examination. Such a rating must be carried out by someone familiar with child psychiatry, since the significance of symptoms varies with age and setting. The first method is in many ways simpler, and yet in a sense it gets more directly at the matter of impairment. This rating could as easily be made by a skilled teacher or a group leader as by a psychiatrist.

The following lists are a tabular presentation of the items about which the questionnaire elicits information. Regarding each of the major pattern divisions, questions have been asked about particular symptoms and, where possible, in which area of life they occur. The ordering of the symptom items is arbitrary and is not intended to convey impressions about severity.

BEHAVIOR OR CONDUCT

General Functioning
Lies
Does bad things all of a sudden
Steals
School
Poor conduct
Absences
Many school changes
Plays hookey
Expelled from school
Attends special school
Has home care (because of conduct disorder)
Social Relationships
Does not get along
Does not participate in group
Teases
Is teased
Aggressive/submissive in group
Neighbors complain
Has run away
Sets fires
Has had trouble with police

Home
Disobedient
Must have his own way
Demands attention
Jealous
Argues with siblings
Hits or hurts siblings
Hit or hurt by siblings
Too good and quiet
Withdraws
Is taken advantage of by siblings
Unaffectionate with parents
Temper and tantrums
Excessively modest (physically)

In reviewing symptoms, the degree of impairment is determined not only by the nature of the disorder, but also by the number of areas in which performance is disturbed. For example, a child who exhibits conduct disturbances only at home with his parents and siblings but who performs adequately at school and is popular with his friends would be considered less impaired in an overall way than a child who creates a disturbance outside his home as well as in it.

DISTURBANCES INDICATIVE OF ANXIETY

General Functioning
Stutters
Bites nails
Extremely concerned with:
  being on time
  having things same way
  arranging clothes carefully
  checking over things repeat-
    edly
  saving things
  washing hands too much
School
  Is afraid of going to school
Social Relationships
  Is shy with other children
  Is afraid of other children
  Is afraid of fights
  Is afraid of adults

Home
Is restless
Is hyperactive
Does not finish what he starts
Does not concentrate on
  homework
Has disturbed sleep
Comes to parents' bed
Has nightmares
Has night terrors
Walks in sleep
Has fears
Fears separation from mother

Although many of these types of symptoms may be noticeable at school and to friends, they are manifest primarily in the home and family setting. Clinically, they are typical symptoms of neurosis and as such the least serious, in our view, of the childhood disorders causing less widespread impairment than other types. This illustrates how evaluation of impairment in terms of areas of functioning can result in determinations consistent with those which are made by reference to the nature of symptoms.

PSYCHOSOMATIC SYMPTOMS

Poor appetite
Has eating difficulties
Has stomach upsets—vomits
Is overweight or underweight
Has diarrhea
Has hay fever
Has asthma

Psychosomatic Symptoms (*cont.*)

Has eczema

Has other allergies

Has headaches

Faints

These allegedly psychosomatic or psychophysiologic complaints have been separated from the group of anxiety symptoms inasmuch as the information may represent actual physical illness. Where the emotional origin has been investigated and appears to have a determining influence on the psychosomatic expression, the items are scored under anxiety.

PSYCHOMOTOR

Delay in:

Smiling

Standing

Sitting

Walking

First words

Sentences

Dressing self

Feeding self

Mispronounces words

Stutters

Other speech defects

Stopped talking after started

Poor coordination

HABIT DISTURBANCE

Has sucked thumb (ever)

Sucks thumb

Bites nails

Wets during day

Wets during night

Is not at all toilet trained

Is soiling

Rocks

Bangs head

Has other unusual habits

Twitches

Masturbates excessively

Habit disturbances have been made a distinct area of questioning apart from psychomotor development because they may sometimes be related simply to neglect or lack of supervision.

MOOD DISTURBANCE

Is easily frustrated

Cries a lot

Rapid change of mood

Is not happy

THINKING DISTURBANCES

General Functioning	*School*	*Home*
Has language defect	Poor grades	Does not concentrate
Does not speak	Trouble getting him	on homework
sentences	to do homework	Daydreams at home
Does not converse	Poor reading	Does not play func-
Does not make sense	Daydreams	tionally with toys
Does not talk	Day-care program	

PHYSICAL ILLNESS

Has had serious illnesses or operations
Has physical or mental handicaps
Has convulsions

The information from this latter section can be divided between illness which directly involves the central nervous system and that which does not. Thus we can score epilepsy, postencephalitis, mental defect, yet at the same time have data on chronic or disabling illnesses of other kinds which may play a role in psychiatric symptomatology by isolating the child from contact with other children or making him a deviant.

Research Methods—Evaluation of Data

No attempt has been made to treat the questionnaire materials in the usual diagnostic way. Diagnosis of psychopathology usually requires more prolonged contact with the child and his parents than is feasible in a survey. Thus we have focused on impairment in functioning as amenable to the significant differential units of psychopathology appropriate for prevalence studies. However, the criteria around which the questionnaire was conceived are admittedly influenced by certain generally accepted diagnostic categories. These are given below along with thumbnail descriptions for each. Also they are used in a tentative and descriptive manner in the case examples presented at the end of the chapter.

Psychoses

Functional (without known organicity, to include schizophrenia, autism)	Withdrawal of affect, bizarre thinking and behavior
Organic	Same as above, but with evidence of differential mental defect and/or neurological signs (i.e., uneven mental defect)
Neuroses	Behavior disorder with predominant evidence of anxiety manifestations
Primary Behavior Disorder	Behavior (conduct) disorder without predominant evidence of anxiety manifestations
Mental Defect (with or without other psychopathology)	Even retardation (i.e., all functions retarded)
Epilepsy (with or without secondary symptoms or behavior disorder)	Especially impulsive and explosive behavior

The rating of impairment from the questionnaire involves five possibilities: no impairment, mild, moderate, severe, and extremely severe impairment. The last category is reserved for children suffering from functional or organic psychoses or severe mental defect. Such conditions are so much more incapacitating even than the destructive behavior disorders that they are dealt with in this special manner. Data from the preliminary investigation of a population of children seen in our clinic suggest that the majority of children fall into the three ratings of mild, moderate, and severe impairment and that disorders usually involve behavioral, neurotic, or situational disturbances. Where organicity is concerned, epilepsy and retardation of variant etiology appear to be by far the most frequent. In other cultures, however, it would be necessary to consider the possibility of conditions due to vitamin deficiencies, parasitic diseases, or indigenous toxic influences which may produce severe or extremely severe clinical pictures. The questionnaire was prepared in anticipation that children with all known disorders would be considered rather than just the disturbances most frequently seen in a clinic.

Placing the child in one of the five impairment categories on the basis of the questionnaire and examination takes into account the nature of symptoms and number of areas in which functioning is disturbed as well as severity of the disturbance itself. Symptoms that are seen for the most part at home but not elsewhere usually constitute mild to moderate impairment by comparison with children demonstrating disturbances in school and social areas. We have also found it helpful to assign numerical ratings for each item of the questionnaire reflecting the nature and frequency of the symptom as well as the child's age, which influences its significance. Such a system forces the evaluator to be specific but at the same time allows the clinical approach of taking into account the meaning of the symptoms as well as the particular areas in which they occur. The final evaluation depends on the various symptom patterns and areas of impairment as well as the total picture in a qualitative and additive sense. In general, ratings with respect to nature and degree of symptomatology check well with ratings on nature and number of areas involved.

Case Materials

The following case illustrations have been formulated on the basis of the questionnaire given to the patient's mother and of clinical write-ups on children who have been under treatment in our clinic. The first cases in the sequence show mild impairment; they are followed by cases in which the degree of impairment is greater. The discussion of each case is designed to demonstrate the rating of impairment and the role that social factors appear to play. Although demographic data are not given in summary form, detailed inquiry has been made about such aspects as well as about how the parents relate to the community and the nature of their expectations about their children.

Case History 1: Female, age 8

Presenting problem and present illness. Stuttering since age 18 months, when she started talking, compulsive traits, minor phobias.

History. One of twins; normal development, though slightly slower than other twin.

Family and social background. Both parents are of Eastern European Chassidic Jewish background and live in rigid adherence to the tenets of their faith. They are located in a homogeneous neighborhood and socialize only within their group. Children go to Hebrew parochial school where Hebrew is first language, English second. In addition to these two languages, Yiddish is also spoken in the home. Father is a mild-mannered, passive, deeply religious man who has held various jobs and changed them often. Mother is the more outgoing, dominant parent, works outside district. Although she keeps all rules of religion she inwardly rebels against them and wishes for a more American way of life.

Psychiatric examination. Quiet, shy, conforming child with variable stutter and some compulsive mechanisms. Of interest: sister is exact opposite of patient—aggressive, undisciplined.

Course in clinic. Psychotherapy with improvement. No changes in home.

Clinical diagnostic impression. Obsessive-compulsive personality, stuttering.

Impairment. Child at all times functions well despite stuttering. Fears and compulsive trends not disabling, good adjustment in special school setting where there are innumerable rules and regulations. Impairment is mild.

Discussion. Family belongs to a small, highly cohesive and organized minority group, remote in many ways from the American community at large. In this family father and two children are still well integrated in the group. Mother conforms only on the surface and departs from it ideologically. It would be interesting to speculate whether the two very different behavior patterns of the children reflect in some way the conflict between conforming and nonconforming, between father's and mother's attitudes.

Case History 2: Male, age 8½

Presenting problem and present illness. First seen when hospitalized for ulcerative colitis of a few months' duration, accompanied by anxiety, withdrawal and overconcern with soiling himself.

History. Second of two children. At time of patient's birth mother very upset because father had to undergo serious surgery for ulcer and intestinal obstruction. Development normal. Moderate sleeping and feeding difficulties during first year. No other psychopathology reported until present illness.

Family and social history. Middle class, Jewish-American. Parents share their home with maternal grandparents. Patient's mother is overly dependent on own mother, who interferes in children's care. Toward patient, mother is overprotective and clinging. Parents' marriage is basically stable, as father accepts the more passive role. Both take part in community, school, and religious activities. Sister, 13, is aggressive, domineering, and overshadows patient.

Psychiatric examination. In the hospital the child was sad, withdrawn, passive, overly adult in speech and mannerisms. Later, elements of depression and withdrawal disappeared and patient presented the picture of an intelligent, moderately passive boy, perfectionistic and slightly compulsive. Doing well in school and in social group though in some conflict with his older sister.

Course of treatment. After a few therapeutic sessions with a woman therapist, mother discontinued clinic visits, claiming patient was becoming worse. Mother appeared unable to tolerate another woman competing for her son's affection. Three months later in the setting of food refusal, nocturnal anxiety, and reading difficulties, mother reapplied for treatment, which was then carried out without interruption by two male therapists. Patient improved considerably.

Clinical diagnostic impression. Psychophysiologic reaction (ulcerative colitis) of recent onset.

Impairment. The questionnaire was given after termination of treatment and impairment was moderate (anxiety symptoms, compulsive traits, and diarrhea much improved).

Discussion. Family is part of a homogeneous community and well integrated within it, participating in most of its activities in reasonable measure. Areas of difficulties are mainly intrafamilial centering around relationship with in-laws. The case is given to illustrate that although intrafamilial and social factors are at work, their importance may vary from case to case.

Case History 3: Male, age 7

Presenting problems and present illness. Multiple fears, separation anxiety, enuresis, nail biting, poor frustration tolerance, mood lability, marked sibling rivalry. Also indulges in potentially harmful impulsive acts and some fantastic lies about material deprivation. Poor performance in second grade parochial school. Difficulties started around age two when first of his siblings was born, became worse at age five when mother suffered miscarriage followed by prolonged hospitalization and when, after that, family moved to a new location.

Past history. Oldest of five children. Normal development except for speech delay which has continued to present. Entered kindergarten age 5½, first grade 6½, each time with marked initial separation anxiety.

Family and social history. Lower middle class Irish-American, Roman Catholic. Father truck driver, often away from home, strict and demanding with children when he is with them. Mother product of an alcoholic and broken home and later foster care. Anxious, confused, overburdened by care of home and children. Handles children inconsistently and demands much of patient who is the oldest. Marriage harmonious at present but disturbed in the past, economic situation marginal. Participation in community activities restricted by housework. No complaints about siblings.

Psychiatric examination. Pleasant little boy, not overly anxious, appearing immature for his age. Speech is often incorrect and poorly articulated. Expressed jealousy of the next oldest brother, spoke of nightmares and fears, denied difficulties in school. I.Q. 86, consistent with level of functioning. Potential may be slightly higher.

Course in clinic. Has been in psychotherapy for several months and mother is seen in casework. Fears and acting-out have improved, separation anxiety and sibling rivalry remain (mother had another child and delivery was followed by complications).

Clinical diagnostic impression. Behavior disorder with neurotic traits and limited intelligence.

Impairment. Most disturbances are centered in and around the home and are of the anxiety type. Some symptoms, however, have reached beyond the home into school and community (neighbors have on occasion complained). Therefore impairment is considered moderate.

Discussion. Patient's symptoms can be viewed as reactive in response to excessive pressures exerted in the home and demands in home and school that are beyond his native ability. Acting-out seems to be a way of getting back at and/or attracting more attention from his mother. The family itself seems marginally integrated into the community, more because of economic and familial pressure than because of inability.

Case History 4: Male, age 11½

Presenting complaints and present illness. Patient referred because of severe asthma since age 3; aggressive behavior in and out of home, sleep and feeding problems, multiple fears and compulsions. Psychotherapy 1956–1959. Asthma improved but behavior problems continued, then worsened leading to revisit in 1960; at that time severe temper outbursts, aggressive acts against girls (not sexual), extreme sibling rivalry with younger sister, very poor school adjustment (social and academic). Asthma very mild and occasional.

Past history (first admission to clinic). Born in Puerto Rico. Normal pregnancy and delivery. Motor development as well as toilet training slightly retarded. Prolonged dependency for self-care on mother and mother substitutes. In early years mother working, patient cared for entirely by succession of relatives and hired help. Some care apparently very poor. Age 5 family moved to New York to obtain better care for patient's asthma. Mother stayed home. Financial situation and housing very poor at first, gradually improving to present. In addition to asthma, had mumps with encephalitis age 6, with no apparent sequelae.

Family and social history. Both parents Puerto Rican, Roman Catholic. Mother middle class, Spanish origin. Father poorer background, has some Negroid features; despite poverty, obtained good education and with help of mother set up own business in Puerto Rico. Move to New York brought loss of status and, at first, income. Father now holds white-collar job in large firm. Father passive, easily frustrated. Mother dominant, overwhelmed by care of home and children, especially the patient; prefers daughter. Lacks outlets. Handling permissive and inconsistent. Good marriage. Parents blame all difficulties on discrimination against Puerto Ricans. Sister: fair adjustment in school, intense rivalry with patient, overly "cute."

Psychiatric examination. 1956: restless, guarded, excessively engrossed in aggressive play activities and fantasies; 1960: preadolescent; relates superficially, talks freely but uses denial constantly; I.Q. 97.

Course in clinic. 1956–1959: play therapy; casework with parents; asthma improved; 1960: recommended drug therapy, not followed through.

Clinical diagnostic impression. Diagnostic impression of severe behavior disorder with psychophysiologic symptoms.

Impairment. Symptomatology is intensive and extensive and impairment is considered severe. Involves all areas (home, school, social).

Discussion. Family appears to have been fairly well adjusted and integrated in Puerto Rico with a certain amount of prestige and means at their disposition. Move to New York for patient's sake brought about a major break with the past, and a loss of both means and status. Despite improvement in their external circumstances and their good command of English, concern with discrimination has been constant and all-pervading. In two successive middle-class integrated neighborhoods they have socialized very little and remained isolated. These feelings have carried over to the children, who consider themselves different and disliked. Both mother and patient see his poor socializing with peers as primarily due to discrimination rather than to his aggressive behavior. Even if patient's difficulties stem in part from earlier years, the above-mentioned social factors and parental reactions must be considered as having a deleterious influence on the patient.

Case History 5: Male, age 9

Presenting complaints and present illness. Autistic behavior, lack of speech and other communication with environment, hyperactivity, destructiveness, insistence on sameness. Lack of toilet and other training. Withdrawal and lack of response go back to first year of life. Hyperactivity, destructiveness, severe temper tantrums date to second year.

Past history. Normal pregnancy and delivery as well as motor development. Few words for short period around age 2, never since.

Family and social history. Both parents Irish, Roman Catholic. Intelligent, hard-working; father more passive, easy-going; mother more aggressive, domineering. Marriage satisfactory. Sister 12, brother 8, very well adjusted. Family is practicing Roman Catholic and participates in church activities as well as in the activities organized by a group of parents whose children have similar problems to patient's.

Psychiatric examination. Age 4, withdrawn, hyperactive, no speech but various sounds, tearing papers or spinning coins in organized ritual fashion. Refuses contact.

Course in clinic. Followed at decreasing intervals for past five years, with play therapy and various medications. Some improvement in contact and manageability.

Diagnostic impression. Early infantile autism. Very poor prognosis.

Impairment. Very severe, all areas extensively affected.

Discussion. Nature of disease and family background seem to preclude influence of any social factors upon its onset and course. In fact family seems to have considerable strength of its own, has produced two healthy siblings despite the difficulties of coping with a child such as patient and has maintained satisfactory adjustment to the community.

Cross-cultural Problems

The applicability of this approach for research in other cultural groups has been borne in mind during the development of the questionnaire instrument described above. The division of inquiry into the areas and aspects of functioning appears to be a fruitful orientation in cross-cultural research even though the pertinent areas would have to be defined in terms of the structure of different sociocultural systems. As mentioned earlier, school performance is the item most likely to need adaptation for other groups where a formal educational system either is lacking or else appears as a rudimentary and qualitatively different institution. The same applies to items that refer to the specific structures of our society—for example, involving policemen as the main law-enforcement officers. For the most part, however, the items seem to be free of cultural bias and would be appropriate to ask as initial questions, allowing for the possibility that some may not be equally relevant to other contexts or that substitutions and additions might be needed. For example, there are no theoretical reasons for thinking that stuttering would not be found no matter what language was spoken. Disturbed feeding patterns could be investigated irrespective of how and what children are fed. On the other hand, the relevance of some of the items in their present form, such as "coming to parents' bed," would depend on the sleeping patterns customary in a given culture and might need to be modified to get at what constitutes sleep disturbance. The section on psychosomatic disorders is the area of greatest doubt and would need to be expanded to cover the physical illnesses prevalent in other groups that may figure in the picture of psychophysiologic expression.

The seeming adequacy of this method as a point of departure for cross-cultural studies does not dismiss the problem that syndromes quite different from those discussed here might be found or that symptoms might have different meaning in different cultures. The test of the method will be in its application. However, the value of organizing data about impairment in terms of the life areas in which malfunctioning occurs and the general applicability of this approach is indicated in the following case of an Eskimo boy evaluated as exhibiting much the same kind of "primary behavior disorder" seen frequently in our clinic.

Case History 6: Male, age 11*

Background. At the time of the observations given below, this little Eskimo boy was 11 years old. His mother died when he was a baby, and his father was extremely desultory in caring for this child and another son. The boy was left to live with first one aunt and then another. The agent for social welfare had repeatedly tried to get government aid but could not because his father and legal guardian, as a job-holder, was considered able to care for his children. At the end of the year the boy was sent to an orphan asylum on the mainland, his father as well as his aunts and uncles being unable any longer to take responsibility for him. The situation was complicated by the financial picture, but the main reasons for his departure were his recalcitrant behavior and unmanageability. In previous years a number of half-breed orphans had been imported from the mainland to live in the homes of Island Eskimos. Children are highly valued in this culture, and such orphans were sought when a couple did not have children of their own. It is also a culture in which the attitude to childhood behavior is tolerant and permissive. The little boy described below was the only known case of an island-born Eskimo child being exported from the group as if he were an orphan.

Anthropological observations. This boy, X, seems to be in trouble with everyone. The schoolteacher says that he continually misbehaves in school, and the other children blame him for any misconduct which occurs around the school. The teacher said that perhaps he would respond to individual attention if anyone could give it consistently, although he isn't considered by the teachers or Eskimo adults to be very bright.

At present he is living with an aunt and uncle who have a large family and both of whom are T.B. patients waiting to go to the mainland hospital. Since X is older than the children in this family, he is expected to do quite a bit of work such as carrying water, but these tasks do not seem out of line with what is expected of other 11-year-olds. The army officers at the nearby installation have taken this family on a relief program. X is the one who goes out to the army

---

* This case presentation was compiled from field notes gathered in 1954 and 1955 by Jane M. Murphy, anthropologist, in the Eskimo study mentioned in Chapters III and IV.

kitchen to get food for the family. The lieutenant says that his manner is very abrupt—"Give me this" or "Do this."

Once I made arrangements with his father to bake a pie for the boy. X delivered a pie crust mix with the comment: "Bake this." Another day he came to me and said: "Give me fifty cents." I asked him what he needed it for, and he said to buy candy bars at the store. Another time he came with a group of boys and wanted some nuts. In comparison to the other boys he seems very aggressive—talking more and laughing in a derisive way. He is known as a pest among the white families for this kind of activity and approach.

During the summer months when there was very little darkness, it was said that X and his "gang" stayed up all night, making noise and nuisance. Following this, arrangements were made for him to go to the other village on the island and to live with a family there. This arrangement was described as an adoption, but it didn't last long and he was soon back in our village with no one in particular to care for him, since the tubercular aunt and uncle had gone "outside." I asked one woman what had happened while he was away that he should be sent back. She said: "He do crying too much over there, and even though he is a big boy he wet his mattress at night."

Before long a widowed aunt took him in. This aunt told me the trouble is that X is "pretty mean and doesn't mind." He fights with the other children, and sometimes he doesn't come home at night and nobody knows where he is. She said that once he had got mad at the other younger nephew she was taking care of and as a consequence he stood out in the storm shed and threw rocks into the house. The aunt said that she was especially afraid about the curfew (an institution established by the village council, which sent around a representative to make sure that children were in their houses by 9 o'clock in order to "keep healthy"). She had told X that he would have to come home at curfew time, otherwise he would be scolded by the council and so would she.

The first night X stayed with this aunt, he was still running around outside when the curfew bell rang. She tried to get him to come in. She talked to him but he ran off, and she ran after him and talked to him some more. Finally she went to get his father. Together they got him to come into the storm shed. Then the aunt fixed him a bed and tried to get him to come inside the house. He still wouldn't come, and finally she gave up and went to bed. In the night she heard him come inside. He slept on the floor beside the door rather than in the bed. He didn't take off his parka or his shoes. In the morning she prepared breakfast for him, but he wouldn't eat it. She asked him why he hadn't come in last night, and he said he was mad at his father who wanted him to live with another family in the village. Finally the aunt went on about her work. X ate what had been prepared and left without saying anything more.

At the end of the summer the social welfare agent arranged for him to go to the mainland.

Summary

Difficulties in establishing criteria for psychiatric disorder in children have been reviewed. Clinical and theoretical considerations lead to the belief that the proper yardstick for such criteria rests in community expectations about functioning. An instrument for eliciting information with respect to the child's functioning has been described. Rating is carried out with respect to nature and number of areas of functioning disturbed as well as the nature of symptomatology. Illustrative case examples have been presented and special difficulties to be faced in planning cross-cultural studies have been discussed.

Notes

1. J. J. Honigmann, *Culture and Personality* (New York: Harper & Row, 1954); J. W. M. Whiting, and I. L. Child, *Child Training and Personality: A Cross-Cultural Study* (New Haven: Yale University Press, 1953); R. R. Sears, E. E. Maccoby, and H. Levin, *Patterns of Child Rearing* (New York: Harper & Row, 1957).

2. A. Kardiner, *The Individual and His Society* (New York: Columbia University Press, 1939); D. C. McClelland, and G. A. Friedman, "A Cross-cultural Study of the Relationship between Child-training Practices and Achievement Motivation Appearing in Folk Tales," in E. E. Swanson, T. M. Newcomb, and E. L. Hartley, eds., *Readings in Social Psychology*, rev. ed. (New York: Holt, Rinehart, & Winston, 1952).

3. G. Gorer, *The American People* (New York: W. W. Norton, 1948); G. Gorer, and J. Rickman, *The People of Great Russia* (London: Crosset Press, 1949); E. H. Erikson, *Childhood and Society* (New York: W. W. Norton, 1950); A. Inkeles, and D. J. Levinson, "National Charac-

ter: The Study of Modal Personality and Sociocultural Systems," in *Handbook of Social Psychology*, Vol. II, Gardner Lindzey, ed. (Cambridge, Mass.: Addison-Wesley, 1954); R. Benedict, *The Chrysanthemum and the Sword* (Boston: Houghton Mifflin, 1946); M. Mead, "National Character," in A. L. Kroeber, ed., *Anthropology Today* (Chicago: University of Chicago Press, 1953).

4. A. Kardiner, *The Psychological Frontiers of Society* (New York: Columbia University Press, 1945).

5. *Diagnostic and Statistical Manual of Mental Disorders*, by the Committee on Nomenclature and Statistics of the American Psychiatric Association (Washington, D.C.: American Psychiatric Association, 1952).

6. L. Kanner, *Child Psychiatry*, 3rd ed. (Springfield, Ill.: Charles C. Thomas, 1957).

7. R. K. Merton, *Social Theory and Social Structure* (New York: The Free Press of Glencoe, 1957); R. Linton, *The Study of Man* (New York: Appleton-Century-Crofts, 1956); R. Linton, *The Cultural Background of Personality* (New York: Appleton-Century-Crofts, 1945).

8. R. Lapouse, and M. A. Monk, "An Epidemiological Study of Behavior Characteristics in Children," *American Journal of Public Health*, vol. 48, no. 9 (Sept. 1958).

Additional Bibliography

Beller, E. K., and P. B. Neubauer, "Patterning of Symptoms in Early Childhood," presented at the 115th Annual Meeting of the American Psychiatric Association, Philadelphia, April 27, 1959.

Escalona, S., and G. M. Heider, *Prediction and Outcome: A Study in Child Development* (New York: Basic Books, Inc., 1959).

McFarlane, J. W., L. Allen, and M. D. Honzik, *A Developmental Study of the Behavior Problems of Normal Children Between Twenty-one Months and Fourteen Years* (Berkeley: University of California Press, 1954).

Mitchell, J. C., "A Study of Teachers' and of Mental Hygienists' Rating of Certain Behavior Problems of Children," *Journal of Educational Research*, vol. 39 (1949).

O'Neal, P., and L. N. Robins, "The Relation of Childhood Behavior Problems to Adult Psychiatric Status—A 30-Year Follow-up Study of 150 Subjects," *American Journal of Psychiatry*, vol. 114, no. 11 (May 1958), p. 961.

Pavenstedt, E., "The Effect of Maternal Maturity and Immaturity on Child Development," United States Public Health Service

Grant Application, September 1, 1959–August 31, 1964 (unpublished progress report).

Wickman, E. K., *Teachers and Behavior Problems* (New York: Commonwealth Fund, 1938).

Part Two

ASSESSING

THE SOCIOCULTURAL

ENVIRONMENT

VIII: Social Science Concepts and Cross-cultural Methods for Psychiatric Research

By Jane M. Murphy

THE purpose of this chapter is to introduce the second half of this volume and to discuss problems connected with developing a conceptual approach to sociocultural environment appropriate for psychiatric research. The book as a whole centers on cultural processes and cultural differences as having some determining weight in the causes and patterns of psychiatric disorders. In Chapter I, a brief description was given of what is meant by "culture." The definition employed may be called the "life-way" view. A shorthand summary of its meaning is to think of culture as the complex of factors which makes a Hopi Indian different from a Navaho Indian, and Indians of the American Southwest different from Bantus of South Africa, from Frenchmen in France, or from Old American stock in the United States.

This definition of culture emerged originally from the inductive, natural history studies of non-Western societies conducted by anthropologists. Most of the first societies investigated in this manner were relatively small and homogeneous tribal groups composed of relatively stable populations. Through the years this concept of culture has proved to be an extremely seminal one, and it holds a firm place in the catalogue of behavioral science ideas.

The culture concept is not without drawbacks and limitations, however. It has raised further questions as well as provided answers. One of the main difficulties now is that the use of the term "culture" has proliferated so extensively in the parlance of social scientists generally that it has come to mean different things to different people.[1] Another immediate problem is that culture can be conceptualized at different levels of generalization. Culture can be writ large as in human culture and writ small as in Hottentot culture. It can be classified according to different criteria and postulated with or without commitment to various theories of origin. To make comparisons between cultural units that crosscut these levels and classifications poses several difficulties.

In view of this state of affairs it is worthwhile to present a brief assessment of the concept in the light of the announced goals of discovering what in the human environment is important in causing or promoting psychiatric disorder. Since these problems have been given close attention in cultural anthropology, it is appropriate to look to the various schools of thought in this discipline in order to sort out the ways of defining and grouping cultures that are significant to the problem at hand.

Schools of Thought in Anthropology

I. CULTURAL EVOLUTION

The classification of culture that draws most heavily on theories about the origin and course of cultural development is the evolutionary paradigm. In this framework, a single culture is thought of as being displayed by all humanity, extending backward by history and forward by prediction to cover all forms of human life and development. The cultural differences characteristic of different groups of people are considered to be dynamic or arrested stages in a uniform process. This view was almost totally rejected by the cultural relativists, who emphasize the separateness of each culture and the necessity of analyzing and assessing each group in its own right without judgments about higher versus lower and civilized versus primitive. It was also uncongenial to the functionalist approach, which tends to minimize the longitudinal history of culture and underscores the functional interrelationships within the cultural pattern exhibited by a living group of people at one point in time.

Despite these varying opinions about cultural evolution, there has been continuing interest in the topic, expressed nowadays in its most unwavering form by Leslie White.[2] White's "culturology" deals mainly with superorganic and superindividual qualities of cultural evolution; that is, culture is conceived as having an inherent evolutionary nature which can be understood without reference to the individuals who compose cultural groups. In this regard "culturology" is at the opposite extreme from the approach of "culture and personality" and is, for the most part, irrelevant to the concerns of cross-cultural psychiatry.

Nevertheless, evolutionary thinking in less structured form has had a profound influence on the way sociocultural environment has been conceptualized as to its importance regarding psychiatric phenomena. This influence has primarily taken three forms.

A. The prevalence of psychiatric disturbances in our own society and our own era has been attributed to the complexity of advanced, civilized life. Innumerable treatises have been written on both sides of this point, such as Freud's *Civilization and Its Discontents*,[3] Goldhamer and Marshall's *Psychosis and Civilization*,[4] and Horney's *The Neurotic Personality of Our Time*.[5]

B. Another approach has been to see different stages of evolutionary development as characterized not by an absence or a prevalence of disorder, but by essentially different kinds of psychopathology. Brill talked of distinctively "primitive" types of neurosis found in some nonliterate groups.[6] Kroeber believed that low-grade paranoia was commonly exhibited in witchcraft-believing groups.[7]

C. At root, all dynamic formulations of culture as a changing and adapting phenomenon are based on the concept of evolution.[8] There is now a sizable body of literature on how the process of cultural change may be stressful and as a consequence productive of mental illness.[9] This has often focused on the idea that transitional periods of very rapid and pervasive changes are disturbing to the psychic equilibrium of the individuals who experience them.

In present-day American behavioral science, the first and second of these influences are largely out of fashion and the third is in ascendancy. Although there is probably a modicum of truth in each orientation, the shift of emphasis from static classifications to cultural processes represents a considerable advance in the conceptualization of sociocultural environment for exploring psychiatric problems.

2. FUNCTIONALISM

The original impact of the functionalist point of view, especially as put forth by Malinowski, was to emphasize the fact that culture is a functionally interrelated constellation of habits concerning economics, religion, kinship patterns, and so forth.[10] This idea was one of the important contributions to insight about the nature of culture. For a time it was so attractive and satisfying as an intellectual approach that all cultures, so long as they were viable and in existence, were thought of as functionally interdependent in their component aspects. Through the years, however, this orientation has been progressively modified to take account of the degrees of "more" and "less" function and of the disjunctures and dislocations between parts sometimes to be observed. Thus the implicit classification of cultural groups inherent in this approach is that of function versus malfunction—integration versus disintegration or organization versus disorganization.

The gradual refinement of the "function" idea applied to cultural processes has led us to a point that has major significance for understanding the psychiatric relationship between man and his environment. Although more work is needed in order to pinpoint the nature of a malfunctioning cultural environment and to establish the criteria by which it can be identified, such a framework offers a valuable approach to sorting apart cultures that are psychiatrically benign and those that are noxious.

3. CULTURAL RELATIVISM

In its strongest form, cultural relativism is essentially opposed to a classification system. It holds that each culture is an island unto itself and that standards of gradation and grouping cannot be applied. In large part this school of thought was a reaction to an oversimplified commitment to theories of evolution. It has had a therapeutic effect on the whole field of behavioral science by calling prejudice and bias into question. It has directly influenced the field of cross-cultural psychiatry by pointing to the difficulties of employing absolute criteria of psychiatric disorders across the barrier of cultural differences.

Nevertheless, this approach also has undergone adjustments and refinements through the years. It experienced a major setback during World War II. However disinclined they might be to make judgments about "good" and "bad" in assessing different cultures, social scientists became fully aware that a culture can go wrong and that it can, if highly organized under a dictatorship, threaten the survival of virtually all other cultural groups. This led to an increased awareness that in some regards absolute standards can be profitably employed to disclose the nature of both human and cultural functioning.

4. CULTURE AND PERSONALITY

Since "culture and personality" was discussed in Chapter I, little needs to be said here except to put it in the context of an anthropological school of thought. Like the others, this body of thought has gone through a number of changes. Originally the coalescence of personality pattern with cultural pattern was thought of as being so firm that one was merely the mirror image of the other.[11] Recently there has been increased exploration of the variations that attend different roles and classes within a culture and of the effects of acculturation and detribalization processes.

The "Life-way" Definition of Culture

Although given different emphasis in different schools of thought, the definition of culture as the "way of life" lived by individuals in particular groups has never been entirely absent from any anthropological formulation of the concept. It is essentially, however, a descriptive rather than a dynamic approach to defining culture. Beginning with a descriptive attitude does not imply that it is antithetical to a dynamic one. Nor does it deny that the dynamics of cultural change are enormously important for this field. If we are to discover what effect change has in promoting disorder, it is evident that we need a concept by which the environment can be described in a meaningful way at different points in time. Comparisons can then be made in order to measure and explain the intermediate changes as they may relate to psychiatric disorders. The "way of life" view of culture—ethnography, that is—appears by all evidence an adequate way to do this.

It also provides a means of organizing information about cultural contrasts so that comparisons can be made between several groups at one time. Here, too, the descriptive "life-way" approach is advantageous. It reduces the possibilities of choosing the wrong groupings or classifications of cultures based on theories of evolution, function, or process that may overlook environmental features important for understanding the individual in a particular social setting. Thus as a point of terminology reflecting this basically descriptive insistence, the search for illuminating comparative material is cast in the first instance as looking for "cultural contrasts" rather than in the civilized-primitive dichotomy or the dichotomies of literate-nonliterate, overdeveloped-underdeveloped, functional and malfunctional. It should be noted, however, that it is exceedingly difficult to refer to "contrast" in the empirical sense without relying on the latter terms.

No one seems likely to dispute that "way of life" is relevant to understanding human behavior. The problem is no longer to prove that culture makes a difference but to find out how and what difference it makes. At the same time, "way of life" is an exceedingly amorphous concept easily used to discuss many types of patterned uniformities—common denominators of behavior and consensus on certain values and assumptions—which may or may not relate to cultural identity in the traditional sense. Customarily we think of culture as being closely allied to ethnic and racial identity as well as national origin, and as being displayed by groups of people living in some sort of definable territorial unit such as a tribe, a community, or a nation.

Writing in the nineteen-sixties, it is apparent that the liveliest issue is whether culture in the sense of ethnic identity or culture in the sense of economic identity is the really important thing about the differences in "life-ways" of human groups. Mediated through the class concept, this has been a major point in the work of Hollingshead and Redlich [12] and of Srole *et al.*[13] regarding problems of psychiatry in a Western culture. It has not yet been undertaken, except indirectly, as a serious question in cross-cultural psychiatry. In the broader concerns of behavioral science it appears to be gaining ground as an extremely potent quality for understanding the human problems of the current world situation. This is to some extent the outcome of the resurgence of welfare concerns which is possible in a period when war is not the total preoccupation. It relates also to the question that, if war comes again, will it be because the instigators are Japanese or German (which was one of the starting-point questions in the national character studies) or will it result from conflicts over economic resources.

The growing concern about the human meaning of economic differences is indicated in a number of current book titles such as John Galbraith's *The Affluent Society*,[14] Barbara Ward's *The Rich Nations and The Poor Nations*,[15] David Potter's *People of Plenty*[16] (interestingly subtitled "Economic Abundance and the American Character"), and Robert Theobald's *The Rich and the Poor*.[17] Among anthropologists the adaptation of concepts under the impact of this new interest is indicated in Oscar Lewis' phrase "the culture of poverty."[18] Arensberg and Kimball sounded the same theme when they said, "There are farmers and there are farmers in Ireland. The small farmer is by all marks of social life a different person from the 'big fellow.'"[19]

An interesting thing about this concern is that variable economic situations are being presented in much the same frame of reference in which variable cultural situations were previously being studied. Economic identity is put forth as having a determining effect on the way people feel, act, and think, as if being high or low on the economic scale were their "way of life." And further, this aspect of "way of life" is presented as overriding the distinctions of being born and growing up as a member of a particular cultural group. The social analysts who stress economic determinism present the economic factor as interacting with and coloring a whole network of other factors—education, occupation, religion, social relations—so that it constitutes a pattern much like what anthropologists mean by culture.

If people are genuinely different in habits, outlook, and emotional response because rich or poor, this fact obviously cannot be ignored in trying to discover what causes, influences, or perpetuates psychiatric disorders. And it seems probable that the concerns of cross-cultural psychiatry will call for better recognition and a clearer conceptual approach to the study of contrasting sociocultural environments in the light of different economic situations. This means that a great deal of work will need to be done on the problem of comparing standards of living and assessing relative deprivation. The character of poverty or affluence—however crucial—still varies significantly as things stand in the world today depending on whether it pertains to a rural slum pocket, an urban ghetto, the Egyptian elite, or the *nouveaux riches* of the American Indian reservation when oil was discovered. For example, what by multiple indices of standard of living many of us would call abject poverty may in a particular sociocultural group be so muted by kinship support, religious dedication, devotion to aesthetics, or other counterbalancing forces that the economic disadvantages lose much of their threat to personality stability. What by the same indicators of living standard would seem to be a secure economic base for one group may in other groups be so weakened by a sense of relative deprivation that their members would have little satisfaction in it. Sudden acquisitions of money and sudden losses may also have special effects that need accurate measurement.

This point about the problem of economic situations in making world-wide comparisons has been dealt with at length because it is current and important, and also because it illustrates an issue about conceptualizing culture that relates to other factors as well.

Having decided to use the "way of life" definition of culture, we observe that many kinds of determining content can be read into it. For example, among the devotees of many religious faiths it is commonly said that religion *is* their "way of life." In describing groups such as monasteries and nunneries, the colonies of Hutterites and Amish, or the Zion Nationalists in Israel, it is evident that religious identity determines the life-way pattern in a manner that it does not in more secular groups. It is likely that, for them, religious determinism could be presented with as much validity as economic determinism in other situations.

Turning from religion to science, we may note that C. P. Snow, in a recent book, has drawn a distinction between traditional culture and scientific culture.[20] He presents a convincing picture of the genuine distinctiveness displayed by a small group of people who, through education, have fundamentally incorporated into their lives the way of thinking involved in the scientific revolution. Although many educated people do not fit this criterion, there is no doubt that he focuses on a differentiation that determines the way of life in such groups. We might call this the culture of scientific identity. Much the same could be said about art determining the way of life in groups who gather in places like Greenwich Village or the Left Bank.

An analyst of sociocultural environment would hesitate to discard any one of these life-way patterns as irrelevant to the concerns of cross-cultural psychiatry, even though putting them forth as *a priori* determinants for classification seems premature (as in the rich versus the poor, the scientific versus the traditional, the religious versus the secular, the artistic versus the Philistine). Getting away from the strictures of cultural determinism should not simply give room for some other kind of equally restrictive determinism to be put in its place. In the changing modern world, there are progressively fewer groups that can be called genuinely homogeneous from the cultural viewpoint, and correspondingly the argument of "there are farmers and there are farmers" has increased cogency.

Initially the most attractive characteristic about the culture concept was that it provided a way of gathering into one term a wealth of data about the patterned uniformities of behavior exhibited by different groups. Even though there is value in having such a shorthand terminology for the complexities of "what makes the difference between a Hopi Indian and a Bantu," it is clear nowadays that culture as ethnic identity does not mean complete homogeneity even when we are dealing with a tribal level of analysis. The culture concept needs to be used in a sufficiently flexible way to highlight variations of the sort suggested above.

The Social Group

In Chapter I, the point was made that "culture" is an abstraction referring to the pattern of life exhibited by a social group that is sufficiently cohesive to constitute a society. Several questions can now be taken up concerning the problem of choosing a group for investigation and defining its boundaries as a unit for analysis and comparison.

There is wisdom in beginning cross-cultural studies with natural groups that are delimited in space and that share a common geographic setting. At an abstract level and for purposes of analysis, people can be grouped according to many of the discrete criteria we have just been discussing such as income, education, occupation, or religious affiliation. It would be a mistake, however, to begin with an effort to relate psychiatric phenomena to any of these factors in isolation. One factor may be dominant here and another dominant there, but the point is to open research with a thorough knowledge of a given social field or territory and whatever empirical intermixing of factors that field displays.

The attempt to focus on the social group as localized in a geographic setting has always been plagued by the meaning, causes, and effects of population drifting. In the modern world, mobility of people is much heightened even in the non-Western areas. This is one more reason to suspect that the cultural group into which a person is born and oriented is not necessarily— certainly not universally—the most important factor in shaping personality and regulating human behavior. Hence in any sociocultural group characterized by large numbers, high rate of mobility, and pervasive institutionalization, it is likely that individuals will be precipitated together on the basis of many characteristics other than cultural heritage.

Many other factors relate to the movements and groupings of people. People gather for the season on the Riviera because they are wealthy. People retire to Florida because they are old. People move to Israel because they are Jewish. Some kind of cult or culture develops under these circumstances—at least while face-to-face relations are maintained. Any one of these social groups might be an appropriate unit for research into environmental influences important to psychiatry. It is also clear, however, that the selective factors of migration would need to be understood.

The problem of mobility is greatly complicated when the factors of selection are less obvious. For example, what accounts for the "coming together" or the "being left together" of people in ghost towns or the city tenement sections in a downtown area when residential areas move uptown? Irrespective of the population dynamics that created them, groups of this kind have empirical validity in the sense of being societies and would obviously be worthwhile units in which to investigate environmental dimensions. As far as psychiatric epidemiology is concerned, the major problem posed is whether inadequate environments produce psychiatric disorders or whether people with psychiatric disorders drift together to form such malfunctioning neighborhoods and communities.

Because they complicate research, the dynamics of social mobility and cultural change require serious attention. People are no more "fixed" in a given social network than they are "rubber-stamped" by culture, and allowance should be made for this in defining and identifying the sociocultural units to be compared in this field. Although the problem of boundaries is far from solved in a concept such as "sociocultural environment," it has many advantages over the straight use of the "culture" concept. Once outside the tribal frame of reference, it is just as difficult to limit and define a culture as it is to choose and delimit units of sociocultural environment. The chief recommendation for "sociocultural environment" is that it is sufficiently abstract to be universally applicable. At the same time its empirical underpinnings are that nearly all human beings live in societies, all societies have a culture, and all human beings exist in an environmental context composed of other human beings who make up the system of social relationships as well as all the nonhuman aspects that fill the environment.

Cross-cultural Methods

It is appropriate now to consider more specifically the problems involved in cross-cultural comparisons. It is our impression that in many scientific fields the methods of "before-after" comparisons in experimental research are somewhat more fully specified and clarified than are the "here-there" comparisons of research in natural laboratories. In cross-cultural psychiatry exceedingly few experimental situations can ethically be designed to produce the kind of evidence regarding cause and effect that can sometimes be achieved in nonhuman research. Probably the closest approximation to "before-after" comparisons we can expect in this field are those between prevalence rates and incidence rates. Thus, perforce, the interests of much of cross-cultural psychiatry require exploration through synchronic comparative analysis.

Almost all work in cultural anthropology is cross-cultural in orientation. This is true because most cultural and ethnographic studies employ our own Euro-American patterns as an implicit point of reference for illuminating cultural differences. In this regard, the cross-cultural approach can be called "a way of thinking" as opposed to a precise methodology.

In recent years, there has been considerable effort to structure cross-cultural research so as to make it an acceptable technique for scientific inquiry. There has been great variation, moreover, in the topics to which cross-cultural techniques have been applied and the manner in which they have been employed. Many aspects of this kind of research have been reviewed by John Whiting in a chapter, "The Cross-cultural Method," prepared for the *Handbook of Social Psychology*.[21] As these methods have been applied in cross-cultural studies of personality, they have been reviewed for the same volume in the chapter "National Character: The Study of Modal Personality and Sociocultural Systems" by Inkeles and Levinson.[22] What is presented here is a brief overview of considerations that relate specifically to the type of research being discussed in this book.

Stemming from the discussion of social group and the "way of life" practiced by the group, it is obvious that an initial problem in comparative analysis is the selection of comparable units of sociocultural environment in which to carry out investigation of psychiatric characteristics. In studies that employ environmental concepts as applying to localized and spatially oriented groups, one of five types of units has usually been the focus of attention: (1) the tribe, (2) the small town or community, (3) the city, (4) the nation, and (5) various groupings of nations. Sometimes these latter groupings have been along continental lines such as in Carothers' *The African Mind in Health and Disease*.[23] More often they are grouped as the Western world or North Atlantic community versus the non-Western world.[24] Each of these five types of units is a natural and historical grouping as opposed to a purely analytic grouping. And even the giants of hemispheric reference—the West and the non-West—are geographic units even though they lack the contiguity we usually associate with cultural unity.

It is immediately evident, however, that these units are vastly different in quality, that they require markedly different conceptual treatment, and that some are more feasible units of analysis than others. They provide, however, a useful outline for taking up the problems of comparative cross-cultural research.

1. THE TRIBE

Thus far the most elaborate use of cross-cultural techniques has involved tribal cultures. The reason is in part that "a culture" is most easily identifiable when it refers to a tribal group. At this level, one can reasonably say that what is reported in a standard ethnography is a bona fide cultural unit, appropriate as one in a series of units to be compared.

Cross-cultural techniques have also been especially pertinent at the tribal level because there are a sufficient number of specific ethnographies to allow the testing of hypotheses for statistically significant results. Such use of cross-cultural materials was enormously enhanced by the construction of the Human Relations Area File at Yale University. This file is a catalogue of existing ethnographic literature, constituting a map of particulars about societies in the tribal world.

There are several landmarks of achievement based on use of the Yale file. For example, there is Murdock's work on relating kinship terminology to social structure,[25] and there are the Whiting and Child endeavors to correlate certain types of child-rearing practices with cultural beliefs about the causes of illness.[26] Murdock's study incorporated information from 250 cultures and Whiting and Child's from 75. These investigations demonstrate a more statistically adequate use of the technique than has been possible in any studies dealing directly with psychiatric questions. This is an outcome of the fact that ethnographic literature traditionally covers topics such as kinship, child-rearing, and cultural beliefs, while systematic coverage on the prevalence and kinds of psychiatric disorders is usually absent.

However, there is a persistent problem involved in reliance on the Yale file for cross-cultural material. This is the difficulty of obtaining adequate representation of nontribal cultures to match the extensive representation of tribal groups. Murdock included "Yankee culture" in his kinship study and Whiting and Child drew on a Chicago study of child-rearing practices done by Davis and Havighurst. For the kinds of topics they investigated, this representation can be considered in some measure adequate. For research concerning psychiatrically important variations in personality structure, it is clear that serious questions must be raised about what is typical of Western culture and how to include cognizance of the variations in subcultural experiences within the Euro-American stream. Where cross-cultural methods have been applied to problems of personality variables and psychiatric symptomatology, attention has necessarily been limited to consideration of only a few contrasting groups.

A classic example of the early use of cross-cultural thinking bearing on a psychiatric theme was Malinowski's effort to find out if the Oedipal conflict has the same psychodynamic meaning among the Trobriand Islanders that it appears to have in our culture.[27] This study holds an important position in the historical development of cross-cultural methods, for it ushered in a period when numbers of anthropologists were concerned about assessing Freudian theories of personality development in cross-cultural perspective. By and large, these studies were directed toward demonstrating the applicability of psychoanalytic theory or testing its universality.

The claim of universality for a given proposition can be disproved by a single case of negative evidence, but rarely are the methods of investigation so unequivocally reliable that further research should be discouraged—especially when one is using as unstructured an approach as anthropological observation. Malinowski found, for example, that the orthodox Oedipal situation does not seem to exist among the Trobriand Islanders, but the meaning of the Oedipal theme in terms of interpersonal dynamics is evidenced between male children and their maternal uncles.

A study such as Malinowski's pointed to several needs which have been given attention in subsequent research. One is for expanding as much as possible the number of contrasting groups to be examined in order to give statistical meaning to results. Another is for a different theoretical attitude, one that is less concerned about testing universality and more concerned about casting hypotheses in such a way as to draw out the relationships between cultural and personality phenomena. Thus, hypotheses are now generally stated in the form: "*If* such and such a cultural practice is in operation, *then* such and such personality phenomena are likely to occur." Another recognized need is for the investigation of underlying dynamics that may be masked from detection by superficial cultural arrangements, such as whether the father or the maternal uncle is the key figure of authority in the family structure.

Between the type of research centering on 100 to 200 comparative units and the type comparing one example of a non-Western group with our own society are a number of cross-cultural studies that can be considered intermediate. Ruth Benedict's study of personality patterns among the Zuñi, Kwakiutl, and Dobuans is an early example.[28] This investigation suffered the statistical disadvantages of being based on general observations rather than on systematic testing of individuals within the cultural groups. It is also open to a criticism that applies commonly to many studies in this field: it drew on generalizations about our own culture and our own personality patterns that have not yet been properly investigated. However, insofar as it concerns comparative treatment of three specific and well-reported groups, it represents a step forward.

The Kardiner and Linton studies of basic personality structures compared the Comanches, the Alorese, and the people of Plainville, U.S.A.[29] One of the chief merits of the comparative approach in these studies was in their specific rather than non-specific representation of a Western culture. Although Plainville is not necessarily typical of Western society, it provides a firmer basis for comparison than would otherwise be the case. The Kardiner-Linton work also involved gathering comparable data through Rorschach testing on samples of individuals within two of their comparative units. Setting aside questions of the validity of the Rorschach for cross-cultural purposes, as a methodological design this, too, is an advance.

The recent work by Florence Kluckhohn and Strodtbeck, drawing on the Harvard Value Study files, has carried forward the methods of cross-cultural comparisons to a point of substantial scientific validity.[30] They and their colleagues designed a questionnaire on value orientations. It was administered to sample populations in five cultural groups in the American Southwest—the Navaho, Zuñi, a Mormon community, a village settled by Texans, and a Spanish-American town. As a consequence they established variations in values understandable in the light of cultural differences. Although this study did not deal directly with a psychiatric topic, it serves in many ways as a model for the use of cross-cultural comparisons in illuminating variations in human behavior as they are displayed in the tribal and community setting.

2. THE COMMUNITY

It is evident by now that "tribes" and "communities" have proved to be useful ways of parceling and bounding units of sociocultural environment for comparative analysis. It is also apparent that comparisons seem to make sense not only between a series of tribes or a series of communities but also in crosscutting to compare a non-Western tribal group with a Western community group. So far this has been the main answer to the need for including examples of cultural variation from both Western and non-Western traditions.

Even without the goal of cross-cultural comparison, "the community" has frequently been the locus for studies in psychiatric epidemiology. This is evidenced in the Hutterite community studies conducted by Eaton and Weil,[31] by Lin's work in Formosa,[32] by Essen-Möller's investigations in Swedish villages,[33] by the Stirling County Study, and by several others. For the most part these studies have been undertaken in isolation from each other and without a common frame of reference regarding criteria and nomenclature of psychiatric disorder or similar methods of collecting data. Nevertheless, interesting experiments in cross-cultural comparison were carried out both by Lin and by Eaton and Weil, using the prevalence findings from various community studies. Although the expected obstacles were encountered regarding the definitions of psychiatric disorder, these explorations outline a way in which comparative analysis will be able to proceed, once the psychiatric problems are surmounted, on the basis of community epidemiology.

It should be noted, however, that for most epidemiological studies the community served more or less as a "given" unit of people in which to make investigations. Very little attention was devoted to exploring the nature of communities as sociocultural environments. A great deal of work has been done on this topic in anthropology and sociology, but only infrequently has it been coordinated with psychiatric epidemiology.

On the social science side, one can point to numerous community studies, such as the Lynds' *Middletown*,[34] Wylie's *Village in the Vaucluse*,[35] Barker and Wright's *Midwest and Its Children*,[36] West's *Plainville, U.S.A.*,[37] the New England communities presented in Homans' *The Human Group*,[38] and Dollard's *Caste and Class in a Southern Town*.[39] However, these are not available in a single catalogue such as the Human Relations Area File. There has also been less tendency among social scientists to apply cross-cultural thinking to community studies than has been the case with ethnographic literature—in part, perhaps, because many of the existing community studies have been conducted in the developed countries where cultural contrast is less marked.

Nevertheless, it seems probable that many of the concerns of cross-cultural psychiatry can profitably be investigated in community settings around the world, and that gradually methods will be worked out for assessing and comparing the sociocultural characteristics of communities, given this world-wide scope.

3. THE CITY

It has long been recognized that there are qualitative differences between the way of life in large, heterogeneous urban centers and that in communities in rural areas. These differences have been referred to by such concepts as Tönnies' "gemein-schaft" and "gesellschaft" [40] and Redfield's "folk" and "urban" cultures.[41] Further, these differences have appeared so over-whelming as to command recognition as probably having psy-chiatric significance. Even though there have been few fully adequate epidemiological studies on this point, it has been assumed that the congestion, impersonality, and pace of urban living are more stressful than rural living and that this would be reflected in higher rates of mental illness.

For the most part, comparative thinking applied to the city as a unit of sociocultural environment has involved rural-urban differences within one cultural stream rather than the broad cross-cultural approach of comparing, for example, Capetown, Hong Kong, Calcutta, and Chicago. Both types of comparative approaches are needed in psychiatric studies, but neither has as yet been fully realized. There are several reasons for this.

One is simply the enormity of the task of comparative studies, involving as they do replication with similar techniques and con-cepts. Thus an ambitious comparative design may peter out in view of the difficulties of doing a thorough and careful investi-gation of the initial unit.

Another problem is the difficulty in presenting urban studies descriptively as "cultural instances." Although sociologists and anthropologists have written extensively on the process of urbanization and the structure of urban institutions, there is no ethnographic map of particulars for cities that in any way ap-proximates the Human Relations Area File. There are a few monumental exceptions such as Warner and Lunt's *Yankee City Series*,[42] but on the whole one would have to rely on documents of history, travel, or literature (Joyce's picture of Dublin in *Ulysses*, for example [43]) in order to get much of the flavor of cultural variation in city living.

As a unit of sociocultural environment, the city has many of the desirable characteristics for comparative analysis seen also in the tribe and the community. It is geographically localized and

can be studied as a social system. It is, however, far more heterogeneous, and so generalizations have to be made at a different
level and with more circumspection. In a city the "way of life"
as a psychological reality in the "culture-personality" sense is
much less readily discernible than in a community. As a matter
of fact, the impact of the city upon its residents has often been
described as *im*personal or *de*personalized, at least as far as modern cities in the West are concerned. These types of differences
make for difficulty in finding common reference points for comparing a rural unit with an urban unit and for comparing a
variety of urban units cross-culturally.

Whatever the impact of the city is, its psychiatric importance
clearly requires thought. But until the analysis of urban sociocultural environments can be conducted with comparable methods and concepts, the meaning of psychiatric comparisons is
questionable.

At the present stage of research in social psychiatry, a number
of epidemiological studies have been carried out in Western
cities; for example the Hollingshead and Redlich work in New
Haven,[44] the Faris and Dunham study in Chicago,[45] Gruen-
berg's investigations in Syracuse,[46] the Midtown Study,[47] and
numerous others. Where cross-cultural studies are concerned,
some attention has been given to non-Western cities. One may
note Yap's work on suicide in Hong Kong,[48] Murphy's investigations of hospital admission rates in Singapore,[49] Scotch's
study of rural and urban differences regarding hypertension
among the Zulu of South Africa,[50] and so on. As in the case of
community epidemiology, none of these studies in urban epidemiology has been sufficiently coordinated to allow psychiatric
comparisons, much less environmental comparisons.

In summary of this point, it seems obvious that since greatly
increased numbers of people in non-Western as well as Western
society are living in centralized and densely populated areas, the
city as a unit for cross-cultural studies should be given more
attention in a comparative framework.

4. THE NATION

As indicated in Chapter I, there was a phase in the history of cross-cultural psychiatry when the national character studies of Gorer, Mead, and others were in a ferment of activity and under much discussion.[51] These were not epidemiological in orientation and were not directly concerned with psychopathology. Rather they were attempts to build from cultural data vignettes of the personality configurations characteristic of Japanese, Russians, Germans, or Americans. Severe criticism has been leveled at these efforts on the grounds that the diffuse and differentiated sociocultural influences within a nation were not properly specified and that the face-to-face study of samples of individuals was not adequate enough to warrant generalizations about personality. The continuing reputation of the national character approach as being unscientific has led to a situation in which national units are virtually dismissed as appropriate in cross-cultural research. It is even somewhat suspect to raise the issue again. However, it appears advisable to discuss the nation as an environmental unit in the context of what this chapter attempts to lay out.

Many of the requirements being suggested here as necessary qualities of the sociocultural units to be compared are met in some nations, especially small nations. Localization in space is almost always involved, cultural homogeneity is sometimes involved, and a system of at least institutional relatedness is inherent in the concept of nationhood. In addition there is ample evidence that people of different national origins practice different life-ways and are committed to different ideologies. In the large, culturally diverse nations such as the United States and Russia, the task of meaningful generalization is exceedingly difficult. To disregard national studies altogether, however, would be to ignore a tremendous amount of apposite and insightful material on the American way of life and that of other nations. The map of particulars regarding nationalities includes vast libraries of documentation from history and philosophy and, where European nations and the United States are concerned, from sociology. Much of this is totally unorganized except by very general library cataloguing devices. There are, however, a few sociologists who have tried to systematize data so that in some respects their presentation resembles a traditional ethnography: Robin Williams' *American Society*,[52] George Stewart's *American Ways of Life*,[53] Lloyd Warner's *American Life*,[54] and Max Lerner's *America As a Civilization*.[55]

In the attempt to draw from this great quantity of information a pattern of personality and behavior that is distinctively American, a frequent course has been to take the leap of intuitive generalization involved in talking about "a typical middle-class American." The social scientists who are extremely concerned about exactness are often heard to decry this phantom creature of the arithmetic mean—like "primitive man" or "Western man"—as among the more disreputable ghosts that still stalk the halls of scientific endeavor. Certainly these summarizations do not do justice to the variability of individuals within a national group. Yet despite the looseness of such discourse, an interplay is needed between these large steps of insight and the small steps of precise empiricism.

There are several reasons, it would seem, why the long-range course of cross-cultural psychiatry should look to better methods, combining approaches of both large and small scope, for international comparisons. One is that in the present situation nations are the main units of governmental administration and decision-making power through which knowledge can be applied. At the same time they are the units by which vital statistics can most easily be gathered and organized. Perhaps most importantly they constitute the crucial alliances of people in the international sense. In making this point we do not intend to return to the original approach and methods of the national character studies but rather to recognize and move toward the goal of utilizing international comparisons of prevalence rates and psychiatric patterns for whatever benefit they may have in planning welfare and the resolution of conflicts.

5. GROUPINGS OF NATIONS AS WESTERN AND NON-WESTERN

The polarization of human groups on the East-West continuum has been referred to throughout this volume. It is extremely doubtful that the empirical approach of epidemiological comparisons between the West and the non-West can ever be achieved. The unity of space and governmental affiliation involved in nationhood is clearly much greater than the unity and shared orientation meant when we speak of the East and the West. Yet equally clearly there are differences that over and over again have been drawn out comparatively: Northrop's *The Meeting of East and West*,[56] Ward's *The Interplay of East and West*,[57] Dean's *The Nature of the Non-Western World*.[58] It is difficult to say what implications these different "world views" may have regarding psychiatric disorder. The probability is that there may be particular patternings or shadings of disorder related to being a member of one or the other orientation.

To investigate such an idea in a comparative framework would seem to require focusing on smaller units of sociocultural environment, selected to represent the broader groupings of society. This brings us back to the points about the adequacy of "tribes," "communities," and "cities" as bounded units of environment.

Psychiatrically Relevant Classifications of Sociocultural Environment

Everything said in the previous section about selecting the environmental units in which to investigate the cultural correlates of psychiatric disorders has been put forth without presuppositions about what is a benign environment and what noxious regarding disorders. A major task of a comparative approach to psychiatry is to develop a scheme whereby we can discover populations or subpopulations that are freer of some kinds of disorders than are other populations. If such low-symptom and high-symptom populations can be found, then the task is to begin winnowing down the associated factors of sociocultural environment to those which may be causal. This is a very different classification problem from that discussed above. There the concern was not whether living in a tribe, a community, a city, or in either Western or Eastern culture was causally related to psychiatric disorders; rather it was to look at the problems of comparability in units of sociocultural environment. However, the processes of detribalization, urbanization, and Westernization have been proposed by many researchers as potentially productive of psychiatric disorders.[59] In such discussion, attention is on *process* rather than *unit*. And it is often the process of cultural change that is intended in the reference to tribe when, for example, one speaks of detribalization.

It is apposite now to describe some of the ways in which workers in this field have attempted to classify culture groups in a psychiatrically significant frame of reference. Among those oriented to genetic psychiatry, attempts have been made to explain the presence or absence of disorder according to a classification of cultures as endogamous and exogamous.[60]

Efforts have been made to group sociocultural units by different kinds of schema regarding social stress. Some of these have been discussed or implied in previous sections of this book. Benedict used the concepts of "discontinuous" and "continuous" cultures, focusing on what she conceived as stressful and nonstressful modes of child-rearing.[61] The Arsenians proposed a paradigm for "tough" and "easy" cultures.[62] Piers and Singer focused on the "shame" and "guilt" dichotomy.[63] Many people have used the ideas of "simple" and "complex" cultures to express the stress differential. Thus far most of these hypotheses about cultural stress have not stimulated empirical research, mainly because it is exceedingly difficult to establish and apply the criteria by which these different classes of cultures can be identified. Most research on stress has centered on more particular factors such as economic disadvantage, broken homes, bereavement, emotional deprivation, role conflict, and rapid acculturation, or on patterns of such factors as in the concept of "social disintegration" employed in the Stirling County Study.

In an effort to assess social stress cross-culturally, all of these specific experiences would need investigation. It is clear, however, that they do not refer to the level of analysis that concerns distinctively cultural patterns such as cultural change, cultural roles, values, and world views.

The topics of role and shared sentiments (sentiments being closely allied to values and basic assumptions) are discussed in subsequent chapters. It is the final task of this chapter to discuss briefly the nature of sociocultural change, especially as it pertains to psychiatric problems.

It should be re-emphasized that the attention given the etiological importance of acculturative stress at this point is not intended to imply subscription to a doctrine of specific causality. To the contrary, the orientation of viewing psychiatric disorders as stemming from multiple causes has been thoroughly interwoven in the topics of this book. But cultural change is especially relevant to the concerns of cross-cultural psychiatry, and it deserves special focus in this context.

One of the most obvious facts about many of the cultural groups to be studied in this field is that they are developing and changing with strikingly great velocity. Already there is much evidence that the technological and ideological shifts involved in these massive revolutions have a toll in human problems and psychic stress.[64]

Before assuming that this evidence points to a genuine cause-and-effect relationship between cultural change and mental illness, a number of qualifications should be registered. It was noted in Chapter I that cultures undergo continuous modification and change. Many changes are a matter of endogenous rearrangements and logical sequences, such as the progression from a digging stick to a plowshare, given the necesssary intervening discoveries. Many involve the slow incorporation of artifacts, traits, or ideas from outside cultures in contact situations. Some changes are imperceptible unless we take a very long historical view. It is doubtful that changes of this order are psychiatrically stressful.

Hence, change *per se* is not necessarily a noxious experience. It is a process that has tremendous adaptive potential, and it is the mechanism whereby progress toward healthier interactions between individuals and environments can be achieved. The Janus-faced quality of change as a process is perhaps best attested by its being fundamental to many conceptions of both therapy and disease. "Making the unconscious conscious," "creating insight," and "strengthening the ego" refer to the kinds of *changes* that are the goals of much of psychotherapy. Where disease is concerned, however, Virchow, referring primarily to the interactions of man and environment in microbial diseases, observed that "disease is life under *changed* conditions." [65] It is clear, therefore, that change is a protean process.

The crucial aspect regarding psychic stress is the manner in which cultural changes occur and their implications for personality and individual functioning. In other words, we need criteria by which to differentiate change that is psychologically stressful from that which is not. This obviously constitutes a large area of unknowns. Many people have given thought to the charting of this question, but few schemes have a demonstrated validity. However, the research experiences upon which this volume draws, as well as the accumulated literature, suggest the following approaches.

The first requirement is for a framework by which to view change as a psycho-social-cultural experience and to specify the intervening connections between these components.

A number of widely accepted principles about the nature of cultural change—viewed from the cultural level—are useful to the clarification of what change means to individuals—viewed from the psychological level. For example, cultural change is never an entirely uniform process as it impinges on the culture carriers. It occurs with different rates and significance in different areas of culture (material versus ideological) and in different segments of the population (men versus women, old versus young, leaders versus followers). Yet changes in one area or segment have repercussions and interlinkings with all the rest. Often it is the disjuncture between lags and spurts within a sociocultural system that creates points of stress rather than an absolute conflict between the old ways and the new ways.

Hence, "differential acculturation" is a valuable addition to the conceptual equipment regarding change needed for psychiatric research. Culture change, as it affects individuals, is mediated chiefly through the role structure of a social system. "Differential acculturation" offers a way of organizing data about cultural change in reference to different roles within a society and of sorting out the changes that implicate motor habits and skills from those which concern the cognitive and affective blueprints for role behavior.

While "role" provides a societal link between culture and personality through which change can be observed and studied, there is further need for concepts and theories to illuminate the ways in which "role" is interposed into the psychological realm of perception and emotion. There are numerous psychological orientations that might be employed—information theory, personal constructs, cognitive dissonance, and so on. At root, however, is learning. It would seem a fruitful beginning, therefore, to specify the processes of "unlearning" and "relearning" and to cast these in terms of role perception and activity.

In studies of cultural processes it has sometimes been valuable to distinguish between "acculturation" and "enculturation." The latter is considered the basic learning and incorporation of the initial culture.[66] Where "acculturation" is involved, some of the same psychological processes are undoubtedly called into play. The complications that make us focus on the learning required in culture change concern the fact that acculturation is by definition an overlay. One of the stress potentials is the possibility of conflict between the groundwork established in childhood and the assumption of different outlooks and procedures that attends change.

The orientations, attitudes, and habits that are laid down during "enculturation" tend to resist change. One reason is that they were implanted at a period in the individual's life when the growth process favors receptivity. However high the motivation for subsequent change, the new learning involves first disorienting and disassociating from the perduring patterns of childhood before the processes of reorienting and reassociating can take place. Rarely is the transformation to the new cultural image complete. Residuals from the past intermix with the importations from the new. This mechanism aids the maintenance of functional equilibrium. However, there are points and possibilities in the change process when personality equilibrium can be seriously disturbed and stress engendered by these complicated needs for maintaining at least minimal stability while at the same time becoming sufficiently free of the previous set to begin learning a new orientation.

The following is a list of selected characteristics of cultural change that are likely to have the effect of damaging personality equilibrium and creating stress. Change is likely to be stressful: (1) when the tempo is accelerated and especially when major dimensions of the change occur within the life span of a single generation, (2) when it involves pervasive reorientation about basic values and assumptions, (3) when it is experienced at the outset of a cycle when few guides and models exist, (4) when there has been little formal training and preparation in the skills and techniques necessary to accomplish the new tasks, (5) if there are serious ambiguities about what change is leading to, (6) if it involves new roles or values that are imperfectly integrated into or incompatible with the rest of the sociocultural system, (7) if it involves expectations that are prone to be frustrated given the pre-existing pattern of life, and (8) if it involves expansion rather than substitution and creates a sense of "overloading."

Although this list is not exhaustive, it gives parameters that would help locate points of stress if one were carrying out a field study of cultural change.

Summary

This chapter has reviewed the concepts of culture and society in the light of requirements for conducting empirical research concerning psychiatric disorders in contrasting cultural groups. It has drawn heavily on anthropology as a source of ideas for studying and comparing the environments of man as they may relate to personality functioning. It has suggested that some types of cultural changes are hazardous to psychic equilibrium and that, given the changing nature of almost every culture known in the twentieth century, this is a factor of considerable moment in comparative studies of mental health.

Notes

1. A. L. Kroeber, and C. Kluckhohn, "Culture: a Critical Review of Concepts and Definitions," *Peabody Museum Papers*, Harvard University, vol. 47, no. 1 (1952).

2. L. A. White, *The Science of Culture: A Study of Man and Civilization* (New York: Farrar, Straus, 1949).

3. S. Freud, *Civilization and Its Discontents*, trans. Joan Riviere, 4th impression (London: The Hogarth Press, Ltd., 1949).

4. H. Goldhamer, and A. W. Marshall, *Psychosis and Civilization* (New York: The Free Press of Glencoe, 1953).

5. K. Horney, *The Neurotic Personality of Our Time* (New York: W. W. Norton, 1937).

6. A. A. Brill, "Piblokto or Hysteria Among Peary's Eskimos," *Journal of Nervous and Mental Disease*, vol. 40 (1913), pp. 514–520.

7. A. L. Kroeber, "Psychosis or Social Sanction," *The Nature of Culture* (Chicago: University of Chicago Press, 1952), pp. 310–319.

8. E.g.: R. Redfield, and J. Stewart, *The Primitive World and Its Transformations* (Ithaca, New York: Cornell University Press, 1953).

9. E.g.: H. B. M. Murphy, "Social Change and Mental Health," *Causes of Mental Disorders: A Review of Epidemiological Knowledge, 1959* (New York: Milbank Memorial Fund, 1961), pp. 280–329; A. H. Leigh-

ton, "Mental Illness and Acculturation," in *Medicine and Anthropology*, I. Galdston, ed. (New York: International Universities Press, 1959), pp. 108–128; G. D. Spindler, "Sociocultural and Psychological Processes in Menomini Acculturation," *University of California Publications in Culture and Society*, Vol. V (Berkeley: University of California Press, 1955).

10. B. Malinowski, *Argonauts of the Western Pacific* (London: Routledge, 1922).

11. M. E. Spiro, "Culture and Personality, the Natural History of a False Dichotomy," *Psychiatry*, vol. 14 (1957), pp. 19–46.

12. A. B. Hollingshead, and F. Redlich, *Social Class and Mental Illness* (New York: John Wiley & Sons, 1958).

13. L. Srole, T. S. Langner, S. T. Michael, M. K. Opler, and T. A. C. Rennie, *Mental Health in the Metropolis: The Midtown Manhattan Study* [Thomas A. C. Rennie Series in Social Psychiatry, vol. 1 (New York: McGraw-Hill, 1962)].

14. J. K. Galbraith, *The Affluent Society* (Boston: Houghton Mifflin, 1958).

15. B. Ward, *The Rich Nations and the Poor Nations* (New York: W. W. Norton, 1962).

16. D. M. Potter, *People of Plenty* (Chicago: University of Chicago Press, 1954).

17. R. Theobald, *The Rich and the Poor* (New York: C. N. Potter, 1960).

18. O. Lewis, *Five Families: Mexican Case Studies in the Culture of Poverty* (New York: Basic Books, 1959).

19. C. M. Arensberg, and S. T. Kimball, *Family and Community in Ireland* (Cambridge: Harvard University Press, 1948), p. 231.

20. C. P. Snow, *The Two Cultures and the Scientific Revolution* [The Rede Lecture, 1959 (New York: Cambridge University Press, 1959)], p. 11.

21. J. W. M. Whiting, "The Cross-cultural Method," *Handbook of Social Psychology*, Vol. I, Gardner Lindzey, ed. (Cambridge: Addison-Wesley, 1954).

22. A. Inkeles, and D. J. Levinson, "National Character: The Study of Modal Personality and Sociocultural Systems," in *Handbook of Social Psychology*, Vol. II, Gardner Lindzey, ed. (Cambridge: Addison-Wesley, 1954).

23. J. C. Carothers, *The African Mind in Health and Disease* [Monograph Series no. 17 (Geneva: World Health Organization, 1953)].

24. E.g.: V. M. Dean, *The Nature of the Non-Western World* (New York: New American Library, A Mentor Book, 1958).

25. G. P. Murdock, *Social Structure* (New York: Macmillan, 1949).

26. J. W. M. Whiting, and I. L. Child, *Child-training and Personality: A Cross-cultural Study* (New Haven: Yale University Press, 1953).

27. B. Malinowski, *Sex and Repression in Savage Society* (New York: Harcourt, Brace & World, 1927).

28. R. Benedict, *Patterns of Culture* (Boston: Houghton Mifflin, 1934).

29. A. Kardiner, R. Linton, C. Du Bois, and J. West, *The Psychological Frontiers of Society* (New York: Columbia University Press, 1945).

30. F. R. Kluckhohn, and F. L. Strodtbeck, *Variations in Value Orientations* (New York: Harper & Row, 1961).

31. J. W. Eaton, and R. J. Weil, *Culture and Mental Disorders: A Comparative Study of the Hutterites and Other Populations* (New York: The Free Press of Glencoe, 1955).

32. T. Lin, "A Study of the Incidence of Mental Disorder in Chinese and Other Cultures," *Psychiatry*, vol. 16, no. 4 (1953), pp. 313–336.

33. E. Essen-Möller, "Individual Traits and Morbidity in a Swedish Rural Population," *Acta Scandinavica Psychiatrica et Neurologica*, Suppl. 100 (1956).

34. H. M. Lynd, and R. S. Lynd, *Middletown* (New York: Harcourt, Brace & World, 1929).

35. L. Wylie, *Village in the Vaucluse* (Cambridge: Harvard University Press, 1957).

36. R. Barker, and H. F. Wright, *Midwest and Its Children: The Psychological Ecology of an American Town* (New York: Harper & Row, 1954).

37. J. West, *Plainville, U.S.A.* (New York: Columbia University Press, 1961).

38. G. C. Homans, *The Human Group* (New York: Harcourt, Brace & World, 1950).

39. J. Dollard, *Caste and Class in a Southern Town*, 3rd ed. (Garden City, N.Y.: Doubleday Anchor Books, 1957).

40. F. Tönnies, *Fundamental Concepts of Sociology*, trans. C. P. Loomis (New York: American Book Co., 1940).

41. R. Redfield, *The Little Community* (Chicago: University of Chicago Press, 1955).

42. W. L. Warner, and P. S. Lunt, *The Social Life of a Modern Community* [Yankee City Series, Vol. I (New Haven: Yale University Press, 1947)].

43. J. Joyce, *Ulysses* (New York: Random House, 1934).

44. A. B. Hollingshead, and F. Redlich, *op. cit.*

45. R. S. Faris, and H. W. Dunham, *Mental Disorders in Urban Areas* (Chicago: University of Chicago Press, 1939).

46. The staff of the Mental Health Research Unit, New York State Department of Mental Health, *A Mental Health Survey of Older People* (Utica, N.Y.: State Hospitals Press, 1961).

47. Srole, *et al.*, *op. cit.*

48. P. M. Yap, "Suicide in Hong Kong," *Journal of Mental Science*, vol. 104 (1958), pp. 266–301.

49. H. B. M. Murphy, "Culture and Mental Disorder in Singapore," *Culture and Mental Health*, M. K. Opler, ed. (New York: Macmillan, 1959), pp. 291–318.

50. N. Scotch, "A Preliminary Report on the Relation of Sociocultural Factors to Hypertension Among the Zulu," *Annals of the New York Academy of Science*, vol. 84 (1960).

51. G. Gorer, "The Concept of National Character," *Science News*, vol. 18 (1950), pp. 104–122; M. Mead, "The Study of National Character," *The Policy Sciences: Recent Developments in Scope and Method*, D. Lerner and H. D. Lasswell, eds. (Stanford: Stanford University Press, 1951); M. Mead, "National Character," *Anthropology Today*, A. L. Kroeber, ed. (Chicago: University of Chicago Press, 1953).

52. R. M. Williams, *American Society: A Sociological Interpretation* (New York: Alfred A. Knopf, 1960).

53. G. R. Stewart, *American Ways of Life* (Garden City, N.Y.: Dolphin Books, Doubleday & Company, 1954).

54. W. L. Warner, *American Life: Dream and Reality*, rev. ed. (Chicago: Phoenix Books, University of Chicago Press, 1962).

55. M. Lerner, *America As a Civilization: Culture and Personality* (New York: An Essandess Paperback, Simon & Schuster, 1962).

56. F. S. C. Northrop, *The Meeting of East and West: An Inquiry Concerning World Understanding* (New York: Macmillan, 1946).

57. B. Ward, *The Interplay of East and West* (New York: The Norton Library, W. W. Norton, 1957).

58. V. M. Dean, *op. cit.*

59. G. DeVos, and H. Miner, "Oasis and Casbah—A Study of Acculturative Stress," *Culture and Mental Health*, M. K. Opler, ed. (New York: Macmillan Company, 1959), pp. 333–350.

60. J. W. Eaton, and R. J. Weil, *op. cit.*; B. J. F. Laubscher, *Sex, Custom and Psychopathology: A Study of South African Pagan Natives* (New York: Humanities Press, 1952).

61. R. Benedict, "Continuities and Discontinuities in Cultural Conditioning," *A Study of Interpersonal Relations*, P. Mullahy, ed. (New York: Hermitage Press, Inc., 1949).

62. J. Arsenian, and J. M. Arsenian, "Tough and Easy Cultures, A Conceptual Analysis," *Psychiatry*, vol. 11, no. 4 (1948), pp. 377–385.

63. G. Piers, and M. B. Singer, *Shame and Guilt: A Psychoanalytic and a Cultural Study* (Springfield, Ill.: Charles C. Thomas, 1953).

64. E.g., E. H. Spicer, ed. *Human Problems in Technological Change* (New York: Russell Sage Foundation, 1952); M. Mead, *Cultural Patterns and Technical Change* (New York: New American Library, 1955); A. H.

Leighton, "Mental Illness and Acculturation," *Medicine and Anthropology*, I. Galdston, ed. (New York: International Universities Press, 1959), pp. 108–128; C. Mertens de Wilmars, and L. Niveau, "L'Influence de l'Evolution Culturelle sur l'Équilibre Psychique," *Mémoires de l'Académie Royale des Sciences d'Outre-Mer*, Vol. XXVII, no. 1 (Brussels: Université Catholique de Louvain, 1961); A. H. Leighton, and R. J. Smith, "A Comparative Study of Social and Cultural Change," *Proceedings of the American Philosophical Society*, vol. 89, no. 2 (1955), pp. 80–88.

65. R. Virchow, in R. Dubos, *Mirage of Health* (Garden City, N.Y.: Anchor Books, Doubleday & Company, 1961), p. 104 (emphasis added).

66. M. J. Herskovits, *Cultural Anthropology* (New York: Alfred A. Knopf, 1955).

IX: The Life History in Cross-cultural Psychiatric Research

By Charles C. Hughes

EDITORIAL NOTES

The present chapter seeks ways of understanding how socio-cultural events affect the functioning of personality. It focuses on life history and role analysis and thus moves away from the more or less strictly epidemiological concerns discussed in earlier parts of this book. It may be helpful, however, to visualize this intensive approach as being articulated with those that are extensive.

If the prevalence or incidence of psychiatric cases were estimated on the basis of a fairly large systematic sample, then, as pointed out in Chapter I, a more intensive investigation dealing with developmental history could be conducted with a sub-sample. Gearing the intensive studies of individuals into the design of epidemiological studies of populations can thus be used to bring about a greater enhancement of understanding than either used alone. This view of the cross-fertilization of the two kinds of investigation may be represented schematically as in Figure IX-1.

What this figure tries to demonstrate is that material derived from surveying or census data is rendered more valuable when supplemented by material derived from deeper exploration with a limited number of people, and vice versa.[1] For example, a life-history investigation of a given person in a given culture may reveal points of stress that appear crucial in terms of subsequent patterns of that personality adjustment. Whether these points of stress are important generally in that culture and society can be discovered only through the extensive methods.

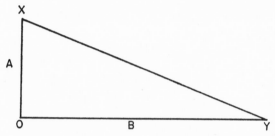

Figure IX-1. Schematic representation of data-gathering techniques. "*A* indicates the amount of data gathered per individual, increasing toward the top, while *B* indicates the number of persons concerning whom it is possible to gather data, increasing toward the right. Thus there is a con-tinuum from studies of one individual to studies of the entire community, with the amount of material that it is possible to gather inversely related to the number of individuals concerned. Personality studies would come at the upper apex of the triangle (*X*), representing considerable material about a few individuals, while census records, containing as they do some facts on everybody, would be at the bottom (*Y*). Between these two extremes come the other forms of data gathering." This figure is reproduced by permission of the author and publisher from Alexander H. Leighton, *The Governing of Men* (Princeton: Princeton University Press, 1946), p. 389.

The life-history investigation may be regarded as a segment in the larger field of "personality study." Such studies are modeled on the methods of investigation and data analysis developed in the fields of psychiatry and clinical psychology, including his-tory taking, intensive interviewing, dream analysis, and projec-tive tests. Although the most voluminous of such studies are undoubtedly those carried out within the framework of psychoanalysis, shorter approaches have also been designed, and in some instances studies have been based entirely on projective tests. The fact that a "complete personality study" is an impossible ideal places any investigation in this field at a disadvantage in the light of the theory that guides it—namely that personality is a whole made up of interdependent parts. If this is so, how can one understand its functioning if one investigates less than the whole and all its parts? The only hope of escape from this dilemma is to suppose that there are levels of understanding, or approximation, and that work can be planned at one or another such level.

In this chapter Hughes suggests that the life history may be considered one such level. On this assumption, he takes up the problems of systematically organizing such data to permit the drawing of conclusions and the making of comparisons. This is in line with clinical procedures used in diagnosis and treatment of persons with psychiatric disorders, but with the considerable difference that the subjects are not selected as psychiatric patients, and even if they turn out to have symptoms, the interest is as much concerned with their capabilities as with their disabilities. The central questions are those of how a person functions as an interdependent system moving through time, and how this functioning is affected by varying environmental conditions.

In addition to problems of approximation level and problems of organizing data, there are, in life-history studies, particular problems of validity. While it is true that for some aspects of personality the subject himself is the only one who can give the information, it is also true that in some respects he may be an exceedingly biased witness. Too much dwelling on this point can lead to a counsel of despair that would result in missing valuable information about human behavior and motivation. On the other hand, one does need to be alert to the problem of distortion and for evidence pointing to its existence. If, to take an extreme example, the subject turns out to be mentally deficient, the use one could make of his life-history data would obviously be limited. Less extreme, but still important, are other types of symptom patterns, which can be expected to introduce more subtle and particular biases. With awareness of its limits, however, the life history is a point of departure for intensive analysis, especially when dealing both with those persons who have no symptoms and with those who have psychoneurotic and psychophysiologic symptoms.

The life story of an Eskimo boy, which Hughes uses as an illustration, comes from the study of an Eskimo village that is now familiar to the reader.

———————————

THE central goal of life-history research is to examine patterns of personality functioning in relation to life circumstances. Associations between some kinds of life experiences and some kinds of psychiatric symptoms are beginning to emerge from field studies.[2] As with any epidemiological finding, however, this is only the first step, one which permits formulation of further, more sharply defined questions. In medicine such questions can often be taken into the laboratory for experimental solution. In social science, however, this is rarely possible and a recourse is assessment of life history with respect to environing circumstances. Thus, in lieu of laboratory manipulation we generally must so design field research that its results will allow, in Claude Bernard's phrase, "experimental *reasoning*" about the observed facts. Synchronic correlations need to be complemented with diachronic associations, and in view of the length of the human life span this task usually requires some form or other of retrospective biographical data.

The purpose of this paper is to consider the place of the life history as a tool in cross-cultural psychiatric research. Despite continuing interest in the life history there still has not developed any large-scale use of it as a basic technique for generalizing about sociocultural environment and personality functioning. To the term "life history" I give an inclusive meaning: an extended account of the events and circumstances, as well as cognitive and affective reactions to these, that make up the recollected fabric of an individual's life. Such an account is usually obtained through a series of direct interviews and can be subjected to various forms of analysis. It treats in more or less detail the main streams of behavior comprising the life-arc of the person.[3]

There are undoubtedly several reasons for the drop in popularity of the life history (as indexed by lack of publication in recent years, compared to the heights of enthusiasm during the nineteen-thirties and forties). Not the least important is the amount of work required to gather data. But perhaps the chief stumbling block to greater research use has been lack of an analytic scheme that is theoretically fruitful and at the same time allows the formulation of a sufficient number of cases that well-founded conclusions might be drawn concerning personality-environmental transactions. Whatever the reasons, it is probably no exaggeration to say that research files contain more unused, unanalyzed data of a life-history nature than any other type. Although these difficulties need to be recognized, we are at a point when the life history should be *re*considered for its help in uncovering the causes in psychiatric disorders.

In cross-cultural research we are continually beset by complications introduced through the notion of cultural relativism. What, in a given bit of behavior, is the genotypic pattern, and what is merely cultural content? In effect, our creation, "cultural relativity," has come home to plague us, for if all behavior is relative to its context there can be no truly comparative categories applicable across cultural boundaries. Does a high level of witchcraft fear in a group, for example, necessarily imply the psychodynamic normality of fear and anxiety? This leads to the further question of the relation between group characteristics and individual symptoms. It is not merely an academic question, nor is it simple of solution. Obviously we need intensive, detailed empirical studies of a range of persons in a group to develop understanding of the meaning and function, for a given person, of any culturally derived beliefs or practices in order to determine their "normality" or "abnormality."

In this task the life history may be of great use. Insofar as what we call "sick" is sick only by reference to some standards of health, we can use biographical materials to help obtain understanding of the nature of nonpathology. What are the features of several inductively derived "typical" life courses in a given group?—not the amalgamated "life cycle" presented as a chapter in most ethnographies. What is the developmental story of the personality in its natural habitat, its confrontation with goals and new complexes of expectation as it proceeds through life, its strategies for problem-solving, adjustment, and adaptation, its mechanisms for maintaining equilibrium? Murray's remarks on this topic some years ago still pertain. He said: "The truth is that until very recently the study of lives—the only possible way of obtaining the granite blocks of data on which to build a science of human nature—has generally been deprecated in academic circles as an undertaking to which no true scientist would commit himself." [4] We have studied segments of lives, but have we on any large scale studied lives?

Beyond, therefore, the epidemiological correlations being uncovered by today's field studies, the next major task is to determine the longitudinal patterns lying behind the association and shaping the response of the individual. Why have some people developed symptoms while others have not, despite the same objective stresses? Psychodynamically does the given association have the same meaning, the same status, in the lives of all the people in which it is found? The present is a precipitate of the past in human personality as much as in any other realm of the natural world, and if we are to lay bare the chain of dynamic factors involved we must inquire beyond this synchronic association. For a human life, and any cross-sectional end product of that life such as a relationship between two elements of personality experience, is a balance of forces; and the stability or instability of a personality, the result of interplay among functional and dysfunctional elements. It becomes important, then, to know the context in which the disordered behavior is occurring —that is to say, the personality in its longitudinal setting. This need for seeing personality in its total chronological span is consonant with the Lewinian insistence on appraising the total psychological "field" in which behavior is occurring.

Certain prior methodological considerations must be met if the life-history technique is to be maximally useful. For one thing, the cases chosen from whom the biographies are taken must be representative in known ways not only of the population with symptoms, but also of the nonsymptomatic group. Quite obviously they should also be in sufficient numbers so that life-history data can be used in corroborating and not only in generating or illustrating hypotheses. Also there is need for a selection in regard to the types of sociocultural events most crucial in the life-arc of the person, and selection in regard to concepts that will elucidate the psychiatric significance of those events.

The following is a suggested analytic paradigm, one which modifies the traditional form of the life history in line with the nature of the problem at hand. The basic principle of scientific conceptualization is selectivity. For our purposes selection needs to occur against the background conception of the total life-arc of the person, its integrative, developmental, and synthesizing trends. We may be selective in regard to two modes or aspects of the life story: (1) the "structural" aspects; and (2) the "phenomenological" aspects. By "structural" I refer to invariant points of reference, shared in the group, for the organizing of individual behavior. By "phenomenological" I mean the subjective responses, the inner world of thought and affect which embroiders the structural points of reference and which is, in the last analysis, the ultimate stronghold of personality uniqueness.

What are the strategic event-sequences that will maximally

show the influence of the sociocultural environment in the life course? The concept of role and analysis of role learning and role playing appear to be of considerable value in this respect, for much of the weight of inherited cultural tradition as well as the effects of social structure impinge on the individual through specific role situations. "Role" may help resolve the diffuseness of a life course into structural patterns that can be easily handled and meaningfully analyzed. At the same time "role" is one of the ways by which people perceive themselves and organize their phenomenological world in terms of a subjective reality.

There is a considerable literature on both role and life history. But there is little that takes the structure provided by multiple and successive role learning and performance patterns over the life course as the point of departure for analysis of a life history, especially in regard to implications for psychiatric disorder.

For these purposes, then, personality (seen in temporal extension as the "life-stream," in Meyerian terms) is considered a collection of interweaving roles—like a hemp rope, or a bundle of cross-country telephone cables. The analogy is not perfectly adequate, of course, for not all roles are operative at any given moment, and some are maintained as part of this image of the personality system only in their potentiality or latency.

As a brief illustration of such "bridging" between the social and the personal, let us look at the role of hunter among the Eskimos. In the past this role was clearly defined and highly honored, and all males were expected to fulfill it. Important not only from the viewpoint of the society in providing economic security for the group, it also was of vital concern in the security system of the men as unique personalities. Its performance gave them the respect of their fellows, the sense of doing what is valued, an avenue for initiative and self-reliance, as well as economic sustenance. Young boys began learning the techniques of hunting as soon as they were able, looking to the day when they would be full-fledged hunters and therefore accepted as "real men."

But what is happening now in most Eskimo communities? Through a series of profound changes in the relationship between the group and the outside world, the traditionally valued role of hunter has a serious competitor for prestige: the wage-laborer. The changed nature of the diffuse ecological relationship with the surrounding world finds expression in new structuring of roles available for individuals. Very often such new roles are far less adequate than former role constellations in satisfying striving patterns for the person and, at the same time, in contributing to the maintenance of the interactional system that is the community. Goals of striving implicated in the role of wage-laborer, for instance, may be restrictive in the areas of satisfaction they offer a personality and also may lead to socially disruptive consequences, such as emigration in search of opportunity. Thus the broad concept, "sociocultural change," can be conceptually translated into role processes that take on vital and immediate relevance for individual psychodynamics.

A scheme of this sort requires preanalysis to determine a role inventory appropriate both to the culture and to research needs. Another prerequisite is that roles be conceptualized at a workable level of generality and inclusiveness—something, for example, in between the role of "woman" and that of member of a particular lineage or subgroup. Further, as a problem in its own right, the criteria for role labeling should be explicated. For example, we should distinguish between characteristics inherent in the role as such, and characteristics serving as the basis for recruitment *to* the role. That is to say, the role of "woman" may indicate very little because it includes a great heterogeneity of behavior, but the fact of being a woman is the main basis for recruitment to the roles of adolescent girl, wife, mother, matriarch, and so on, which can be specified in terms of rights, duties, and goal-seeking patterns.

If we are to organize the gathering of the life-history data around the series of roles appropriate to an individual of such and such a type, what about a scheme for analysis that will bring out the relevance of these data for mental health? As intimated above, the position taken here follows a theoretical framework that emphasizes the ceaseless striving of the individual toward manifold goals, and the malfunctional effects of interference with certain types of those goals. Such a position takes its start from three fundamental postulates found in Leighton's recent frame of reference:

I. All human beings exist in a state of psychological striving.
II. Striving plays a part in the maintenance of an essential psychical condition.
III. Interference with striving leads to a disturbance of the essential psychical condition.[5]

The types of goals believed to be maximally relevant to the mental health of an individual are grouped into ten categories, listed as follows with relation to the manner in which the sociocultural environment may be of importance in fostering the development of psychiatric disorder:

I. Sociocultural situations which interfere with sentiments of physical security foster psychiatric disorder.
II. Sociocultural situations which interfere with sentiments of securing sexual satisfaction foster psychiatric disorder.
III. Sociocultural situations which interfere with sentiments bearing on the expression of hostility foster psychiatric disorder.
IV. Sociocultural situations which interfere with sentiments of giving love foster psychiatric disorder.
V. Sociocultural situations which interfere with sentiments of securing love foster psychiatric disorder.
VI. Sociocultural situations which interfere with sentiments bearing on obtaining recognition foster psychiatric disorder.
VII. Sociocultural situations which interfere with sentiments bearing on the expression of spontaneity (positive force, creativity, volition) foster psychiatric disorder.
VIII. Sociocultural situations which interfere with sentiments of orientation in the person regarding his place in society and the place of others foster psychiatric disorder.

IX. Sociocultural situations which interfere with the person's sentiments of membership in a definite human group foster psychiatric disorder.

X. Sociocultural situations which interfere with sentiments of belonging to a moral order and of being right in what one does foster psychiatric disorder.[6]

With the data of the life history gathered in a semistructured way in terms of this bridging concept, concomitant roles can be organized more or less chronologically to show sequence and pattern. They may then be analyzed in terms of the essential sentiments listed above to determine whether, and in what way, the roles played by the individual throughout his life have created situations of serious interference with striving or have developed patterns of security that are now being seriously disrupted by current circumstances. Looking at a series of such case histories chosen from both patients and nonpatients, one may, and theoretically should, be able to see different patterns of role involvement between those individuals who manifest psychiatric symptoms (on the basis of sociocultural determinants) and those who do not. Such an illustration of the specific manner in which this environing whole has affected the course of development will at least take us into the area of elucidating sociocultural causes of psychiatric disorder.

Life-history Analysis

To illustrate how the above scheme might work, I take for analysis a portion of the life story of a young St. Lawrence Eskimo male. The story deals with the formative years of childhood and early adolescence. The document in hand is actually an autobiography of more than 200 full-size pages written under financial contract over a period of several years. In this respect it does not conform to suggestions for gathering the original life-history data in terms of role categories. That, however, may be disregarded in view of the heuristic clarity of the document in illustrating the phenomenological and developmental facets of role learning and performance. In any analysis of an extensive series of life histories, the detailed behavioral examples to be given below would be omitted and only summaries of relevant data included for examination of associations between life experiences and psychiatric status. In this pilot assessment of the method, however, such examples are helpful.

The subject of the life history, whom I shall call Robert, is now in his twenties. He was resident in the village during most of the year of the 1954–1955 investigation. In linking his life story to the psychiatric studies reported in earlier chapters, we should note that he did not fall into the sample to which the psychoneurotic inventory questionnaire was administered. And at the time of the survey, he had left for tuberculosis hospitalization on the mainland so that it was impossible to procure such additional data as were obtained in the other cases for whom life-history materials are available. In the population-wide study, however, there were no indications from informant interviewing, medical records, the minutes of town council meetings, or recorded observations that he evidenced any recognizable psychopathology.

Thus as far as the rough mapping of the epidemiological features of the Eskimo population indicated, this life story concerns a relatively normal person. This is said with considerable reservation, not only in the light of the approximate methods used but also because the subject is still young and the full effects of the experiences described in his autobiography have obviously not been lived out yet. The presentation of his life history is thus an effort to illustrate an analytic technique and not to demonstrate the linkages between sociocultural experiences and a psychological state known definitely to be either pathological or nonpathological.

Until the mid-1950's the St. Lawrence Islanders were still very much oriented to remaining recognizably Eskimos—albeit with some importations from the white man's world. As indicated in the earlier chapters about these Eskimos, the decade following World War II brought successive changes in their economic situation, social structure, and sentiment systems. Of extreme importance were increased contact with the white man's world, including schooling of the young; increased economic and political dependence on the mainland; a high level of stressful factors of many types; new opportunities to participate in and practice the new culture; and the common-sense observations about the superiority of the white man's goods and practices over some of the Eskimo ways.

Robert's life experiences span the massive sociocultural changes occurring in his environment. He spent many of his early years with his family in an isolated hunting and trapping camp, where the outdoors, the movements and habits of animals, the changing face of the sea soon began to have meaning and lifelong appeal for him. The family also had a house in the central village of the island, where they journeyed for supplies and aid. A few years later the family went there to live for several months at a time to enroll the children in school. It was in this way that the author acquired his formal education on the island —up through grade four—although the schooling itself was obtained in a piecemeal fashion owing to the family's frequent return to the hunting camp.

In the village during and after World War II the author began to experience the new world moving in on the island. A critical and undoubtedly irrevocable step in this opening of a new way of life occurred in the fifties, when the author was taken to the Alaskan mainland with a serious case of tuberculosis. The hospitalization lasted for several years, during which time he was exposed again to many far-reaching acculturational influences, including further formal schooling.

The life history up to this point (it is still being written) comprises first memories through early adolescence—the time in life when a person in this culture passes from indulgent infancy and the beginning of childhood, through the increasing responsibility-training of later childhood, and into apprenticeship for the pre-eminent role of able-bodied adult male in this culture: hunter of sea mammals.

A prerequisite in using the analytic paradigm suggested above is an inventory of roles found in the culture. The list suggested below is partial; a full compilation would include the roles of both males and females and old as well as young persons. In this instance, "role" is defined as a cluster of socially shared ideas and sentiments that focus on a definable activity capable of being performed by a single person. It is different in this respect, for example, from the "role of the family." The role inventory appropriate as an analytic background for this life history can be

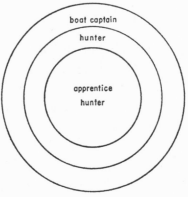

Figure IX-2. Role "nesting" as illustrated by Eskimo apprentice hunter, hunter, and boat captain

divided into three classes: (1) technological roles, which deal with the handling or manufacturing of "things" (material objects), whether or not in the context of interaction with other people; (2) social roles, which center on goals deriving from human relationships with or without the involvement of "things"; and (3) ideational roles, which involve the manipulation of ideas, beliefs, and commitments with or without the involvement of people and/or things.

Two other points may be noted about role analysis. The first is that of role "nesting." For example, in this particular society a young man is first of all an apprentice hunter, then a full-fledged hunter, then boat captain. The one role, boat captain, implies that the person filling it has already passed through the roles of hunter and apprentice hunter. Conversely, however, the role of apprentice hunter does not imply that of boat captain. This "nesting" is illustrated in the accompanying diagram, Figure IX-2. Other examples of this phenomenon can also be found, but it is by no means characteristic of all roles. Another point is that roles can be divided between those which are relatively focused or relatively diffuse in their behavioral requirements. The distinction is important, for a diffuse role does not lack psychological reality—as, for example, when a person experiences a sense of role identity in being an "Eskimo" in a white Alaskan city versus a "white man." An inventory of relevant roles for men in the St. Lawrence Eskimo culture is as follows:

TECHNOLOGICAL ROLES

Focused	*Diffuse*
Hunter	"Able-bodied man"
Ivory carver	
Trapper	
Fisherman	
Carpenter	
Boat-maker	
Storekeeper	
Postmaster	
School janitor	
Tractor driver	
Reindeer herder	

SOCIAL ROLES

Focused	*Diffuse*
Son-father	Clansman
Son-mother	Villager
Grandson	"Young person"
Sibling	"Old person"
Husband	
Father	
Grandfather	
Collateral kinsman	
Councilman	

IDEATIONAL ROLES

Focused	*Diffuse*
Elder	Pagan
Deacon	Christian
Shaman	Schoolboy

It is clearly impossible in the space of an illustrative exercise to examine all these roles in terms of the analytic paradigm. Therefore I will choose one example from each of the three areas delineated above as they pertain to Robert's life history. The roles selected are: (1) hunter (or, more appropriately in this case, apprentice hunter), (2) son (to a father), and (3) schoolboy.

Although each role will be examined separately, it is relevant at this point to note the close empirical linkage between the role of apprentice hunter and that of son. This is a function of a specific cultural setting in which much of the technological learning for subsistence roles is carried out in the family rather than in vocational or professional schools. Similarly the role of schoolboy is empirically intertwined with that of son and apprentice hunter. The degree to which this may be psychodynamically important in creating conflicts for an individual comes out below.

ROBERT AS SON TO HIS FATHER

I shall begin with the logically most prior role, that of son. Robert is the eldest son in a family that eventually was to have three sons and two daughters born alive, although only a sister was still alive in 1954–1955. In general terms, the role of son in this culture is one in which the individual emerges from a favored early childhood to begin learning the adult male roles from his father as soon as he is physically strong enough and mentally able. This means a long period of dependency on the initiative and control of an older person, a situation which may lead to feelings of resentment and covert hostility. In adult life the relationships between sons and fathers are characterized (in terms of cultural directives) by a heightened sense of interpersonal reserve and lack of a jocular or teasing quality. Such sentiments develop gradually and slowly, however, and in the early years they are set in a context of indulgence and demonstrative affection.

Several different behavioral patterns are persistent throughout the role of son in the portion of the life story examined here. One is Robert's careful tutelage by his father in activities appropriate to the adult male—hunter, ivory carver, trapper, household provider, and guardian in the father's absence. Another behavioral pattern is that of care and solicitude, coupled with a rigorous discipline and clearly defined action-reward or action-punishment sequences. There is also a consistent emphasis on development of a moral sense and of conscience—with its existence illustrated dramatically by occasional youthful revolt with consequent feelings of guilt and the justness of punishment.

Against the ten categories of essential striving sentiments considered crucial to personality functioning, the subject's experience in terms of his role as son can be appraised. In the analysis to follow I will consider the manner in which a role conceived as a "sociocultural situation" of a perduring type may, through promoting sentiments in each of these categories, foster either psychiatric illness or psychiatric health.

Physical security. The subject experiences no marked physical deprivation such as maltreatment in his role as son. The father, although a poor man, consistently tries to provide physical essentials and maintains a thrifty and prudent behavior in caring for his family. The principal frustrations occurring are those of relative deprivation, with Robert wondering why his father will not allow him to purchase luxury goods in the store when money occasionally comes in. But Robert does have sufficient food, clothing, and housing, although these are of a relatively inferior quality to those of some other villagers.

In another important respect Robert's experiences in the role

of son are conducive to psychiatric health, for his father dili-
gently teaches many of the arts and skills necessary for achieving
physical security. On a dog-team trip across the island, for example, Robert's father taught him several things about how to
stay alive in this environment:

My dad pointed out the way we were to take and told me the names
of the places. He told me that I will be traveling by myself in the
time to come and it is the time to study the way now. All I can learn.
Finally we stopped on top of a hump to wait for the others. I stood up
and looked all around and tried hard to study the places, but what
drew my interest the most was the wild beauty of the surrounding,
that was covered with the white snow. Spotless white country,
seemed to have no end at all. Again waited a long time. This time Dad
showed me how to use the compass that we always took along
whenever we go on the long trip. I thought the compass just pointed
out the village or the camp. For the first time I learned that it points to
the North at all times and we have to figure out the way by it. Not
just follow it. He said that it is the most precious instrument for
traveling.

The worries and long-range concerns about physical security
that Robert expresses tend to be shared by most other people in
the group, and there are no persistent expressions of frustration
over these problems arising from the subject's particular situation as a son.

Sexual satisfaction. This aspect of personality dynamics is
relevant in the son-father role mainly in terms of instruction and
attitudes about sex. The data do not disclose any severe problems in this area. They may have existed, of course, but if so we
have no way of assessing them since none are manifest in the
document.

Expression of hostility. Robert's life story gives no evidence
of deep-seated hostility toward his father, but he does tell of
events that may be interpreted as indirect expressions. This point
needs to be seen in the context of cultural patterns regarding
aggression. From observation it appeared that parents were

extremely tolerant of minor acts of physical assault and "sassing" from children up to about the age of ten. After that a pattern of quiet obedience was enjoined, and commonly adolescents appeared to be reserved and self-contained. More important, however, the cultural ideal was clearly that a son should not harbor hostile feelings toward his father, an ideal that in Robert's case may well have been reinforced by his rather youthful and dedicated acceptance of the Christian faith.

In his life story there are two occasions when Robert beats his father in a race, after which he teases him and expresses pride in his own accomplishment. Also Robert reports his regret that his father does not smoke, feeling that this sets him aside as less of a man than others in the village. Later Robert disobeys his father's injunctions about smoking, which may also be evidence of some hostility being expressed. Any deeper rebelliousness toward his father is probably repressed and may be important psychodynamically although latent. As a matter of fact, however, a strong theme in his life story is the opposite—the expression of respect and affection for his father rather than hostility.

Giving love. The role of son is one that involves considerable scope for the giving of love, and in this case, as indicated above, Robert expresses love through emulation and support of what his father does. From his earliest years he tries to be like his father, do what his father does, is sorry when told that he is too young or otherwise unable to follow his father. There is, however, the aforementioned cultural injunction against open demonstration of affection in the later years, but this does not seem to be psychodynamically an interference with the giving of love. The latter is strikingly illustrated in one passage in which Robert describes his father's return to a temporary camp following a period of possible danger during the early days of World War II when all adult males remained on guard duty to protect the village against a possible attack by the Japanese:

One of my brothers rushed to say, "It's Daddy! It's Daddy!" I didn't believe him. But a delightful sight met my eyes as a dog familiar to me, our old gray-brown lead dog, came into the view of the opened door. I'm still not sure it's Dad. I have a thought somebody might have borrowed that lead dog, 'cause many people liked it and often borrowed it. And I didn't want to be disappointed but was curious enough to go out and find out who the visitor was. I slowly stood up from the front of the old oil barrel camp stove. As I looked outside of the door I found all our dogs, but who was the driver? He looked like Dad but I'm still not sure—still digging up for truth in case it might be only my imagination. Those dirty little rascals clinging to him were brothers of mine. I had a great desire to do the same in that instance, but I'm too grown up. I'd be embarrassed. Just the old Eskimo ways again. Sure enough, it was Dad.

Securing love. In a manner similar to opportunities for giving love, the role of son is also important in creating situations for the receiving of love. Again this may become veiled or disguised in later years as far as open demonstrativeness is concerned, but it nonetheless can exist at a profound level, as it did for Robert. His father's love was manifested in many ways. Care, solicitude, careful instruction, gentle rebuke, learning by experience in a context of a warm, loving human relationship— all these accumulated experiences added up to a feeling on the part of the subject that he was, indeed, the object of love and affection from his father:

When I and Dad were working doing ivory carving, I did the sanding and polishing. I worked hard there when I felt like doing it. I knew if we got them done, Dad would get something from the store. I didn't know it much, but my Dad was preparing for further teaching in how to provide for the family which I was going to do in the near future. And I was getting the experience of ivory carving. I learned I needed patience, work, and care. Once in every short while I asked, "How is this? Isn't it done yet?" And then Dad asked me, "What do *you* think of it?" I would say, "Maybe it is all done now." Because I was always sure I had gotten it right and got it done. But it wasn't done at all. Sometimes at a glance he would say, "Look at that part. You haven't done it yet." So I had to work all over again. Then I showed him again: "There! I'm sure I got it done now." But still more he would say, "Wait, wait. You haven't done this part," or "Little more polishing here," or "Remove the scratches here." Sure enough, I hadn't touched that part.

He was a good teacher that way. It was just to get me started for the thing. Later on I always made sure I'd done the work so I wouldn't have to be bothered by it. What helped me do the work better was a sort of reward I got from Dad. It was that I liked to see him look pleased when he saw the work was well done.

Obtaining recognition. In the son role there are numerous opportunities for recognition, such as praise for being a good son, for following the father's directions and desires, for learning to behave as a provider-surrogate for the family, such as in the following passage:

Now I had learned to use our tools well enough that Dad could trust me for some of the work with our boat. He got some wood ready for me to saw and plane, telling me how to do, what next to do, and so forth before he could go to work down at the Civil Aeronautics Authority. I did as he told me to do. Often at noon he came home for lunch to see all of the work done. Then he would say, "Fine. You have done the work well." Then give me some more work to do. I always did it with much pleasure, because he made me feel good when he was pleased with my work and told me how good a help I was to him.

Expressing spontaneity. After early childhood there is restriction and control placed on spontaneity between father and son. While it is definitely not one of the "joking relationships" found in this culture, the role does not entirely inhibit impromptu behavior. Robert relates several instances in which he acted impulsively toward his father and engaged in childish pranks as well as constructive activities. An example occurred one day when he had accompanied his father hunting. Being left alone for a moment while his father was off scouting for animals elsewhere, Robert grabbed his father's rifle and shot a seal, despite the latter's warning not to handle firearms because he was too young. His father, although very happy with the result, nonetheless pointed out the disobedience involved. Such an incident occurred several times in the life story.

Orientation in society. Perhaps more than any other role that of a child provides opportunities for learning one's place in society and the place of others. Constant reference to "your family," "your relatives," and other people in the village and instruction about how to behave toward them or how they should behave reciprocally help create a conceptual network in which the subject feels that he knows where he belongs. Robert's father acted in many contexts as tutor regarding how to be a good, valued son, as well as a respected member of this Eskimo society. The sociocultural setting in which Robert lives is changing, however, and it is no longer entirely sufficient for a young person to be a good Eskimo in the traditional sense. Such a situation has ample potential for intergenerational conflict and could seriously disrupt the father-son relationship, and a parental attitude of clinging to the past could markedly interfere with the process of orienting to the current situation. In Robert's case, however, his father is supportive and strongly encourages his son to become educated:

I didn't know if I would like it in the school. But if I wanted to learn I must have some, and my parents wanted me to learn, too, because they knew by themselves it's real hard if we don't learn those three: read, write, and speak English. Our parents said we [the children in the camp] must have some school somehow.

To be educated thus becomes part of his duty as a son, together with becoming a good hunter. At times the double aspiration promoted by his father creates fairly profound conflicts in the subject's own mind. Eventually he works out a compromise, as will be illustrated below.

Membership in a group. The role of son obviously implies a group context, if only of two persons. In this case such a dyadic group did exist—a feeling of community and intimate social bond between Robert and his father based on their common experiences in hunting, trapping, and caring for the family. But the family group that subsumed the father-son relationship was also one to which Robert felt a strong attachment and involvement. Beyond this there were his other relatives, particularly his father's brothers' families (the "patriclan" which comprises the relatives of primary importance in this society). Over and over again in the life story he expresses joy at seeing his cousins, sadness at their departure or prolonged absence, and profound grief at the death of his father's oldest brother:

At some length of time a very awful bad news reached us from my father's oldest brother. He had passed away. A sorrow hit us hard. For some days I couldn't go to stay with my cousins. I couldn't bear to see their sorrow, in fear they would make mine worse. It was so bad, it's not easy to describe on paper or by words. He had been an uncle to me—good as a father. So his death was a bitter sorrow. For a long time at nights I cried myself to sleep. I didn't pay much attention for my daily working. So was poor Dad. He was moody, but kept on as always. When I got brave enough to bear my sorrow, I returned to my cousins. We bore one another's hardship. That made it a little easier for us. His last words to me stood out very clearly now in my mind. No wonder he had given me his words. He might have known that he was to depart soon.

More than this, however, there are sentiments of membership in another group—that of school boys—which is strongly supported by Robert's father. The only obstacles in terms of identification with this group are those injunctions by his father not to be always wandering around with his set of friends, wasting his time in idleness. This does not assume much importance in the total life context, however.

Belonging to a moral order. Again, in interaction with his father, Robert very early acquires ideas about the moral nature of certain types of behavior and receives definite instruction in the ethical code of his society. He internalizes certain behavior as commendable and feels guilt if he violates those codes and thus learns to take initiative for doing things he knows should be done:

Now I took what I had laid up for myself by being naughty. Before I could eat or go to bed, I had to get done or receive what was for me. Dad would roar at me that froze me solid with fear. He would say, "Get that thing done," or "Go get some water" before you go to bed or eat. I would make excuses but none worked, because Dad knew none of them have much truth in them—as plain as daylight. I started on what he told me to do, trembling or even with a big lump in my throat and a sharp pain in my heart. More and more, little by little, I learned to realize I was receiving what I very rightly deserved. And there was no way of escaping except by doing them. And my parents didn't mean any bad for me. They were only giving me my lesson, to teach me to live the right way. The lessons I would need just within a few years from the time I was living; because I was to take over to provide for the family—our growing and increasing family.

ROBERT AS AN APPRENTICE HUNTER

There are many types of satisfactions for Robert in his role of a young hunter, and one major and continuing conflict. The conflict is that with the role of schoolboy. Robert is drawn to each role, but they are largely incompatible insofar as being in school means that one cannot be out hunting for most of the year, especially during the exciting spring hunting:

After a day or so the Bering Sea was white with ice. The men went hunting. I went to school. I didn't do any good that day in school, because it was hard for me to put my mind in what I was to do. Instead, my thoughts went with my Dad to hunting. I wanted to make believe that I was shooting a seal, mukluk, or even a walrus. But I dragged myself around in school all morning. Every little chance we got, my friends and I got together and chatted about hunting. We told each other if the weather was good on Saturday we would ask our Daddies to let us go with them out hunting. We talked on until a rough, gruff voice or a high-pitched voice called, "Boys! Get busy." After the usual classes we would be excused for lunch. I was poor in my work in the class, but who cared? It didn't bother me. All I wanted was being released from unpleasant sissy school.

Robert ultimately reaches something of a solution for the immediate situation by proposing to his teacher that he be allowed some time out of school for hunting if he will do extra lessons. This does not resolve the long-range implications of the conflict —which, indeed, may be said to epitomize a major theme for the entire society in changing from a hunting, subsistence culture to one entering into the modern world.

Robert is strongly drawn to hunting. Even as a five- or six-year-old he attempts to follow his father out on the ice and to handle the hunting weapons. He wants to be thought of as a "man" in order to be allowed to hunt. The hunter is still the prestige role of his culture, the cynosure of social approval. Such prestige is reflected even in childhood, as when Robert receives approbation from his schoolmates who were not allowed to go out hunting. It is this role which underscores his acceptance and support by several different groups, beginning with the family.

Physical security. In view of the physical hazards involved, the role of hunter requires constant attention to preventing accidents and death. It is not known how much the hardships of hunting may have influenced Robert's later development of tuberculosis. As a role it can be thought of as cutting two ways: it subjects the person to extraordinary dangers and at the same time it may provide some protection against disease by body building.

Also this role is the main avenue to physical security in terms of providing food, heating, and light, some clothing, and traditionally even part of housing insofar as walrus skin was used. Thus if hunting is poor, as it frequently is, physical security in these larger senses is threatened. If hunting is successful, the role is pre-eminently that of satisfying such needs:

My boots were soaked badly, too. I was glad when I took them off and toweled off my sweating feet, followed up by washing up. This refreshed me better than anything else. Around the wooden eating platter I was proud and self-satisfied to tell the good hunting story with my Dad to the happy family. Mom was pleased of me to become a real help in providing for the family.

The lack of satisfaction when no animals were sighted or killed and when there were tiring hours of waiting in the bitter cold is equally poignant:

A brisk cold wind cooled us off quickly and my hope faded away along with the warmth of my body. Until "No hope, no hope" seemed to tick, tack, tick, tack in rhythm to the beating of my heart. Slowly, or it seemed slow, the water froze to a glassy crust of ice. My feet got colder and colder. I closed my fists in my mittens to keep them warm. I kicked and jumped up and down and everything to keep warm. Less and less I paid attention to the glassy spot that had been a wide crack. Now and then I brushed off the white frost that formed on my fur ruff from my breathing.

Not a bit of hope or interest was left in my mind. It was all boring, and cold, plus my growling empty stomach. I began to imagine getting into our warm little house and a good warm boiled meat and some nice hot tea. But I tried hard to push that out of my mind, and tried to think of something better, because of those thoughts made things worse for me. But they kept coming. . . . It was all phooey for me. What a day. Time dragged—even must stuck. . . . I hung on to my patience the best way I could. The idea of going home became a very strong desire. But just as much I wished there would be something to shoot at. It was hard to let a long day pass without shooting at something. I thought of shooting those black specks on the ice just for the fun of it, and to satisfy my want. But it would be just a waste of precious bullets.

Sexual satisfaction. Sentiments in this area are not directly relevant to the role of apprentice hunter, and no data exist in the life story that would possibly indicate a connection.

Expressing hostility. The role of hunter affords extraordinarily good opportunities for the discharging and catharsis of hostile impulses in a possibly productive manner. The animals sought and ultimately killed can serve as indirect targets for much accumulated and often repressed hostility deriving from other life-situations. Robert's life story contains considerable material on the excitement and tensions involved in the hunt, and the satisfactions and apparent release following success. It seems very possible that even for an apprentice hunter the role admirably serves as a channel for such expression.

Giving love. Through the instrumentality of the hunting role love can be expressed intangibly through persistence and hard work in the group effort and tangibly through the voluntary giving of the products of the chase to other people. Robert expresses affection and loyalty to other people through both these means. As mentioned previously, he identifies with his father in the hunting role; he similarly strives to belong to the fraternity of hunters and be accepted by them. He also feels much satisfaction when he is able to give meat to other people, not only his own family. A traditional Eskimo custom was for the apprentice hunter to give the first animal or bird killed, or the skin of the first fox trapped, to an old person in the village:

I kept my face down as we worked unloading the meat onto the shore, while they told the story over and over. One of the others bragged to my Dad, "We have a new rifleman today; and a sharpshooter, too." He offered the skin to my father proudly. Dad accepted the skin, and we gave it away to an old man, as is the old custom. We still kept the custom for its common goodness. He was pleased, and so was I. It is always my best pleasure to do that.

Securing love. The role similarly affords occasion for receiving love through praise for work well done, for being a successful hunter and for being generous with meat. One of the traditionally most honored social roles is that of the generous man; to be stingy with the goods of life is an unforgivable breach of custom, one that if carried too far might result in the miser's own death in times of scarcity. Robert receives such approbation for his attempts to learn and perform well the role of hunter:

I was coming home from a duck hunt one morning. It was a lucky night, and I was tired from carrying my ducks for a long walk from the south of the lake. It was early in the morning. I threw the bunch of ducks in the door and I sat down on a crate outside to rest. When the family woke up Dad asked me if I didn't get anything. I proudly told him,"Plenty ducks." He was pleased, saying, "Fine. We'll have a feast then." Mother was more glad and pleased. She was going to make goodies of those ducks.

Negative evidence for the extent to which the hunter's role affords a channel for the securing of love is found in remarks and feelings about males who do not hunt. In the culture at the time the story was written, the onus of explaining why he did not hunt lay with the individual; the culture still expected a man to hunt and rewarded him accordingly.

Obtaining recognition. Only if the individual is unsuccessful is there interference in achieving recognition through being a hunter (and, in a bizarre way, even a proverbially unsuccessful hunter can achieve recognition of a sort). Social approval accrues to the role from all quarters of the society: father, family, extended family and lineage, schoolmates and peers, elderly hunters, and the village as a whole. And it is not just the traditional prestige system that focuses on this role; much of the transitional cultural system also underscores its importance, not so much because it is economically most vital but because it is an indicator of a man's worth and courage. The enviable quality of the role in Robert's life is seen in the reaction of his schoolmates:

Most of my schoolmates were there when I got back from hunting. They asked me, "How come you didn't come to school?" I lied to them, again just to protect my secret with my teacher [who had asked Robert not to tell others because they, too, would want to go out hunting with their fathers and miss school]. At first they didn't believe me when I told them about my seal. . . . Almost every one of them treated me like an old hunting companion, and I felt that way, too. But their questions were kind of tough; but every time I told them that I ran away from school. They said, "How are you going to face the teacher?" I just said, "I don't know," and pretended to be afraid.

Expressing spontaneity. Hunting is an activity in which creativity and volition can be given vent insofar as alternatives must be appraised and selected, decisions made, and tactics carried out to a successful conclusion. The young hunter begins very early to acquire the habits of thought which, set against a background of regulated and scheduled behavior, will result in actions appropriate to a crisis or unanticipated situation. He cannot be wholly an automaton, although certain procedures must partake of this characteristic. In the life story there are several instances in which, through the role of hunter, Robert engaged in impulsive behavior, acted on a desire of the moment, and did so in a fashion that brought social rewards. He remembers going out hunting without his father's permission, accompanying an older hunter whom he had deceived into believing that the outing had been given parental sanction:

When I got home Dad talked to me while we ate. "You deserve a good scolding and punishment, but I'm going to let that go, since you have done lots of good one way. But you should have let Mom know about it—and the worse is fooling her." I told him I did that because she might not let me go. And she wouldn't have let me go. Dad said, "From now on don't go hunting or anything without letting us know about it before you go or do anything. We will let you go when we feel it's all right for you to do it." Now I felt real good. And they were very pleased with the meat that I'd brought home.

Orientation in society. The hunter is the principal expression of the traditional male ethos of the culture. Through constant repetition in behavior and precept this becomes internalized in Robert from his earliest years. Even before he is six years old he agitates to accompany his father hunting:

Every time they are going hunting in the boat I go to my father and say, "I'm a man now. Isn't I old enough?" My father would answer, "Well, be a good boy and wait a little while longer. Help your mother or aunt with their work." Then I help them get ready and watch them go.

The sense of belonging to the fraternity of hunters is also strong in Robert as he describes one of his first trips out over the winter ice on foot. Group cohesion is reflected in a common recognition of the implicit dangers of the situation, the constant instruction of the young, and the lighthearted camaraderie after the tension of the hunt has relaxed:

After we had finished hunting and were ready to go home, my Dad told me to draw my own seal. Oh! I felt proud as a person could be with my rifle across my back and an ice tester in hand and drawing a seal. When I looked around I was surprised to see every hunter heading toward the shore. Soon we joined the rest, and it was a long line of hunters drawing their catch home. We joined after the last hunter. Men were surprised to see me hunting. Everyone said good things for me, praising me for good hunting. I felt swollen and chapped, but proud. The hunter next to us stepped aside and told my father to get in ahead. He said, "You have a young hunter to take care of. Get ahead." So we did. It went the same thing until we were next to the leader. He told us to get ahead, too, but my Dad wouldn't. Some of the hunters teased me that I was a little pup training to be a hunter. I thought that was real funny, so we laughed.

As we walked the men chatted and told stories. I had to half run to keep up. Sometimes my seal got stuck on some ice and I had to tug at it to free it. The man behind me helped, with a smile, when the seal was freed so suddenly that I nearly plunged forward and became the laughingstock of the group. But I didn't mind a bit. I was too thrilled to mind a thing.

Although within the context of the role of hunter itself there appear few obstacles to orientation in the society, when that role is considered in its larger setting the profound conflicts between the traditional and modern world emerge. Recognition of this situation is a recurrent theme in Robert's life story, but the question of whether to be a hunter or have a job is postponed for a few years:

That spring when the spring hunting came around it was, as every year, the happiest time of the year for me. It meant to me fun in hunting. The best part was good-by to tedious, old, sissy school. That was my biggest mistake, but it wasn't at that time, because it was more necessary for me to have more hunting experiences than school. In fact, every boy needs the knowledge of hunting, since it's our chief source of living.

Membership in a group. Robert's sentiments of belonging to the group of hunters of the village, his importance to his family as a hunter, and the approval given by school peers for this role have all been illustrated in the preceding excerpts.

Belonging to a moral order. Far from interfering with sentiments about belonging to a moral order and being right in what one does, the role of apprentice hunter creates a keen sense that one is doing what is culturally most commendable and praiseworthy. Robert indicates several times that he feels he made a "mistake" not to be more interested in schooling, and yet he reiterates throughout that hunting is just as important.

ROBERT AS A SCHOOLBOY

Several aspects of the role of schoolboy have been previously touched upon. Most obvious is its conflict with the role of apprentice hunter. At the same time education is highly valued in this group as preparation for mastering many of the new situations confronting a modern Eskimo. For Robert, schooling had both these positive and negative aspects. At one point he indicates that he was a pet student of his teacher, which is possibly a reflection of the interest and motivation he brought to the learning situation. He openly acknowledges the importance of schooling for his future life, and he takes considerable pleasure in belonging to a group of peers in the school.

But adjustment to this situation is not without difficulties. When he first began school he felt timid and shy at meeting new people. This is manifested in other situations as well, and there is perhaps a projective aspect to some of the hesitancies he expresses about other people's perceptions of him. In the first two or three years there is also conflict over being separated from his own family while they remain in the hunting camp and he lives with a paternal uncle's family in order to attend school. But, with time, these situations change and he feels accepted by his fellow schoolmates and respected and liked by the teacher. He also finds the role one in which he can obtain special recognition for his talents. That the role was congenial to his long-term personality structure is perhaps best evidenced by his later life, and dramatically expressed by the remarkable life-history document which he was to write.

Physical security. The long-range aspects of the role in terms of providing physical security are indicated when Robert realizes that he must study if he is to get a good job. The advantages of education for salaried jobs are apparently clear even to a youngster:

The first thing we did in school was spelling. That I liked quite well. Then on to correcting the words we had misspelled or left out. Followed by arithmetic, which I thought was the worst part of school. The only thing that kept me doing it was our teacher who said we "must learn it that we might become the storekeeper; if we do we would use what we learned now. If we don't learn it the people will laugh at us and we would be a no good storekeeper. But if we learned we would be a good storekeeper that the people would like us to be their store man." At that, I imagined myself seated behind the counter selling everything. Then I would think I must study arithmetic.

In the short-term view, however, Robert often becomes frustrated at the restrictions against hunting created by the role, thereby reducing his share in providing for the physical security of himself and his family. But in some ways the role of schoolboy may be said to function in a protective fashion, through keeping the child out of dangerous situations and away from exposure to intense cold and wind before he is able to withstand it. Also, Robert experiences some relative deprivation over his poor clothing compared to his classmates', but this does not seem to be a significant interference with striving.

Sexual Satisfaction. Again as with the other two roles, one can say very little in regard to sentiments in this area. The only indication of a sexual interest arises when Robert discusses his friendship with a girl in school and the overtures of help and affection which they display. This theme is not picked up again, but it should be remembered that the document stops just at the time Robert was entering adolescence.

Expression of hostility. Insofar as discipline and regulated behavior are crucial elements in school training, there is little leeway for the expression of hostility in this context. Robert gives no instances in which he is forced to swallow his resentments in the classroom situation or before the teacher. Some behavior possibly interpretable as hostility is indicated, however, in Robert's statements about how other school children teased him about his poor clothing or his scholastic achievements. His reaction to such comments is one of trying to avoid situations in which this comes up, of feeling that the others have no right to torment him in this fashion, and of being glad when some of his friends come to his rescue. If this is hostility, it is exceedingly indirect, as was also the case in the son-father relationship, and it seems probable that the inhibition of hostile feelings and the possibly damaging effects, psychodynamically, of such repression constitute a theme to which a personality analyst would be sensitized in watching Robert's future development.

Giving love. The giving of love is translated in this role in diffuse terms. It is expressed in "ganging" behavior, in sharing of experiences with peers, and in conforming to his parents' desires that he attend school and study hard. Also, in the context of this role he finds "special" friends, one of whom is a girl, as mentioned above:

There on my desk I found a little folded piece of paper. Picking it up, I looked at the next person in front of me, so I could see it was from her. She was my special classmate. She looked especially pretty because I had been without seeing her for quite a while. But I looked down on my desk, avoiding her eyes. Then I looked in my desk. It was nicely straightened up and clean. Then I looked up at her again. She was still looking at me. Then she whispered, "I cleaned it for you." I could feel my face warming up and thanked her for it. "How many walrus did you shoot? I heard that you are a shooter now," she spoke up again. "A few of them. Yes, I started shooting," I told her awkwardly, and then I was tongue-tied.

Securing love. The obverse of giving love is the securing of love, and many of the same behavioral patterns are relevant. His parents' approval of his attention to school studies is of key importance in this regard, but also important is the affection and solicitude coming from his teacher, as well as acceptance by peers:

I rode back from camp on the sled and we went right to our little house. All my old schoolmates were there to meet me. They had been writing to me all winter and sent me packages. Oh, we had lots of things, lots to tell each other. Yet we didn't much hear from each other because mostly we spoke at the same time. Our little house was overflowing with visitors who wanted to welcome us; it was good to be with old folks again.

Obtaining recognition. A salient characteristic of the school-boy role is that of creating situations for Robert to obtain recognition and reward for work well done, and he is apparently a gifted student:

The next few days we got our promotions. Now that included me. Boy, oh boy! That made me feel like somebody special. I knew well what promotion meant. It was really something good and not very good at the same time. The good part of it was that we were more respectable by our fellow schoolmates, and the praise of our parents. The other part was more and harder work to do. At the close of the school for the day I asked our teacher to let me take my books with me for homework, but that was not the real reason why I asked. It was I wanted to show them off to my folks. He let me. I proudly showed them off and as I had promised, I stuck my nose in some of them that evening before bedtime and did some work. And Dad liked looking them over.

Expressing spontaneity. The requirements of classroom conduct impose restraints on spontaneity, but they are sufficiently confined to the classroom, from which there are periodic releases, that they do not offer serious interferences. In another way one can view education as a means of increasing the volitional potential of an individual by expanding intellectual horizons and increasing knowledge of creative possibilities. This latter appears to have occurred in Robert's case, one expression of it being that he wrote hunting stories for his teacher in order to be allowed to go hunting on some of the school days. In all, Robert seems to have managed his early life so as to afford him spontaneity of expression in several ways, such as in conniving a sanctioned release from school and by capitalizing on his creative writing abilities.

Orientation in society. Education in the broad sense, either informal or institutionalized, is the chief way of learning one's place and that of others in society, quite aside from its benefits in technical training. In this case, as indicated earlier, education is preparing Robert for a life unlike that of the adult members of his group; new moral sanctions as well as new techniques follow from exposure to school. Most of these do not become focused as conflicts in Robert's mind at the time covered by the life story.

Also the interferences with sentiments of orientation to society arising over the conflict with the hunting role are ameliorated by another consideration: the entire society of which Robert is a part is beginning the process of change at the time he is going to school. In this respect, school plays a key role in preparing young people for gaining a place in the society that will be of importance to them as adults, even as rigorous training in hunting techniques prepared the youth of the previous generations for a life in another type of society.

Where Robert is concerned, the incompatible pull between hunting and education lacks the cruciality it had for many other Eskimos because he does well in both, values both, and has the sympathetic support of both parents and teacher:

The first thing in the school was spelling in the afternoon. My mind was too far from that. I didn't do any good in spelling. I had plenty of words that I had to work over. Next came arithmetic. I was worse in there. After the class was sent back to their seats and desks, our teacher wanted me with him for a moment. I sat by him at his big desk. My heart hammered against my chest. I knew he was a rough person. But to my surprise this time he was very gentle. He spoke to me at almost a whisper. He started, "I don't know what is wrong with you. You have been our best student in your class, but all of a sudden you fall back. Surely something is wrong with you. If this goes on I'm going to lower your grade to the next lower grade. But if you tell me what's wrong with you, I will do my best to help you over that thing that's bothering you." I was stunned very much. I couldn't find a word to say. All I said was, "I don't know." Then he told me to be back at my desk and get busy and he added, "We will talk this thing over later on."

When I sat back at my seat, I put my opened book in front of me and pretended to be busy. Others just in front of me and one to my back poured on some questions, but I couldn't hear any. I sat there thinking, thinking, and thinking until I dreamed up an idea. I made up my mind to write a note to the teacher before going home. It was not going to be the first time that I wrote him a note. Several times I'd been doing that to get help from him over any rough spots. But this time it was going to be a special note. So I got busy and wrote a note and read it over; then tore it up, and made another note. And I went on until I thought I'd done it best.

The note read: "Dear Sir, I want to go hunting very much. Please, shall I go with my father tomorrow? That is my trouble. Please answer me. Robert." Then I waited for a chance, putting my note between the pages of my book. When the teacher left his desk for a moment, I wadded up some scrap paper and walked to his desk, pretending to be getting rid of my trash. And I dropped my folded sheet of paper where he could see it. When he returned to his desk,

I watched him with the corner of my eye. I saw him pick up my note. After he read it, he glanced at me, and started writing something. It was near time for us to go to the other room for our ivory carving class. When he stood up from his desk, I fixed my eyes on my book. My heart beat as if it would break out through my chest. I even sweated a bit. As he passed by he dropped a folded sheet of paper on my desk. Without drawing any attention from other students, I opened it carefully. I read it, holding it in the page of my book so I would look as if I were busy reading my book. The note read: "Please see me after your ivory carving class. We will talk this thing over privately. Thank you."

At last 4 o'clock came. As soon as I put away my work and tools in their proper places, I went to see my teacher. He said he wanted this privately. My heart started beating harder and harder. He asked me to sit in front of him while he sat down in his chair behind his big desk. Then he began: "I want you to learn in school very much. We need you here. We can hardly spare you just a day." I kept silent as a mouse. "But I have been thinking about it this afternoon. If you're thinking too much about hunting, you won't do any good in school. Does your father want you to go hunting with him?" I answered, "I don't know. But I'm sure he wants me to learn about hunting, and I want to go hunting more than anything else." He asked me, "Are you tired of school?" I said, "No, I'm not, but I like hunting very much." He said, "Oh, I see. Tell you what. If your father really wants you to go hunting, I will let you go. But I will give you extra homework, and I wish you will write a story about your hunting every time you go hunting while in school." I hated to write stories, but I said, "Yes! Yes! I will do that." "Now remember—I will let you go hunting only once a week. Again I said, "Yes." Now I was full of joy, but I had to work on my father, now that I was cleared with my teacher.

Just before he excused me he told me not to tell any one of my schoolmates. He said, "Be sure to remember to keep this thing within yourself only. If you tell them they will want to go hunting, too, and hunting will take away their attention from school, as it has done to you. Now you may go, but take your books with you." Oh, boy! My mind was so full of good stuff, I started to run; but I stopped short when I ran across a thought that wised me up. If I ran

I might attract people's attention, and make them ask me what I was so excited about. So I slowed down my legs. But my thoughts were in a big hurry and way ahead of me.

In the following afternoon I wrote a short story of my hunting and my teacher rewrote it and he was pleased with it. When he found all of my works satisfactory he said he would excuse me every Friday from that time on. But I became the envy of my schoolmates and gave my teacher a hard time. After a few weeks he was losing his school boys.

Membership in a group. Both directly and indirectly the schoolboy role facilitates and strengthens Robert's membership in various human groups. He is, of course, a member of the schoolroom class, and after his first period of shyness and hesitancy about entering into the network of relationships involved in that, he begins to feel accepted and a part of the undertaking. He also joins his schoolmates in groups that play and have recreation together outside of school hours—doing everything from getting together to talk about hunting, to skating on a small frozen pond or engaging in illicit cigarette smoking. Also Robert remembers his classmates' reactions when he appears at the Christmas program dressed in a new suit of clothes:

As soon as we pulled off our parkas the other children gathered all around us and "ohed" and "ahed." I felt proud all right and somehow I felt full; they hadn't done this to me before. I hadn't been in such good clothes before. I tried hard to smile but couldn't; and I couldn't find a word to say.

The schoolboy role interferes, of course, with his membership in a boat crew. Disappointment is lessened, however, by the attitudes of the boat crew members themselves, who strongly support the need for Robert's getting an education and are willing to accept him as a full-fledged member whenever he is able to hunt with them.

Belonging to a moral order. There are no serious interferences in this respect deriving from the role of schoolboy. Quite the contrary, there is strong support for the idea that Robert is doing the right thing to get educated and to study hard. He himself internalizes this sentiment at an early age and he receives consistent encouragement from others:

Another thing I wanted to have was to learn how to read and write, mostly how to talk English. But I had to have some school to learn any of these, and there wasn't no school of any kind in our camp. We would have to get our school in the village, and I wasn't sure I wanted to be in the village. The schoolteachers wanted us to have some school too. They sent us old books and some school material, but without a teacher they were useless. To us the books were nothing much more than to look at the pictures in them, and the pencils and papers were nothing but to draw pictures with them. But some of our parents had been in school a little bit. It was too bad, cause they lost what little they had learned, because they didn't have much time for reading and writing, or they weren't too interested in that. But they gave us what they had learned, such as how to say and write the numbers and alphabet. And they had done something to me by that. At least they got me started and increased my interest in learning. Uncles and Dad decided to go to the village after trapping season closed in March every year, and came back to the camp before the snow melted. So we could have school that way.

Moreover, school teaches the basic structure of a moral code in specific ways. One time, after the school children had been dismissed to help with the unloading of the annual supply vessel and had thereby earned money for themselves, the teacher commended their behavior. Robert describes this:

After the ship had come was payday—the happy part of the time when we were supplied. I was surprised when I found out that my pay was more than half as much as my Dad's pay. With the money I got us some nice looking red sweat shirts. I proudly gave the shirts to my brothers. When everything was settled down once more, we started to school again. I proudly wore my new red shirt that I had got myself. Our teacher made a short speech that made everybody happy and himself, too. The speech concerned how we had been loyal to the school safety rules and how hard we had worked. He said that he was very glad to see that we had earned our own school clothing. Oh, I hadn't felt so proud before.

Concluding Remarks

Several questions must be faced in a concluding review of the material and technique presented here. Is this a fruitful way to analyze life-history data when the problem is that of examining the longitudinal intersections between sociocultural environment and personality? Does it accomplish the purposes of showing how factors originally external to the person are incorporated into personality processes and function in either a beneficial or injurious manner in regard to maintenance of psychiatric health? Insofar as the pattern of analysis presented here may be helpful, to what extent is it a product of the particular document used? What crucial personality patterns or themes might be left out through use of the role and sentiment concepts? Finally, does the amount of time involved in an analysis of this sort militate against its use on a large scale, so that we can use only relatively few life histories as examples of depth processes, not having enough to use as statistical instances to deal with hypotheses?

It seems to me that the method is useful in showing the manner in which patterned models for behavior deriving ultimately from the cultural environment (e.g., role of hunter, schoolboy, son) become important as motivating forces in a single personality. Moreover, the process extends over a period of several years in which the person is growing, developing, and broadening the cognitive and emotional context into which these segmental roles fit, charting long-term objectives in life. Some aspects of these three particular roles take on crucial significance for the person's self-esteem, his feeling of acceptance by others, his sense of security and substance in life. They are therefore vitally centered in the personality system. But they are similarly critical foci of activities that must be accomplished if the society is to remain an integrated system in its own right. In its present situation, for example, hunting must be done and new incumbents recruited to fill the role in order to provide for the group. The sociocultural significance of the role of son, incorporating as it does many "enculturation" or "socialization" processes, thus performs functions essential to group continuity. Since education is increasingly important for the group's relationships to the white world, the role of schoolboy is similarly vital in sociocultural terms.

I have no doubt that the document used here for illustration is a statistical anomaly, and that if one were to attempt a similar analysis on a series of cases from a population there would not be comparably full material. This difficulty might be ameliorated somewhat through the original gathering of life history in terms of roles, with a concomitant direct attempt always to obtain perceptions of situations recounted and expressions of feelings. An advantage to purposefully structuring the responses in this way is that of achieving some measure of comparability in the basic documents, which is one of the major pitfalls in the life-history approach. The disadvantage in such structuring is posed by the question: What is left out, when one segmentalizes personality into constituent roles, that might be of overriding importance psychodynamically? Intimations of a possibly significant theme in Robert's personality were found throughout the document—his timidity with people and his projections about potential hostility or antagonism to him. This sentiment is possibly an expression of a general insecurity. Perhaps also it is a function of his youth, although when the subject first became known to me nearly ten years after his life-history document ends there was still something of this diffidence and anxious straining to do the right thing in his human relationships.

One way of guarding against ignorance of important sentiments of this type would be to obtain full-length life histories in the traditional manner and then subsequently to segmentalize them into roles as I have done for this one. To do so, however, would probably defeat the purpose of research economy. On the other hand, if a sufficient number of trained assistants is available there is much to be said for obtaining full documents, the most important asset being that the analyst sees the personality more or less as a whole in its uniqueness of experience and perception before he analyzes it in parts.

The problem of the length of time required for analysis by the method proposed here is a real one. I selected three key roles. With a life history from an elderly person there would be a larger number of roles that should be similarly analyzed. It might be necessary, therefore, to limit the analytic process to selected roles. The difficulty, of course, is that of making a wise *a priori* selection of the key roles. These decisions could, however, be guided by the sociocultural investigations that are prerequisite to any intensive work.

A way of speeding up the process of analysis and presentation would be to have trained semiprofessionals index relevant passages throughout a life-history document. They could also be trained to help in the gathering of the data in the first place. It is clear, in any case, that to adapt this approach to any statistically sufficient scale, several people would need to participate in gathering and analyzing the data. As far as I know, no attempts have been made to use life-history materials in a statistical design, and it seems probable that with trial, expeditious maneuvers would come to light.

To me the most important finding in this exercise has been that a large, diffuse environmental process affecting the society as a whole—sociocultural change involving increased interdependence with the white world—can be translated into specific role terms and conflict situations which take on meaning for mental health. This is not to say that this attempt has been a "personality" analysis in which patterned sequences of behavior and thought were traced and related to a theoretical framework. That was not the purpose. But it does mean, I think, that we have seen how several crucial strands of Robert's personality during its unfolding years are intertwined with the network of external social relationships and cultural sentiments of which he is a part.

Notes

1. A. H. Leighton, *The Governing of Men* (Princeton: Princeton University Press, 1946), p. 389.
2. L. Srole, T. S. Langner, S. T. Michael, M. K. Opler, and T. A. C. Rennie, *Mental Health in the Metropolis: The Midtown Manhattan Study* [Thomas A. C. Rennie Series in Social Psychiatry, Vol. I (New York: McGraw-Hill Book Company, 1962)]; T. S. Langner, and S. T. Michael, *Life Stress and Mental Health: The Midtown Manhattan Study* [Thomas A. C. Rennie Series in Social Psychiatry, Vol. II (New York: The Free Press of Glencoe, 1963)]; D. C. Leighton, J. S. Harding, D. B. Macklin, A. M. Macmillan, and A. H. Leighton, *The Character of Danger: Psychiatric Symptoms in Selected Communities* [Vol. III, The Stirling County Study of Psychiatric Disorder and Sociocultural Environment (New York: Basic Books, 1963)]; A. B. Hollingshead and F. Redlich, *Social Class and Mental Illness* (New York: John Wiley & Sons, 1958).
3. This view of life history has been markedly influenced by A. H. Leighton, and D. C. Leighton, *Gregorio, The Hand-trembler* [Peabody Museum Papers (Cambridge, Mass.: Harvard University Press, 1949)].
4. H. A. Murray, "Introduction to Volume I," in *Clinical Studies of Personality. Case Histories in Clinical and Abnormal Psychology*, 2 Vols., A. Burton and R. E. Harris, eds. (New York: Harper & Row, 1955), p. 15.
5. A. H. Leighton, *My Name Is Legion: Foundations for a Theory of Man in Relation to Culture* [Vol. I, The Stirling County Study of Psychiatric Disorder and Sociocultural Environment (New York: Basic Books, 1959)], p. 421.
6. *Ibid.*, pp. 423–424.

Additional Bibliography

Allport, G. W., *Becoming: Basic Considerations for a Psychology of Personality* (New Haven: Yale University Press, 1955).

Deutsch, M., "Field Theory in Social Psychology," in G. Lindzey, ed., *Handbook of Social Psychology* (Cambridge: Addison-Wesley, 1954).

Hughes, C. C., with the collaboration of J. M. Murphy (formerly Hughes), *An Eskimo Village in the Modern World* (Ithaca, N.Y.: Cornell University Press, 1960).

Inkeles, A., and D. J. Levinson, "National Character: The Study of

Modal Personality and Sociocultural Systems," in *Handbook of Social Psychology*, Vol. II, Gardner Lindzey, ed. (Cambridge: Addison-Wesley, 1954).

Kluckhohn, C., "The Influence of Psychiatry on Anthropology in America during the Past One Hundred Years," in *Personal Character and Cultural Milieu*, Douglas Haring, ed. (Syracuse: Syracuse University Press, 1956).

X: Society and Sentiments in Two Contrasting Socially Disturbed Areas

By Seymour Parker and Tom T. Sasaki

EDITORIAL NOTES

Much of the background for this chapter has already been sketched. The topic continues to be the sociocultural environment, but examined from a somewhat different point of view. Like the last chapter, this one deals with a concept that is useful in mapping the interface between person and environment. Where previously the focus was on "role," here attention is given the notion of "sentiment." The concept of sentiment was employed in the Stirling County Study.[1] It has also been alluded to at various points in this book. Sentiments, like values and attitudes, are the recurrent compounds of belief and feeling by which people psychologically structure the sociocultural environment. They are the emotionally toned constructs that define "what is," "what ought to be," and "what is desirable" and thus relate a person to other people and to objects in his environment. Salient sentiments are commonly shared throughout an interacting group, and it is possible therefore to use the idea of "sentiment" to organize information about the way in which the social environment is perceived by a group of people living in it, and its meaning to them in terms of personality functioning.

On the more strictly environmental side of the intersection between individuals and environment, the concern of this chapter is still with culture and with cultural change. The question asked now, however, is whether there are effects characteristic of sociocultural disintegration. That is to say, are there psychological reactions that occur as a result of sociocultural disintegration more or less regardless of either culture or acculturation?

In this aspect, also, the chapter at hand draws on a concept that has been referred to elsewhere in this book and that was previously used in the Stirling Study.[2] "Integration" and "disintegration" have as referents the processes of functioning and malfunctioning of social groups. Disintegration is conceived as a comprehensive pattern of ineffectiveness consisting of various combinations of deleterious factors. As indicated earlier, it was feasible to identify this process in the Stirling County communities by the criteria of poverty, secularization, and cultural confusion. When the process of disintegration reaches an extreme it is characterized by a state of pervasive breakdown in the interaction patterns of a group and may be indexed by such phenomena as ineffective leadership, a high frequency of broken homes, poor communication, increased hostility, and little control of crime and delinquency.

This matter is of some interest because one of the propositions put forward in the Stirling Study is that sociocultural disintegration is conducive to psychiatric disorder in a major way, and that in many circumstances the difference between integration and disintegration will be greater in its psychological concomitants than will the difference between two culturally contrasting but well-integrated social systems.

It was suggested in Chapter VIII that, depending upon *how* and under what conditions acculturation occurs, cultural change is an environmental process that also may be associated with increased prevalence of psychiatric disorders. This chapter follows the same line of thought in proposing that cultural change is mainly productive of psychic stress when it is part of a disintegrating complex, and that, conversely, acculturation may not be associated with a greater tendency to psychiatric disorder when it does not involve disintegration.

Of course no single study can settle this point. In the present chapter, however, Parker and Sasaki seize an opportunity to compare two groups, each with a different culture and each disintegrated. The first is a collection of rural depressed pockets in the Stirling County area of Northeast America. Epidemiological estimates of psychiatric disorder suggested a much higher prevalence than in the surrounding population.[3] The second group is a Navaho settlement at the edge of a boom town in the Southwest. No epidemiological studies were conducted there. Nevertheless it was possible to make a comparison of the sentiment patterns in the socially disrupted Navaho community to see whether primarily they were like those characteristic of Navaho culture generally or like those of the disintegrated community in the Northeast. The results provide a basis for additional thought on disintegration as a process that may have certain uniformities—including certain types of psychological reactions stemming from complexes of similar sentiments—despite cultural differences.

THE rapid pace of technological and social change that has occurred in wide-flung areas of the world since World War II has stimulated both theoretical and practical interest in the "human relations" concomitants of these phenomena. For the development of theory, it would be important to know more about the extent to which transcultural patterns of human behavior can be derived from the varied "natural experiments" in social change. For example, to what degree do cultural differences, in populations experiencing change, influence reactions to roughly similar social processes usually associated with industrialization and urbanization? How will acculturation be affected by such differences?

Practically, we need to understand the mental health implications of social change, and how they vary in different situations. For example, a number of studies have indicated that migration is associated with an increase of mental illness.[4] However, other studies dealing with this relationship have shown that in some situations migration does not appear to be associated with an increase in mental disorder,[5] and even that the two are negatively correlated.[6] Similar apparent contradictions have arisen in research dealing with the mental health and mental illness implications of other sociocultural factors such as status mobility, social isolation, and early socialization experiences. Clearly, more information is needed about the extent to which the variance in any set of epidemiological findings can be explained by a particular variable, and also to what extent (and the mechanism through which) the variable becomes operative in different sociocultural contexts.

Closely associated with mental health is the problem of the development of anomie, often found in populations experiencing rapid social change. This phenomenon has profound ramifications, not only for mental health, but also for economic development and political change. These are but a few of the areas to which cross-cultural studies of social change can make a contribution.

This paper attempts a preliminary comparison of the sentiments held by peoples in two very different societies—a group of Navaho Indians living in the semiurban setting of a small town in the Southwestern United States (1953), and three pockets of economically impoverished and socially disorganized rural slum communities in Maritime Canada (1949–1952).[7] Areas are designated as "socially disturbed," for example: (1) when social life and organization are felt by the local inhabitants to be inadequate to satisfy many of their needs and wants, (2) when social life is perceived as a departure from a more satisfying state of affairs that existed in the past, and (3) when social life is characterized by a high incidence (compared to neighboring communities) of drinking and intoxication, promiscuous sexual relations, crime and delinquency, and physical violence.

Given these gross similarities in both groups, it will be interesting to see what other similarities arise, notwithstanding the divergent character of the cultural backgrounds in the two situations. Problems of comparison often arise in cross-cultural studies owing to manifest differences in cultural beliefs and practices and in value systems. In this connection, we have found the concept of "sentiments" to be helpful. Leighton defines the term "sentiment" as a "representation of predominant ideas that are colored with emotion and feelings, that occur and recur more or less consistently. . . ." [8] Thus, this concept has both cognitive and affective aspects and provides a conceptual device for understanding the manner in which an individual integrates his perceptions, evaluations, and overt reactions to his environment. Although the locus of a sentiment is always within an individual, sentiments that are shared by members of a group provide a communication matrix that permits the integration of interpersonal behavior. Because of this dual aspect, the concept of sentiments serves to bridge the gap between sociocultural and personality processes.

In the course of this paper, when the Navahos or people in the rural slum communities are described as having particular sentiments, we mean that these sentiments are held by the majority of individuals in the subgroup, and also that they provide a cultural climate within which group members relate to each other and to their external environment. Although unconscious motivational elements may frequently underlie a given sentiment, the basic idea contained in it can be consciously formulated. There are, of course, considerable variations among people in the degree of abstraction and the mode of conceptualization of the behavior under consideration. In this sense, a sentiment may be regarded as a conscious aspect of personality functioning.

Although sentiments are derived and inferred by the social scientist from observations of concrete behavior, they are abstractions of patterned reactions to types of social situations and can be employed in comparing common modes of reaction to different cultural settings. In one of the areas studied, for example, a wide variety of authority situations appears consistently to invoke feelings of hostility and of being exploited. Reactions to authority figures are a function of unique aspects in the personality that is reacting and also are a function of the cultural meanings associated with authority situations. These shared meanings contribute to the perception of such specific social situations, illustrating one way in which "sentiment" offers a convenient device for bringing the concepts of personality and culture into a coalescing framework. Thus a sentiment is a statement concerning the relationship between two levels of conceptualization.

The data presented in this study were gathered while the authors were associated with two research projects directed by Alexander H. Leighton. One of the authors of this paper (Parker) was a Research Anthropologist on the Stirling County Study in Nova Scotia (1950–1952) and on the Navaho project in the Southwest (1953). The latter project was concerned with studying social change among Navahos in an area affected by sudden technological developments. The other author (Sasaki) was Assistant Director on the Navaho project from 1948 to 1954. A considerable body of data pertaining to the sentiments in the rural slum area in Nova Scotia was gathered by field workers on the Stirling County Project beginning in 1949. It was upon this material that the present study was built. An examination of these data impressed us with certain interesting parallels (and differences) between the Southwest and the Nova Scotia situations.

In spite of numerous differences between the two populations (many of which are not discussed in this paper), it seemed to us that there was a large area of convergence in some of the salient sentiments. This led to the decision to do a systematic comparison of the outstanding sentiments in both areas. After a preliminary mapping of some of the sentiments, we returned to our respective field situations in order to search for data that would elucidate these initial impressions. By means of interviews with key informants, occupying different positions in the social structures of their respective communities, the preliminary broad outline of sentiments became progressively focused on pertinent target areas. These were further "firmed" by additional interviews and by participant observation in the communities. This more focused research enabled us to modify previous ideas and to incorporate new ones in the final formulation. It also provided insight into some significant sentiments that were peculiar to each of these groups. As will become clear, sentiment 7 pertains only to the rural slum areas, while sentiment 8 characterizes the Navaho subgroup (see pp. 350–351).

At this stage of the research into the system of sentiments characteristic of these two areas it was desirable to "cast a wide net" in order to follow the thread of consistencies in cognition and affect as they operated in a variety of situations. For this reason, and also in order to obtain a deeper understanding of the *function* of any particular sentiment in the social life of the areas, the use of highly structured research techniques was regarded as premature. It should be noted that these comments on research methods pertain only to the data under consideration in the present paper; other kinds of techniques were employed on the larger projects from which this study emerged.

An examination of the present and the recent past of the town Navahos and the inhabitants of the slum settlements indicates a number of broad similarities in the social processes to which they have been exposed. The following presentation will include a brief description of the two communities and a comparison of some of the sentiments they hold.

The Communities

THE RURAL SLUM COMMUNITIES

The rural slum area consists of three communities located near the shore of St. Elizabeth's Bay.[9] Its total population includes approximately 400 people. In the past, these people were caught between two contrasting value orientations, religious beliefs, and languages—those of the French Acadians and those of British Isles derivation. Although this occurred some time ago, the effects are readily observable today. Present-day values and norms consist of a pale, watered-down version of elements of both cultures. Language skills in both idioms are remarkably poor, and religious practices and beliefs are attenuated.[10]

During the nineteenth century and the beginning of the twentieth, these settlements had a thriving economy based on the lumbering and ship-building industries. Prosperity supported the belief among the local inhabitants that governmental intervention of any kind in economic matters was unjustifiable and incompatible with individual initiative.

By the beginning of the twentieth century, there were alarming signs of economic depression and decay. Steam-driven steel hulls and the coming of the railroad were responsible for the decline of the local ship-building and shipping industries. In addition, the virgin timber lands were all but exhausted by 1910. Since the end of World War I the area has experienced chronic depression. Most of the small family woodlands were depleted, and the commercial timberland that remained was bought up by large concerns. Today, sporadic employment may be had in a few small lumber mills or by cutting timber in the backwoods. Both of these occupations are extremely seasonal and yield a submarginal income. Periodic unemployment has become virtually a "normal" state of affairs. The philosophy of self-reliance has been replaced by a deep sense of inferiority and dependency. Such governmental aids as "Mothers Allowance" and unemployment insurance have become expected supplements to income.[11]

In past years, when this area was economically and socially thriving, families tended to live in rather close proximity and to cooperate in economic pursuits. As lumber resources dissolved and shifts took place in family residence, cooperative patterns disappeared. The transition to wage labor accentuated this tendency.

Traditional kinship and neighborhood relationships were further disturbed when existing sources of economic livelihood were swept away and chronic depression set in. At this point, many of the families that had provided leadership for the community's activities migrated to seek better opportunities. As the area came to be regarded as a rural slum and its residents defined as inferior, "misfits" and maladjusted persons drifted in from other places. Group cohesiveness and communal activities declined to such a point that they barely exist today. Visiting patterns are weak and relationships between kin and neighbors are rent with mutual suspicion and hostility.

With the decline of the economic and social life, organized religious activities also suffered a severe setback. There are no full-time clergymen in the depressed pockets. Having accepted the stigma of inferiority and being fully aware of the disdain with which residents in neighboring communities regard them, most of the rural slum dwellers are ashamed to go to church because they feel that they are not wanted there. They are usually identified by their poor clothes and idiosyncratic speech, and are derisively referred to as "monkeys" or by similar terms. They are aware that many of their common experiences are defined as "sinful" by clergymen and religious laymen. Common-law marriages, premarital and extramarital sex relations, excessive drinking, bootlegging, and petty theft are not unusual. Symbols of respectability such as a savings account, a nice home, and good clothes are difficult, if not impossible, for these people to attain. In retaliation for being branded as immoral, lazy, and degenerate, they regard the majority in the religious community as "hypocrites" and "snobs."

Another serious handicap to participation in religious activities results from the nature of the social organization in these communities. The lack of cooperation and patterns of mutual help between neighbors, together with the high level of suspicion and hostility, makes it difficult to organize religious functions.

Almost invariably the inhabitants of the depressed settlements are regarded by residents of the surrounding region as mentally, morally, and genetically inferior. This definition operates in almost every situation in which these people interact with outsiders. These stereotypic expectations themselves are, to some extent, instrumental in calling forth the responses that are condemned as immoral. Thus, a vicious circle of reciprocal behavior is set up from which it is difficult for either the slum dweller or his neighbor to escape.

Very few informal social relationships exist between the rural slum inhabitants and persons in the surrounding district. Friendships and home visiting between the people of the two areas are relatively rare. Even relationships with their kinsmen in neighboring communities have become attenuated.

On the formal level, most of the inhabitants of the depressed neighborhood interact with "outsiders" in a subordinate-superordinate relationship. They take such jobs as common unskilled laborers, domestics, and handymen. During the election period, they are given "rum and a free ride" by the local politicians. Children attending the county schools usually carry the stigma of their home with them. They are regarded by other children as unintelligent, dirty, and immoral.

These settlements have been described as progressively deteriorating over a period of several generations. The following description of the Navaho community illustrates the impact of recent technological and economic changes which resulted in better wages and increased contact with white men, but which also led to consequences similar, in some ways, to that found in the Nova Scotian rural slum.

THE NAVAHO SETTLEMENT

The Navaho settlement consists of roughly 200 people living on the outskirts of a growing industrial town in the northwest part of New Mexico. In addition to these Indian families, a number of Navahos commute to town daily from nearby parts of the reservation. Rich findings of natural gas and oil account for the very rapid development of the community since 1949. Because Navahos came to town primarily for work, most of them have been living here only for a few years. At present more than 90 per cent of the Navaho male working population consists of truck drivers and unskilled laborers on construction jobs. Owing to meager occupational skills and low job seniority, they are usually the first to be fired and the last to be hired.

Perhaps as many as 50 to 60 per cent of the Navaho adult females work as domestics, laundresses, or dishwashers on a part-time basis. Their services can be obtained at a lower rate than that paid to Negroes and Spanish-Americans for comparable work. This creates antagonism between the Indians and these other groups.

Many Navahos still have economic interests on the reservation. For both economic and other reasons, there is considerable movement of Navahos between the reservation and the town.

Two important changes that have come about as a result of the transition from the traditional Navaho economy to a wage-labor system are as follows:

A. In the traditional Navaho economy, women usually owned or controlled more of the economic resources than the men. In their new urban wage economy, this has been reversed.[12] Men have replaced women as the main economic prop of the family. The ramifications of this important role change are manifold and stress-provoking.

B. Traditional Navaho economic activities were based on a defined system of mutual-help patterns within the Navaho extended family, and even within the clan. These cooperative activities formed the core of a more elaborate system of obligation and responsibility woven into the fabric of their social organization. This network of obligations and cooperation has been seriously shaken by the individualistic and impersonal nature of the urban wage economy.

In traditional Navaho life on the reservation, there is little distinction between kin and neighborhood relationships; people who are living in proximity are usually related by kinship ties. Within these extended families and outfits, social interaction is governed by traditionally accepted modes of behavior and mutual obligation. Although social control mechanisms among the Navahos were never as strong and all-embracing as in some neighboring Indian groups (for example, the Pueblos), the individual usually lived his life among kinsmen and remained clearly aware of his obligations and responsibilities to others. The Navahos living in town find themselves in an anomalous situation of being involved in two sets (sometimes overlapping) of residence relationships. In town, the Indian community consists of two concentrations of families living in small huts or tents with relatively undefined and fluid settlement patterns. Families will put up their tents wherever they can obtain space—relatives or friends do not concentrate in one locality. Except for some sporadic church attendance, the town Navahos engage in no formal associations and show almost no tendencies to organize for mutual benefit. Although many consider themselves to be permanent town dwellers, they take little interest in community affairs or in their urban neighbors. Psychologically, most of their "significant others" are on the reservation. Although Navahos have always been helpful to strangers, their traditional organization provides for no set of accepted patterns of behavior toward those who are neither kinsmen nor clan relatives. Western abstract attitudes such as "neighborliness" have little meaning for the Navaho. Generally, aside from relations within the nuclear family, the closest ties of the town Navahos are not with those with whom they daily interact, but with kinsmen on the reservation. It may be said that the town Navaho lives in two worlds—usually at the margin of each.

Navaho religion, unlike religious systems in the Judeo-Christian tradition, does not depend heavily on abstract moral precepts and ethics. It consists of "ways of doing things" within the framework of a traditional social organization. In a sense, it can hardly be said to exist apart from social organization. The shift from the traditional Navaho life on the reservation to an urban setting (where this social organization is rapidly disintegrating) has made it almost impossible for the religious system to be carried over into town life. Town Navahos are becoming increasingly involved in two religious systems—Christianity and Navaho ceremonials in which they participate when they visit the reservation. The reasons Navahos give for not following their traditional ritual practices in town are: (1) many ceremonials can only be performed in hogans—since there are no such traditional houses in town, practices cannot be carried on effectively; (2) most of the kinsmen of the town Navahos are still living on the reservation—since it is necessary for kinsmen to participate in many of the rituals, they must be conducted on the reservation; (3) very few Navahos in town have the knowledge necessary to conduct religious rites; (4) some religious ceremonials are effective only if carried out in places that are involved in traditional Navaho mythology; and (5) Navahos feel that white people would ridicule them if they conducted religious rites in town.

It is safe to say that a very high proportion of urban-dwelling Navahos (perhaps as many as 90 per cent) return to the reservation at least a few times a year to participate in religious ceremonials. This includes many Navahos who are members of a Christian church. Most of the "converts" to Christianity see no contradiction or harm in participating in both Christian and

Navaho religious practices. In fact, this is felt to double their chances of receiving divine aid.

The teachings of Christian missionaries in the area contribute to the stress and conflict among the younger Navahos who attend church and/or mission schools. Local missionaries (for the most part) teach that Navaho religion is a cult of ignorance and superstition that "comes from the devil" and that those who take part in it are doomed to damnation. In sermons, many Navaho practices (e.g., marriage, use of economic resources, sexual mores) are contrasted with "Western" practices, and are labeled as inferior and primitive. Probably, as the town Navaho becomes progressively involved with Christianity, the conflict of choosing between two ways of life will become more serious.

The town-dwelling Navahos sustain two sets of relationships that, to some extent, are kept separate in feeling tone and form of interaction. They maintain contacts with the non-Indian ("Anglo," Spanish-American, and Negro) population of the community as well as with kinsmen and friends on the reservation. Interaction with the former is usually impersonal and pragmatic. This is typified by dealings with merchants and employers. Government employees (both at the local and the federal levels) are treated with deference because of the power they wield and the favors they can dole out. However, they are frequently regarded with suspicion and resentment. This is especially true of the local police force, which is perceived as exploitative and prone to discriminate against Navahos. Although Navahos are aware that they are not held in high regard by the population of the town, this has not seriously deflated their concept of self. The Navahos tend to feel that the non-Indian segment of the town is outside their moral community and circle of significant others. Among the children and the young adults, conflict arising from the prevailing "Anglo" definitions and evaluation of the Navaho people and culture is more serious.

Summary of the Social and Cultural Changes

In both instances, the changes noted above had (and are having) extensive ramifications for role alterations, family life, and virtually all aspects of living. It is of particular interest that the direction of the economic change is different for both groups. In the rural slum communities, the shift has been from prosperity to economic marginality. Contrasted with this, the Navahos are making a transition to a higher material level of living.

Both the Indian and the rural slum populations occupy the lower rung of the status-prestige hierarchy in their respective communities. Many of the subcultural peculiarities of both these groups are characterized as "ignorant," "degenerate," and "inferior" to the cultural values and practices of the dominant society.

The Navahos in the mainly "white" urban setting are, at present, experiencing the push and pull of conflict engendered by an acculturative situation. Although it is too early to predict the results of this process, certain trends indicate similarities to the Maritime communities. Language skills are rapidly declining, especially among the younger Navahos. Although about three-quarters of these people speak some English, it is mostly of a halting and broken nature. Religious conflicts are increasing, and Navahos often engage in both Christian and traditional Navaho religious practices.

With this brief outline of the sociocultural changes in the depressed rural communities and among the town-dwelling Navahos, we are now better prepared to examine some of the similarities and differences in their pattern of sentiments.

Sentiments in Two Socially Disturbed Areas of Contrasting Cultures [13]

1. *People occupying positions of power and authority are exploitative, and thus are to be feared and distrusted. However, one must be deferent when interacting with them.*

With but little variation, this sentiment applies to both the population in the rural depressed area and the community of town Navahos. Many bitter lessons have taught these peoples that authority figures—economic, religious, or political—are to be feared and distrusted. Employers use them for intermittent jobs, laying them off in a manner that appears to them arbitrary, and religious leaders threaten them with divine moral sanctions; for the most part they feel that political leaders are interested in them only for their votes. The government is the source of power that imposes, among other things, restrictive laws on hunting, land ownership and use, timber-cutting, and production of alcoholic beverages, and provides punishment by law-enforcement agencies.

On the other hand, deference behavior must be shown to these "higher-ups," because the people living under depressed circumstances depend heavily on these same authority figures for their survival. Lacking land to exist as independent farmers (even if they had the necessary agricultural skills), lacking sufficiently developed skills to offer successful competition on the job market, lacking enough education to deal with complex problems of modern existence, they depend on these authority figures for the few benefits they are able to exact. Political bosses provide patronage and jobs such as road work; economic bosses provide jobs and credit; religious leaders control access to the blessings of supernatural favors; and the government provides the pensions, family allowances, welfare, and other benefits.

While the sentiment generally applies to both areas, it arises out of somewhat different kinds of experiences. In the slum communities, development of this sentiment begins in infancy in the family arena. There, the father is the authority figure, and the child learns early that he is likely to displace his hostility and aggressions on the children for frustrations he has experienced elsewhere. Punishment is seemingly willful, harsh, arbitrary, and unjust. Uncertainties about authorities are generalized, and the difficult circumstances of adult life provide ample ground for reinforcing early distrust.

Among the town Navahos, this sentiment stems from their long experiences with "Anglos" mentioned earlier. The Navahos have been exploited by some unscrupulous traders, have heard belittling remarks about their native institutions, and have, at times, been subjected to unfair treatment by the police force. The unpredictable and often confusing manner in which government policies have been carried out on the reservation is too well documented to require expansion here.

2. *Nature and the world around are full of threats from dangerous supernatural forces such as witches and ghosts.*

Although members of the depressed rural communities frequent the woods while hunting or lumbering, many of them seem to be very fearful of evil forces lurking in this environment. These fears, possibly augmented by projections of antisocial hostile impulses, are nurtured and fed by an interest in sadistic and bloody "comic" books and pulp magazines.

Stories are common about ghosts (especially of individuals who met a violent end) haunting the woods or returning to their homes. Apparitions make their presence known by knocks on the walls and other weird signs. The motivation for these nocturnal perambulations is usually revenge. There are stories about "forerunners" or omens of evil, and there even have been several cases of alleged witchcraft in the area.

In their attitudes toward organized religion, these people emphasize impressively the more punitive rather than the rewarding aspects of supernatural powers. God might strike one blind, or cripple one. The devil is an ever-present source of trouble and pain. Religion provides but a weak force for moral improvement. However, the extent to which it is operative rests on the fear of divine punishment rather than internalized concepts of intrinsic goodness or badness.

Witchcraft fears among Navahos on the reservation seem to

be the strongest where social disorganization is most severe.[14] Among the Navahos who live in the vicinity of the town, violence stemming from witchcraft accusations has not infrequently occurred. Several diviners, hand-tremblers, and star-gazers are available to Navahos for diagnostic purposes. The diviners, besides having the purported ability to diagnose illnesses, make prophecies, and recommend singers and sings, also "point" to persons presumably responsible for causing illness by witchcraft.

In their contacts with missionaries, the Navahos have added a new dimension to their own supernatural world. Such new and relatively little understood concepts as hell, heaven, and divine wrath frequently provoke anxiety in believers.

> 3. *Human success and getting ahead in life are beyond the control of the individual. The main forces behind social and material success are "luck" and "pull."*

The concept of getting ahead through one's own efforts is not well developed in the rural slum area, nor is it felt that if one is good he receives God's help. The major forces thought to be responsible for economic success are "luck" or "pull."

In a questionnaire administered to workers from the rural slum areas, a frequent response concerning how the working man can get ahead was that it was only possible through "luck" or by "knowing the right people" and not by hard work and initiative.

Among town Navahos, this sentiment also prevails. However, social and material success lack precise definition and social consensus. Navahos do not usually wish or expect to mingle socially with "Anglos," nor are "middle-class Anglo" valuations on items such as good homes and furniture important to them. Success in this "alien" situation is measured largely in the accomplishment of immediate ends: getting a job, being the last fired, buying a car, and finding a friend are all measures of success accomplished by means of "luck."

On the reservation, the goals, and means of achieving them, are fairly clear-cut. The Navahos behave in traditionally defined ways to achieve socially valued ends. The means-ends relationship is defined within the context of their value system and beliefs. On the other hand, the town Navahos are still unable to link one item of behavior with the other insofar as they relate to means and ends.

4. *Concerted activity toward long-range goals is futile. Short-range gratifications are the main things worth striving for.*

This sentiment is implied in those stated earlier, and expressions of it are numerous. In general, there is very little anticipation of, planning for, or aspiring toward distant goals. In the depressed settlements, pensioners sometimes "drink up" a considerable portion of their check money the same day they receive it. The liquor bottle provides immediate gratification and freedom from worry about the consequences of momentary extravagance.

The work situation offers many overt expressions of this sentiment. Local men are regarded as irresponsible; they do not appear at the appointed place for work, or they work at a job long enough to pay for food, settle pressing bills, or buy liquor and then quit until their needs force them to work again. Statements frequently heard are: "Let someone else work for a while; I've got my share," or "I've got enough for now; I'll give someone else a chance."

The roots of this sentiment differ in the two areas. In the case of the slum communities, there is a long history of depressed circumstances which breed such sentiments. Among the town Navahos, the sentiment is partially a carry-over from their reservation-oriented values. The reservation Navaho is "industrious in order to accumulate possessions—within certain limits." [15] He also will "stop work when he is comfortably off, or even sooner, partly for fear of being called a witch if he is too successful." [16] Both the level and content of the Navahos' achievement motivation differ from "Western" motivation in this regard.

The general patterns of spending hard-earned money, even aside from the patterns of liquor purchase, reflect this sentiment. Rural slum women who work in shellfish plants spend their checks on "flashy" impractical clothing which provides momentary gratification. They neglect nutrition and medical care because they do not satisfy obvious and immediate needs, and live on inadequate diets such as boiled cabbage or pancakes with molasses, with occasional baked beans included. Navahos subsist on coffee and bread when they are out of work, and at other times gorge themselves with mutton.

5. Physical labor is a necessity for satisfying immediate needs —it has no intrinsic value.

In sharp contrast to the surrounding communities, the attitudes in the "depressed rural pockets" toward work reflect this sentiment. In the past, the entire region was largely characterized by the attitude that work *in itself* is a good thing. This value is now lacking, and in its place one finds the pervasive attitude that work is largely a matter of being exploited in an unpleasant and difficult kind of activity. However, it must be endured periodically for short-range gratification and in order to keep alive.

Expressions of this sentiment are numerous, sometimes overlapping with those about attitudes toward employers. Lumbermill workers sometimes cut machine driving belts so that work will be lightened for a while during repairs, young people are increasingly reluctant to engage in sustained hard work, and malingering on the job is fairly frequent. "Putting in time" and "one job is the same as another" are other commonly heard comments.

Similar patterns of overt behavior and verbal expressions are found among the town Navahos. On the reservation, "industry is enormously valued," and "faithful performance of duties" is given a high place in the enumeration of virtues.[17] Contrasted with their situation on the reservation, where relatives and friends constantly scrutinize behavior, Navahos in the town are among relatively indifferent neighbors.

6. *Upward mobility, on the part of a member of the in-group, is considered equivalent to rejection of the in-group.*

Any indication of striving for success and upward social mobility is interpreted as a threat to the notions embodied in some of the prior sentiments, e.g., success is not due to individual efforts or worth, but to "luck" or "pull." These serve to minimize the stress resulting from failure to "make the grade." Also, successful upward mobility tends to "ally" the mobile person with authority figures. As long as it is felt that uncontrollable forces keep people "down," the loss of self-esteem can be reduced. However, when a member of the group successfully challenges the idea that these forces are insuperable, the rest must either attack the individual or experience self-deprecation.

Expressions of this sentiment are frequent in the rural settlements. Self-improvement is ridiculed, and predictions of failure are constantly made about those who actively attempt to improve their economic or social position.

The town Navahos participate in *three social worlds:* the reservation, the town "tent city," and the wider town context. The standards of success in each of these are measured differently and are, to some extent, compartmentalized in the Navaho's mind. In the first two situations, traditional attitudes toward outstanding individual economic success, and the responsibilities it entails, probably act as a brake on upward mobility.

Several Navaho families in town have "made the grade" in the white world. They live "on the right side of the tracks," and participate in the social activities of the "Anglo" world. Because of this, they are frequently labeled "agency Indians," and are said to be "going the white way." In recent years, some jealousies have developed among those who have cut themselves off from Navaho society and who speak out without hesitation about the behavior of "blanket Indians." As against the feelings of futility which the people in the depressed pockets have about upward mobility, the town Navahos strike hard at what they believe will improve their standing—namely, education for their children.[18]

> 7. *Residents of the depressed rural communities are morally and mentally inferior to people in neighboring communities.*

These people are excluded from full participation in the occupational, educational, and social activities of the communities surrounding them. They are unable to secure or hold good jobs, as can their neighbors, unable to achieve as high a level of education, and unable to participate in the social and institutional activities of the type characteristic of the surrounding region. The explanation used by outsiders who consider themselves living in "respectable communities" is that the people of the depressed areas are mentally and morally inferior to most people. What is more important, the people of these depressed areas themselves have partly incorporated this prevailing definition of their inferiority into their collective self-image. This concept of self has an inhibiting effect on their motivation to improve.

Expressions of this sentiment are numerous and easily accessible on an overt level. They take two forms, depending on the context of the relationship between the observer and informant. The most frequent and initially accessible level is manifest when the observer is defined as an outsider of superior status. In this situation there is often a continuous round of belittling comment and gossip about the neighbors, friends, and relatives of the informant. The second kind of expression is where the informants themselves openly state that they, too, share these undesirable characteristics of inferiority. This second level of manifestation is only reached after the informant becomes convinced that the observer knows the situation too well to be fooled into believing that the informant is really dissociated from those whom he belittles, or when the informant is in a situation where he pours forth many ordinarily suppressed thoughts and feelings, e.g., while under the influence of liquor.

Some expressions of hostility may be due to residual feelings that cannot be expressed easily within the community because of the already very tenuous nature of friendship and cooperative bonds. There is the fear that even these will be disrupted and shattered by any strong overt expression of hostility.

The attempt to dissociate oneself from the neighborhood context is frequently encountered when one meets a person from the depressed area away from his home. When such a person is asked where he comes from, he usually gives a vague answer, denoting a region or the nearest community that has high status. It is only after a great deal of pressing and narrowing-down that one learns that his actual residence is in the slum area.

8. *Situations are to be evaluated according to the definitions as set down either by the white or Navaho way of life.*

An outsider is constantly impressed with what seems to be paradoxical behavior among Navahos. They attend native religious ceremonies as readily as they attend Christian rites. They go to white doctors, and then have curing ceremonies conducted by their own medicine men. Medicine men and diviners send patients to hospitals as often as they recommend sings or other native practitioners. They are intensely concerned about their role obligations in their own social situation, but in their relation with "Anglos" apparently similar obligations are often overlooked.

There are indications, however, that such "contradictory" behavior is becoming less clear-cut as acculturation experience increases. The Navahos' attempt to incorporate white middle-class values creates considerable confusion. The whites place a high value on good housing and furniture; the Navahos do not earn enough, nor do they have a clear conception, by middle-class standards, of what a "good" house is. Whites stress cleanliness; Navahos live in the poorer section of town, where running water is difficult to come by. Missionaries preach that Christianity and native religion are not compatible; the Navahos, under constant derogation, are beginning to become ashamed of their own religion.

Certain situations that are dichotomized on the reservation are becoming less so among town Navahos. They still believe in sings, but the shacks and tents in which they live are not considered appropriate settings for them. Furthermore, town Navahos have few friends and relatives in town to help pay for such curing rites, not to mention the difficulties in finding a singer. To return to the reservation for ceremonials is becoming more difficult because relatives and friends are in similarly dire financial straits. Therefore, town Navahos are beginning to rely more and more on white man's medicine, and to give up their attitude that curing rites are at all necessary.

Navaho children are the chief victims of this growing confusion and multiple standards. At school they see themselves in a situation where standards are set by white children. At home the Navaho children find behavior and housing conditions far "inferior" to what they experience in school. Their clothes appear relatively shabby, their speech is noticeably inferior, and they look different.

Summary and Conclusions

The coincidence of overlapping sentiments among the two groups we have examined indicates broad areas of similarity. This is true in spite of the fact that the actual cultural patterns of these societies are widely divergent. Although differences were apparent in the description of some of the more outstanding aspects of the social environments and historical backgrounds of these people, a certain similarity of experience along the continua of broad social processes was noted. Both populations have been involved in a rapid acculturative process, have encountered rather sudden economic and technological changes, and occupy the lowest socioeconomic stratum.

Although this paper has not been specifically geared to a discussion of mental health problems, we have provided some pertinent background data for a consideration of the cultural context in which these problems occur. Rapid social change creates a fertile breeding ground for such problems. However, the outcome of the challenges posed by social change will be, in part, determined by the pattern of sentiments held by the population involved in the phenomenon.

At this time it might be fruitful to discuss some of the differences between the Navahos and the rural slum dwellers that are potentially related to mental health and illness. The previously discussed significant reference groups of these peoples are important determinants of their feelings of self-esteem and personal worth.

At a number of points in this paper the issue of reference groups in these two populations has been discussed. For purposes of understanding the psychological stresses to which these people are exposed it is crucially important to know, not only their actual position in their respective societies, but also their value frame of reference.[19] With whom do they compare themselves? In a large measure, this will determine the nature of their self-concept, their level of aspiration, and their evaluation of their own achievement in various areas of life. Although both populations occupy the lowest socioeconomic stratum in their communities, the implications of this fact for their mental health are very different.

The people in the depressed pockets are almost universally defined as inferior (intellectually, physically, and morally) by those in their larger community. For the most part this definition has been adopted as their own concept of self. Their only frame of reference for judging their lives and achievements is the "respectable" elements of society. These standards are held up before them in the schools, in the churches (which are attended sporadically), and in all the popular media of mass communication. It is not surprising to find that the people in the depressed pockets exhibit a plethora of self-devaluations. Closely related to this is a feeling of powerlessness to manipulate and control their external environment, which always appears "to be doing things *to* them." This further contributes to a drastic lowering of levels of aspiration, which is clearly seen in the frequent apathetic reactions to the challenges with which they are faced. Although the standards used for self-evaluation are those of the larger society, the norms of behavior and goals of the latter are not sufficiently meaningful for the slum dwellers to become part of their motivational system, or serve as an effective means of social control.

Let us briefly compare this description with that of the reference-group behavior among the town Navahos. Here the situation is more complicated and (at this point in time) probably less psychologically stressful. Although the Navahos occupy the lowest socioeconomic stratum in their community, their frame of reference for self-evaluation and appraisal of their material achievements stems from life on the reservation. As yet the small Christian sect has not brought about large-scale conversion. The majority of Navahos return to the extended family on the reservation for their religious ceremonials. Many of them still own property on the reservation and have hogans there for their use. Although this becomes less true as time passes, Navaho adults in town do not appear to evaluate themselves by white standards. Clearly the jobs that they occupy and their economic situation are not thought of as inferior by their reference-group. Although other conflicts occur because of their marginal position, the self-image of the town Navaho has not been debased nor have they exhibited any lowering of their levels of aspiration. In evaluating the future development of this Navaho community the study of their reference-group values is important.

There are some indications that conflict and self-devaluation are becoming serious problems among the young people. It is questionable whether the two worlds can be kept apart much longer. Insofar as the social-isolation theory of schizophrenia is valid,[20] one could predict that there is less schizophrenic withdrawal among the town Navahos than among the rural slum dwellers.

The differential impact of social change on the sex roles in the two groups also has relevance for psychiatric problems. Past social changes in the rural communities served to remove the father from the home for varying periods in his pursuit of a livelihood. The dwindling of economic resources further undermined the male in his attempt to perform his family roles. On the other hand the women were increasingly employed as domestics, and as hands in some of the local fish processing and packing plants. In such a situation it is likely that the male might develop serious confusion about his sex role and doubts about his "masculinity." This situation provides fertile ground for such problems as sexual impotence and possibly various forms of sexual perversion and promiscuity.

In this regard, the impact of social change among the Navahos has been very different. First, it should be noted that the Navahos' sentiments concerning "masculinity" and "femininity" were traditionally very different from those prevailing, for the most part, in the Western world. The Navaho woman on the reservation usually owns a great deal of property and has always provided a considerable portion of the family's income. In terms of decision-making within the family, the woman's position was at least equal to that of the man. In town, the woman's traditional role is weakened. Her husband now provides the main support of the family. If he deserts her, or fails to provide income for varying periods, her subsistence and that of her children are seriously endangered. No longer can the automatic support of the extended family be counted on in such a situation, as it was on the reservation. Clearly the town Navaho wife has become much more economically dependent on her husband. At the same time, sentiments carried over from traditional Indian culture ill-adapt her for this increased and enforced dependency. In this connection, it is interesting that a rise in antisocial behavior among Navaho women in the town community has been notable. On the other hand, the changes for the male have been a mixed blessing. He now finds that his wife and family are completely dependent on him. Social workers and law-enforcement agencies often plague him when he becomes delinquent in assuming his new responsibilities. To what extent has his recent increase in status position within the family compensated for the burden of new responsibilities and independence? Certainly this would be an important area of investigation in a mental health study. Conversations with some of the local physicians in the community indicate the possibility that psychophysiological complaints of various sorts are on the increase among male Navahos. Also of relevance here is the fact that Navaho males did not associate their "masculinity" with mastery over females and being the sole support of the family. This would lessen the probability of sexual malfunctioning when other aspects of the male role are disturbed.

Our data allow some interesting speculation about differences in the types of psychiatric symptoms that might be found in the two groups. We have already spoken about the possibility of greater self-devaluation and sexual problems among the rural slum dwellers. Also, the lack of clear-cut norms of behavior and greater disorganization of the family among the rural slum dwellers is likely to yield a higher proportion of "psychopathic personalities" among their psychiatric disorders. On the other hand, the traditional concern in Navaho society with physical health problems, plus the relatively tighter social control in the Navaho community, may produce a relatively greater amount of psychophysiological complaints among these people. The considerable degree of normlessness among the rural slum dwellers with an accompanying high degree of antisocial aggressive behavior in their environment may also potentially make for frequent symptoms of paranoid ideation.

In some respects, the Navaho town community today is in a position similar to that of the depressed Maritime communities during the latter part of the nineteenth century. Whether or not they will evolve in the same direction depends on a complicated set of factors, such as the economic destiny of the area, the attitudes and behavior of the larger "Anglo" community toward this group, and the internal resources of these people to cope in a progressive fashion with the disorganizing tendencies of rapid social change, and the fate of the reservation Navaho community. Any sudden or sharp barriers preventing the town Navaho from identifying positively with the larger community of reservation Indians will probably have serious consequences for his self-respect and will ultimately reduce his chances of becoming a contributing member of the dominant society.

Notes

1. A. H. Leighton, *My Name Is Legion: Foundations for a Theory of Man in Relation to Culture* [Vol. I, The Stirling County Study of Psychiatric Disorder and Sociocultural Environment (New York: Basic Books, 1959)], especially ch. 7 and App. A; C. C. Hughes, M.-A. Tremblay, R. N. Rapoport, and A. H. Leighton, *People of Cove and Woodlot: Communities from the Viewpoint of Social Psychiatry* [Vol. II, The Stirling County Study of Psychiatric Disorder and Sociocultural Environment (New York: Basic Books, 1960)], especially ch. 3, 4, 5, and 6.

2. A. H. Leighton, *op. cit.*, especially ch. 6; C. C. Hughes, *op. cit.*, especially ch. 2.

3. D. C. Leighton, J. S. Harding, D. B. Macklin, A. M. Macmillan, and A. H. Leighton, *The Character of Danger: Psychiatric Symptoms in Selected Communities* [Vol. III, The Stirling County Study of Psychiatric Disorder and Sociocultural Environment (New York: Basic Books, 1963)], especially ch. 11.

4. See: B. Malzberg, and E. S. Lee, *Migration and Mental Disease* (New York: Social Science Research Council, 1956); Ø. Ødegaard, "Emigration and Insanity, A Study of Mental Disease Among the Norwegian-born Population of Minnesota," *Acta Psychiatrica et Neurologica*, Suppl. 4 (Copenhagen, 1932); A. Weinberg, "Mental Health Aspects of Voluntary Migration," *Mental Hygiene*, vol. 39 (1955), pp. 450–464.

5. See: C. Tietze, P. Lemkau, and M. Cooper, "Personality Disorders and Social Mobility," *American Journal of Sociology*, vol. 48 (1942), pp. 29–39; A. B. Hollingshead, and F. Redlich, *Social Class and Mental Illness* (New York: John Wiley & Sons, 1958), p. 245.

6. See: Ø. Ødegaard, "The Distribution of Mental Disease in Norway: a Contribution to the Ecology of Mental Disorder," *Acta Psychiatrica et Neurologica*, vol. 20 (1945); M. H. Lystad, "Social Mobility among Selected Groups of Schizophrenic Patients," *American Sociological Review*, vol. 22 (1957), pp. 288–292; R. J. Kleiner, and S. Parker, "Migration and Mental Illness: A New Look," *American Sociological Review*, vol. 24 (1959), pp. 287–290.

7. Although we use the designation "community" to describe these settlements, it is doubtful that they have enough internally cohesive formal or informal structure to merit the appellation.

8. A. H. Leighton, *My Name Is Legion*, pp. 26, 233, and 257.

9. St. Elizabeth's Bay is a pseudonym used in order to protect the identity of community residents.

10. For a more detailed description of the overall characteristics and history of the depressed communities and the surrounding area see: C. C. Hughes, *People of Cove and Woodlot;* see also A. M. Macmillan, and A. H. Leighton, "People of the Hinterland," in E. H. Spicer, ed., *Human Problems in Technological Change* (New York: Russell Sage Foundation, 1952). The latter is a description and analysis of one area in particular.

11. The "Mothers Allowance" is a sum given to families by the government of Canada at the birth of a child.

12. L. S. Hamamsy, "The Role of Women in a Changing Navaho Society," *American Anthropologist*, vol. 59, no. 1 (Feb. 1957), pp. 101–111.

13. The formulation of sentiments of the rural slum communities was originally undertaken as a working memorandum by the staff members of the Stirling County Study. Those who were mainly responsible for the original formulation were C. C. Hughes, A. M. Macmillan, S. Parker, R. N. Rapoport, and R. N. Wilson. The statement of the sentiments that appears in this paper departs slightly from the original version. A more complete discussion of this material appears in C. C. Hughes, *People of Cove and Woodlot.*

14. C. Kluckhohn, "Navaho Witchcraft," *Peabody Museum Papers*, Harvard University, vol. 22, no. 2 (1944).

15. C. Kluckhohn, and D. C. Leighton, *The Navaho* (Cambridge, Mass.: Harvard University Press, 1946), p. 220.

16. *Ibid.*, p. 222.

17. *Ibid.*, p. 220.

18. Although some parents in the rural slum area express a desire for

their children to obtain a decent education, there is very little evidence that they actually strive or make sacrifices to achieve this end.

19. It may be pertinent to note here that Clausen and Kohn, in a recent study, found that those in the lower socioeconomic class in their population did not yield a higher rate of "functional psychoses" than those in the strata above them. This finding is contrary to those of previous epidemiological studies. For the details of the Clausen and Kohn findings, see: J. A. Clausen, and M. Kohn, "Relation of Schizophrenia to the Social Structure of a Small City," in B. Pasamanick, ed., *Epidemiology of Mental Disorder* (Washington, D.C.: American Association for the Advancement of Science, 1959), pp. 69–94.

20. S. K. Weinberg, "A Sociological Analysis of a Schizophrenic Type," *American Sociological Review*, vol. 15 (1950), pp. 600–610.

XI: Psychophysiological Symptoms and the Status of Women in Two Mexican Communities

By *Thomas S. Langner*

EDITORIAL NOTES

This, the final chapter, describes a study in which one of the "approaches" discussed earlier was employed in cross-cultural epidemiological research from which substantive findings can be presented. Chapter IV focused on the possibilities of using a scorable set of test questions (the HOS) in a non-European culture. The particular emphasis of that chapter was on feasibility, and an exploratory field trial was made with a small sample of Eskimos. Evidence was gathered from multiple sources in order to estimate validity, and effort was made to detect influences that might be characteristic of culture and situation rather than of psychiatric disorder.

The present chapter has to do with the same kind of instrument—the Twenty-two Item Score used previously in the Midtown Study and familiar to the reader from the discussion in Chapter IV. The context of this study remains exploratory, but a different set of questions is taken up. Setting aside the matter of indicator validity, this investigation is concerned with the administration of the questionnaire to large numbers of people in a different culture and its employment as an integral part of a research design that attempts to test a hypothesis.

The investigation was conducted by Langner in two Mexican groups in 1959. The two groups were selected for contrasts of a variety of kinds. The Mexican project followed Langner's work as a sociologist in the Midtown Study.

In regard to analysis of the sociocultural environment as well as in the use of the Twenty-two Item Score this report takes off from the Midtown Study. A central notion is that of "status." In the forerunning metropolitan research, the distribution of psychiatric symptoms in the population was found to vary significantly with socioeconomic status; the lower the position on the socioeconomic scale the more likely that the individual was psychiatrically impaired. In the Mexican study there is continued emphasis on socioeconomic status; however, Langner extrapolates from this to an investigation of status differences between men and women. It is customary to view "status" in this latter regard as closely allied to "role." The similarities and differences between the two concepts are pointed out in this chapter, and Langner uses "status" to refer to "relative position in a hierarchy." It is of interest, however, to recall the conceptualization of "role" employed in Chapter IX. Where previously "role" was conceived as a valuable device for intensive analysis of life experiences, here a rather comparable idea—"status"—is used extensively. "Status" is employed as a way to generalize about the "role" or "position" of all women in a given cultural group *vis-à-vis* all men of the same group.

This approach allows the application of epidemiological techniques. The hypothesis guiding this investigation is that low status, either in the socioeconomic scale or in the social hierarchy of men and women, is stressful and conducive to the development of psychiatric symptoms. Research results concerning this proposition are given in the following pages.

THIS paper is concerned with the use of a psychological screening questionnaire in a cross-cultural situation.[1] The general hypothesis to be tested was that persons of low status report a greater number of psychophysiological symptoms than those of high status. There is already considerable evidence that persons of low socioeconomic status report a greater number of these symptoms than people of high socioeconomic status.[2] In light of this, it appears worthwhile to ask further questions about the relationships between symptom prevalence and other kinds of status: for example, do women whose status is greatly inferior to that of the men in a given community report more symptoms than women in a community where the two sexes are more equal? Mexico City and a provincial town in Mexico were chosen as communities offering maximum contrast in the position of women. Thus a natural situation was selected that would approximate an experimental design.

This report will cover the development of the general hypothesis. It will define the term "status," which is central to the hypothesis. Descriptions of the two communities, the screening device, and the field procedures will be followed by the presentation of statistical data and interpretations.

A General Hypothesis

Many studies have found that a large proportion of persons in treatment for various types of disorder are of low socioeconomic status.[3] People of low income, having little education, and engaged in unskilled labor, comprise the greater proportion of those now in treatment in mental hospitals and clinics.

What about those in the community with emotional disorders who are not in any kind of treatment? Recent population surveys in Midtown Manhattan and Stirling County have shown that a large segment of the general population can be considered to show some psychiatric impairment or disorder. Most of this segment have not sought or received therapy of any kind. The surveys found again that the low socioeconomic portion of the community was contributing most heavily to this large pool of untreated mental disorder. In addition, the Midtown Study found that persons of low socioeconomic status report a greater number of *psychophysiological* symptoms than do those of upper status. A score based on twenty-two of these symptoms was highly correlated with two clinicians' ratings of overall psychiatric impairment (tetrachoric $r = .80$). Our concern in this paper will be with the prevalence of these psychophysiologic symptoms.[4]

Why is socioeconomic status related to mental disorder? Any hypothesis to be formulated must hinge on the meaning and implications of the word "status." It is defined in *Webster's Universal Dictionary* as "standing or position as regards rank or condition; as a man's social status." Although the same term is often used to denote a "socially defined behavior pattern" or a collection of rights and duties, this latter meaning is reserved in the presentation here for the word "role."

A "role" can be thought of as the dynamic aspect of a status. "When he puts the rights and duties which constitute the status into effect, he is performing a role." [5] There are some advantages, however, in using the term "role" (rather than status) for the *abstract pattern* of rights and duties, and the phrase "role performance" for the *actual behavior* of an individual. The term "status" is now generally reserved for designating "relative standing" (Webster) or *relative position* in a hierarchy. Benoit-Smullyan suggests three criteria for differentiation between individuals: status (relative hierarchical position), situs (membership in a social group), and locus (socially defined function in an organized group, or *role*).[6] He clearly makes a distinction between status and role.

Status or ranking of individuals may be made on the basis of economic, political, or prestige criteria. Socioeconomic status is based upon economic standing and various prestige criteria such as education and occupation. Higher education and the professional and skilled occupations are generally accorded higher prestige. Social status is a judgment of the rank of an individual on the basis of a value hierarchy.[7] Thus the specific cultural prestige rankings of the economic sphere itself, as well as occupation, education, skin color, reading habits, dress, and other characteristics, combine to determine the individual's status. Secure status must rest on a nonambivalent value system that assigns stable rankings to various behaviors or characteristics. The importance of the subjective cultural values in determining "status" as opposed to more objective measures or criteria constituting a "class" or category of persons (such as income, relationship to the means of production, height, or weight) was clearly recognized by Max Weber:

In contrast to the purely economically determined "class situation" we wish to designate as "status situation" every typical component of the life fate of men that is determined by a specific, positive or negative, social estimation of honor.[8]

Since subjective "social estimation" may vary radically between cultures, nations or regions, *status itself must also vary between cultures*. Objective measures, however, should yield comparable "classes" of individuals who have some characteristics in common despite cultural differences.

Socioeconomic status is only one of various status ranking systems. Age is another criterion of status, by virtue of the prestige attached to various age levels. Age ranks show a wide range of status variation within and between cultures. The status of the aged is low in the United States as compared, for example, with that of traditional China or Europe. When the West Germans referred to Chancellor Adenauer as "Der Alte," they indicated respect.

Since time immemorial, sex has been another criterion of status. There are few cultures past or present that accord more prestige and power to women than to men. Hence sex, age, and socioeconomic position are all variables commonly used in the hierarchical ranking of individuals.

Low socioeconomic position is not the only low status associated with increased risk of mental disturbance. Larger proportions of Midtown residents showed some psychiatric impairment of functioning within each age decade from the twenties through the fifties.[9] While physiological changes may account in part for some of this rise in impairment with increasing age decades, the large proportion of impaired individuals in their fifties also may be partially due to loss of status. This proportional increase in impairment with age is independent of socioeconomic status, which in itself tends to diminish among the older age groups.

If low socioeconomic status and low age status are both associated with a greater risk of mental disturbance, other low statuses might show a similar association. In particular it can be hypothesized that in a culture where women were accorded low status they would have more symptoms of mental disorder than men. Conversely, women who have equal status with men would resemble men closely in regard to the number of their symptoms.

Why do persons of low status seem more likely to exhibit symptoms than those of high status? Many hypotheses could be invoked to explain this relationship. Perhaps people of low status are actually subjected to more environmental stress. For example, persons of low socioeconomic status may have to work harder and longer with less food, clothing, and shelter than others. Older people, particularly those over sixty in the United States, tend to be of low socioeconomic status. Their earning power is drastically curtailed; they are more prone to the deteriorative diseases; and many have suffered the loss of spouse and friends. It is difficult, however, to support the argument that women are exposed to more stress than men.

A less probable explanation of the status differentials in symptom prevalence invokes heredity or endowment. This position holds that the poor are genetically deprived, the aged are fated to deteriorate, and women are physiologically or mentally inferior to men, *hence* their almost universally low position. This argument does not, however, account for the upwardly mobile children of the backwoods or slum areas, the active octogenarians, or the increasing leadership of women in our society.

A third relevant hypothesis is that low status inhibits the development or maintenance of ego-strength. In its broadest definition, ego-strength is synonymous with ability to resist stress. More specifically, it involves adaptive ability, planning for individual survival, conscious control over the self, and conscious attempts to control the environment. Strange as it may seem, this "enlightened self-interest" does not automatically function as part of natural human endowment. On the contrary, it seems to flourish only when the individual has been exposed to love, affection, and attention.

While love and attention are most important in the rankings of siblings, prestige status soon becomes important in the lives of most Americans. This is clearly shown in accounts by Bernice Neugarten of the prestige ranking systems of young school children.[10] She found that children from poorer families—regardless of their dress, habits, behavior, intelligence, or classroom performance—were perceived by children of wealthier families as sloppy, dirty, mean, and stupid. Socioeconomic status, worship of youth, disparagement of the aged and minority groups—all these rankings soon become an integral part of the child's value system. In the adult world, the emotional benefits derived from prestige, signs of deference, conspicuous consumption, career, and success may abet, and perhaps even replace, the function of love and affectional bonds. Although attention is a poor substitute for affection, whether received from one's family or society in general, it may sometimes be the only nutriment available for perpetuation of the self.

It seems clear that prestige status—derived from various roles such as executive, athlete, or debutante—becomes an important source of attention and perhaps even affection after early childhood. Status is accorded to people who play these roles by the "significant others" in one's life: friends, associates, and the community at large. After affection provides the soil for the development of ego-strength, status may in effect provide continued nutrition.

Ego-strength may be evaluated indirectly by assessing an individual's "self-image." It is generally agreed that how a person feels about himself is to a large extent the product of what others have felt about him or toward him. Their estimate of him is largely reflected in his estimate of himself. This process starts with parents and siblings and continues with peers, teachers, neighbors, work associates, and finally with society as a whole. To say that his self-esteem as an adult is partly a reflection of the esteem of others would be accurate. If, however, he were merely a mirror-image of the demands, values, and opinions of others, he would exhibit the "pseudo-self" which Fromm feels is an important criterion of neurosis.[11]

In initiating this work, it seemed to me that persons of low status would tend to exhibit a negative self-image, while those of high status would be more likely to have a positive self-image. Self-image was, in turn, assumed to be indicative of ego-strength. Without love, attention, and status, the processes of adaptation and planning would be abandoned. Instead withdrawal, resignation, fatalism, physical violence, alcoholism, and addiction would be utilized as ways of meeting life stresses.

An initial assumption (which later proved false) was that people project their individual self-images onto persons of their age-sex position in general. For example, I assumed that a woman who does not hold herself in high esteem will agree that "men are more intelligent than women" or that "women's place is in the home."

As mentioned above, evidence has already been gathered indicating that low socioeconomic status and low age status tend to be associated with increased psychiatric impairment and the multiplication of psychophysiological symptoms. Perhaps this is related to the low *prestige* of older people and of the poor who are uneducated and employed in manual labor. A logical further step was to investigate the low prestige of women to see whether it related to symptomatology and some measure of self-image. If a group of women could be found whose prestige status was equal to that of men, they could be compared in terms of symptoms and self-image with a group of women in a community where women had low status.

This hypothesis about sexual status is a corollary of the general hypothesis that low status is associated with increased psychiatric disturbance and a negative self-image. An opportunity for research came into view when I read Miguel Covarrubias's book, *Mexico South*.[12] This describes the community of Tehuantepec, where there is a remarkable equality between women (Tehuanas) and men (Tehuanos). Would these women with high status in their society exhibit fewer symptoms *in relation to men* of the same community than the more typical lower-status women of a "control" community such as Mexico City? Would the Tehuanas also have a better "self-image"? Thus Tehuantepec and Mexico City were chosen as contrasting communities in which these hypotheses could be tested.

Status of Women in Mexico

In Mexico City there prevails a pattern of women's status typical of countries with a history of Spanish colonization. The woman is sheltered during adolescence. She is placed on a pedestal and courted, her "honor" defended at any cost by her brothers and father. After this brief period in the limelight, she marries and is then expected to take responsibility for a household. She undertakes the education and religious training of the children and often contributes full or partial economic support of the family. Extramarital activity on her part is strongly condemned by the society and might expose her to physical punishment by her husband.

The man, on the other hand, is not condemned for having extramarital affairs. He may even have a *casa chica*, that is, a second family composed of a mistress and her children, whom he supports. The plight of women in Mexico City has been described by Rogelio Díaz-Guerrero, a Mexican psychiatrist and psychologist.[13] He conducted a survey of symptoms among residents of Mexico City, and concluded that the women had many more symptoms than men because of their low position in Mexican society.

While the role of "asexual drudge" is a relatively common one among the married women of Mexico City, quite the opposite is true of the women of Tehuantepec. Their independence is well known. The anthropologist-artist Covarrubias reports:

> The relations between the sexes are natural and uninhibited, free of the puritanical outlook on sex of the Indians of the highlands, and of the Spanish feudal concept of the inferior position of women, so characteristic of other parts of Mexico. . . .
>
> The frankness of Zapotec women, their rather loose use of strong language, and their social and economic independence give them a position of equality with men, and a self-reliance that is unique in Mexico.[14]

My own experience with the Tehuanas, while limited, reaffirmed this picture. They had no apprehension at being interviewed or observed by a strange man, even though husbands and sons were away in the fields. In addition to this independence, women seemed to be the "social cynosures" of the community. For example, during the daylight hours of a two-day fiesta there were few men available to dance with the women. While the men were working in the fields, Tehuanas danced in pairs and drank beer and native liquors. The festivities did not stop simply because many men were absent. The older men played in the band, while the few younger men and children clapped their hands in rhythm. The ladies then formed a chain, each placing her hands on the waist of the woman in front of her. They danced in this fashion for the rest of the afternoon, making colorful patterns in their embroidered velveteen dresses.

An anthropologist's observations and my own brief impressions indicate that the position of women in Tehuantepec is higher than the position of women in Mexico City. The main hypothesis to be tested is that this position, or sexual status, is related to a particular range of mental disorder as measured by psychophysiological symptoms. Presumably, the women of Tehauntepec, having higher sexual status than the women of Mexico City, would report fewer symptoms on the average.

It would be ideal if the average number of symptoms reported by the Tehuanas could be compared directly with the average for women in Mexico City. This would be a comparison of the absolute (as opposed to the relative) levels of symptomatology. Such a direct comparison, however, makes an assumption about the comparability of women in a complex metropolis and a rural town. Such an assumption is called into question by many factors, not the least of which is that one location has a heterogeneous culture while the other has a consistent tradition. In addition we are actually interested in comparing the status of women relative to men in each community. We should therefore also compare the sex difference in the average number of symptoms in Tehuantepec with the sex difference in the average number of symptoms in Mexico City. Put in operational terms this means finding the difference between the average number of symptoms of men and women in Tehuantepec, then doing the same for residents of Mexico City. After that, the difference between those two differences is calculated, thus providing a statistical comparison of the relative sex differences in symptomatology in the two cities.

Two Cities

Mexico City lies in a great basin surrounded by mountains except to the north. It is 7,349 feet above sea level, and the climate is temperate. The rainy season lasts from June through September.

The population of this cosmopolitan manufacturing center is now about 4,000,000. The people are almost all Catholics. With the exception of some North Americans and Europeans, the population is descended from Indians and their Spanish conquerors. While the national language of Mexico is Spanish, many Indian tongues are still spoken. The city is a complex of parks and boulevards. Architecture varies from old Spanish structures to radically modern buildings. Transportation by bus, streetcar, and taxi is available. Hotels, elegant restaurants, museums, opera, and theater make Mexico City the Latin-American equivalent of Paris.

Tehuantepec, in the state of Oaxaca, is small by contrast. In comparison to many other Mexican communities, however, it is sizable. It is located fifteen kilometers from the Pacific coast, several hundred miles southwest of Mexico City in a jungle area called the Isthmus of Tehuantepec. Tehuantepec is one of three main towns on the Isthmus and has a population of about 14,000. It is situated on the Pan American Highway at a bend in the wide river named Rio Tehuantepec. The surrounding area is covered with lush tropical growth, much of it under cultivation. Coconut palms and fruit trees grow in great profusion. By contrast the rest of the Isthmus is either desert or jungle.

Although Spanish is spoken, the native tongue called Zapotec is still in common use. Traditional customs are preserved, and in each of the twelve wards or *barrios* there is a constant round of fiestas, elaborate wedding ceremonies, and Saints' days. The *barrio* fiestas are promoted mainly by the women, who vie for leadership. Husbands generally comply or are shamed into complying.

The Tehuantepec houses are small and mostly made of adobe brick. They have back yards surrounded by tightly woven stick fences and covered with a loose palm thatching. These areas are cool during the intense midday heat but light enough to permit work. A few buildings and churches are of Spanish architecture. Being practically at sea level, the city is extremely hot and the rainfall is even greater than in Mexico City. There are, however, long dry spells, which threaten corn, fruit, and other crops. The precariousness of life under these circumstances may partially account for the group solidarity and reciprocity exhibited by these agricultural communities.

The Questionnaire

An interview to be conducted in the home of each respondent was chosen as a practical method of gathering data on sex differences in symptomatology. The limited time available for field work was a major consideration in choosing the questionnaire survey method. This procedure yields data that are comparable between individuals and appropriate for statistical treatment. The survey used a five-page questionnaire. The questions were precoded for IBM analysis so that the interviewer, in most instances, needed only to circle the code number next to the answer coinciding with that given by the respondent.

The questionnaire consists of four major sections: (1) demographic or "background" variables; (2) psychophysiological symptoms comprising the Twenty-two Item Score; (3) miscellaneous psychophysiological and psychoneurotic symptoms; (4) attitude questions concerning male dominance and the family.

The questionnaire survey was introduced as a study of health in the community. Following this questions were asked concerning age, schooling, family income, type of work, and marital status. The interview then shifted to questions about health. These were the twenty-two questions about psychophysiological symptoms often associated with psychoneurosis.

These questions had been tested during the Midtown Study on 139 hospitalized and clinic psychiatric patients and on a screened "well" group of 72 persons, each of whom had been interviewed for half an hour by a psychiatrist. Of approximately 120 items so tested in the Midtown Study, these 22 had the highest validity (distinguished best between known sick and known well). The items and their ability to discriminate between patients and "wells" are given in Table XI-1.

Table XI-1. Twenty-two Item Score *

Item	r	V.V.	CR
1. Feel weak all over	.76	2.46	10.00
2. Can't get going	.66	2.21	13.33
3. Low and very low spirits	.76	1.88	6.94
4. Hot all over	.47	1.70	8.70
5. Heart beats hard often	.63	1.61	6.05
6. Appetite poor	.75	1.51	5.00
7. Restlessness	.57	1.51	13.08
8. Worrying type	.52	1.42	8.62
9. Shortness of breath often	.75	1.40	5.00
10. Nervous often	.79	1.38	7.65
11. Fainting (more than a few times)	.74	1.38	7.65
12. Trouble getting to sleep often	.65	1.23	7.09
13. Sour stomach	.52	1.16	6.04
14. Memory not all right	.65	1.14	3.93
15. Cold sweats often	.60	1.14	3.93
16. Hands tremble often	.50	1.14	3.93
17. Clogging in nose	.49	1.14	5.53
18. Personal worries get me down physically	.67	1.02	6.03
19. Feel somewhat apart even among friends	.41	.95	5.54
20. Nothing turns out right	.56	.87	4.17
21. Headaches often	.54	.60	2.68
22. Wonder anything worthwhile, agree	.52	.48	2.65

* From Thomas S. Langner, "A Twenty-Two Item Screening Score of Psychiatric Symptoms Indicating Impairment," *Journal of Health and Human Behavior*, vol. 3 (Winter 1962), p. 273; used by permission. Criteria for selection of items: r = tetrachoric correlation of item with the Mental Health Impairment Rating assigned independently by two psychiatrists to each of 1,660 respondents; $V.V.$ = validity value based on comparison of 139 sick and 72 screened well; $CR = t$ test of significance (Critical Ratio) of difference between the percentage of 139 sick and 72 psychiatrically screened "well" giving the pathognomonic answer. All items are at .01 confidence level or better.

It seemed pertinent to include ten additional questions which had already been used in a survey of residents of Mexico City by Díaz-Guerrero.[15] These covered various other psychoneurotic and psychophysiological symptoms.

A group of questions pertaining to the Mexican family and attitudes toward male dominance had also been used by Díaz-Guerrero. These were modified somewhat and incorporated into the questionnaire. Disagreement with a "male dominance" statement such as "men are more intelligent than women" was considered to indicate an attitude of "female equality." Attitudes of "female equality" were assumed to be a measure of each woman's individual self-esteem. The assumption was made that a positive correlation existed between a woman's individual self-esteem and her opinion of the status of women in general. Presumably, the woman who felt men were no more intelligent than women would hold her own intelligence in good esteem. If she also felt that women's place was not in the home, and that men shouldn't "wear the pants" in the family, then she would have a generally more positive self-image than women who agreed with such statements. Women with a positive self-image (as measured by the "female equality" items) were expected to exhibit fewer psychophysiological symptoms.

The interview contained a total of forty-nine questions, and was conducted in Spanish. Its administration averaged one-half hour per person. Explanations of items not clearly understood were made in Spanish in Mexico City and in Spanish or Zapotec in Tehuantepec. There were three revisions of the Spanish translation of the questionnaire prior to the field trip, and a team of interviewers with a survey supervisor was organized.[16]

Some changes were necessary in listing categories of demographic data. An intimate knowledge of the social structure is required to define meaningful levels of schooling, occupation, and different marital statuses. For example, the number of families abandoned is so large that a category for this circumstance was added to the list of marital statuses in order to avoid including them under "divorced and separated." The categories of literate and illiterate were added to the levels of schooling. A fair proportion of people, particularly in rural areas, have had no schooling but can read and write. These were labeled *alfabeta*.

Another sizable group have had no schooling, and in addition cannot read or write. They were labeled *analfabeta*.

Sampling

The sample in Mexico City is based on "place name" neighborhoods. The neighborhoods were sampled to assure a wide socioeconomic range of respondents. Ideally, a random sample of city blocks would have been chosen, and respondents selected randomly from these blocks. In view of limitations of time, and the lack of adequate block statistics, a sample of neighborhoods was substituted. No recent data were available on the exact socioeconomic distribution of Mexico City by city blocks. Developing this would have been a major project in itself. As an alternative a large number of "lower class," "middle class," and "upper class" areas of Mexico City were marked on a block map. In order to categorize an area as lower, middle, or upper class, all four interviewers had to agree on the socioeconomic level.[17] If there was disagreement, as in two or three instances, the area was not covered. The interviews were to be distributed equally among the three socioeconomic levels. The apportionment of interviews to areas within each level was left to the discretion of the interviewer supervisor. In each block chosen, an approximate sampling n was used so that all sides of the block would be covered. The results are indicated in Table XI-2, showing the districts covered and the number of interviews in each district and socioeconomic category.

Within each dwelling unit the respondent was chosen by means of a table of random numbers, from persons aged twenty to fifty-nine in the household. Thus the interviewer had no choice as to the sex, age, or personality characteristics of the respondent. The only exception was that all "foreigners" (Germans, Italians, North Americans, and so on) not born in Mexico were excluded. This was done in an attempt to get a homogeneous sample suited to testing the main hypothesis of the study. The latter rests on the assumption that in Mexico City the traditional Spanish-Colonial attitude toward women is maintained. Northern European and North American attitudes might vary somewhat from this pattern. After selection of the appropriate respondent, the interview was conducted in the home.

Table XI-2. Number of interviews in Mexico City by district and social class *

District	Interviews
Lower class	
Legaria	26
Río de la Piedad	24
Bellavista	21
Tizapán	21
Mercedes Gómez	4
Galeana	5
Total	101
Middle class	
Roma Sur	25
Condesa	15
Narvarte	25
San José Insurgentes	10
San Pedro	22
Mixcoac	3
Total	100
Upper class	
Morales	26
Guadalupe	24
Coyoacán	37
Anzures	19
Total	106

* Five cases were dropped because of incomplete interviews; thus, for Mexico City, the total sample used in analysis consisted of 302 cases.

The sampling in Tehuantepec was conducted in much the same manner.[18] However, the areas of the city (*barrios* or wards) were ignored, and a sampling *n* of every twelfth dwelling unit chosen. At this time it was expected that 200 interviews could be collected. Thus every twelfth dwelling unit would properly have covered the entire city. An average of six persons to a dwelling unit was estimated. With a population of 14,000, approximately 2,400 dwelling units needed to be sampled. Owing to the voluntary status of the interviewers, the press of their duties in the Public Health Clinic, and the short time available for data collection, only fifty-nine interviews were completed. These interviews did, however, constitute a random sample adequate for statistical comparison, even though somewhat smaller than originally planned.

Streets were marked out on a map radiating from the Public Health Clinic, which was the work place of the two Public Health nurses who did the interviewing. Seven of the fifty-nine interviews were conducted in my presence during a two-day training period. The same random number chart (as in Mexico City) was used to select respondents within the dwelling units. Every twelfth unit (counting both sides of the street) was enumerated, and a random person between twenty and fifty-nine years of age selected. If no age-eligibles lived in the unit, the eleventh and thirteenth units were enumerated until an age-eligible respondent was selected. Owing to the large number of people residing in each house, only one or two households had no age-eligibles.

The final samples drawn from both cities show some bias in favor of women (see Table XI-3). While women actually outnumber men, the sample exaggerates this fact.[19] The prolonged absence of men as itinerant workers and, in rural Tehuantepec, their work in the fields during the entire day may have contributed to the bias. In addition, it is possible that some of the interviewers misunderstood the random number selection chart, while others might not have desired to return late at night in order to interview the man of the family.

The average age of the men and women in Tehuantepec and Mexico City does not vary radically. It ranges between thirty-two and thirty-nine years. Only one category is radically deficient in the sample. This is Tehuanos in their twenties.

Table XI-3. Sample characteristics: age and education by sex, income, and residence (in per cent)

| Variables | Tehuantepec | | Mexico City | | | |
| | | | Low income | | High income | |
	Male $N = 18$	Female $N = 41$	Male $N = 38$	Female $N = 97$	Male $N = 67$	Female $N = 100$
Age						
20–29	5.6	39.0	23.7	32.0	46.3	21.0
30–39	50.0	31.7	28.9	35.1	20.9	40.0
40–49	22.2	12.2	26.3	13.4	19.4	25.0
50–59	16.6	12.2	21.1	19.5	13.4	14.0
No answer	5.6	4.9	0.0	0.0	0.0	0.0
Average age *	(38.0)	(32.4)	(39.5)	(36.8)	(34.7)	(37.6)
Education †						
Illiterate	33.3	51.2	18.4	27.8	0.0	1.0
Literate	61.1	46.4	31.6	45.4	7.5	6.0
Primary	5.6	0.0	34.2	18.6	23.9	34.0
Secondary	0.0	2.4	15.8	8.2	68.6	59.0

* The average is based on frequencies in the full eight age categories, each of five years' span.

† *Illiterate (analfabeta); Literate (alfabeta)*, but no schooling; *Primary (primaria completa)*, up to 2 years of high school; *Secondary (escuela superior)*, includes 3 years of high school or more; all secondary, preparatory, college, and professional schooling.

Despite a somewhat exaggerated sex ratio, the age distribution of the sample is fairly even (see Table XI-3).

The educational distribution of the sample shows marked differences by sex, residence, and income. Men, residents of Mexico City, and those of high income show more years of education and less illiteracy.

Findings

1. *In a community where women's prestige status approaches that of men, women report slightly more symptoms than men. In a community where women's status is low, women report considerably more symptoms than men.*

The average number of complaints reported (that is, from among the symptoms listed in the Twenty-two Item Score) was

calculated according to sex, residence, and income. This information is presented in Table XI-4.

Table XI-4. Average number of symptoms (Twenty-two Item Score)
according to sex, residence, and income

	Average no. of symptoms		No. interviewed	
	Men	Women	Men	Women
Tehuantepec (all income is under $32 per week) *	3.56	4.70	18	41
Mexico City, low income (under $32 per week)	5.18	7.27	38	97
Mexico City, high income ($32 per week or more)	3.66	4.80	67	100
Mexico City, total	(4.21)	(6.06)	(105)	(192)
Midtown, low income † (under $50 per week)	3.84	4.06	49	145
Midtown, high income ($50 per week or more)	2.27	2.93	622	777
Midtown, total	(2.38)	(3.11)	(671 ‡)	(922 ‡)

* The modal family-income bracket in Tehuantepec was 100–109 pesos,
with a midpoint of 104.50 pesos, or $8.36 per week. The range was from
50 to 799 pesos, or $4.00 to $63.92 per week. There was only one family
with this top income, *all others* receiving $24.72 or less. The $32 figure
is used as an approximation for making comparisons with Mexico City.

† Only 32 people had a "family income" of under $25 per week in
Midtown. While this group would have been more comparable to the
Mexico City low-income group and the Tehuantepec sample, only six
men were involved, too few for calculating an average score. The
radical differences in income range between the cities could not be completely corrected. For example, the proportion with income under $25
per week was 1.9 per cent in Midtown, 45.7 per cent in Mexico City, and
100.0 per cent in Tehuantepec. The "under $50" group, the next avail-
able category, comprising 12.1 per cent of the Midtown sample, was
therefore chosen for comparative purposes.

‡ Sixty-seven people did not know or would not reveal their income
(2.8 per cent of the women and 4.9 per cent of the men).

A low-income group in Mexico City (with a "family income"
under $32 per week) was selected to match the range of income
in Tehuantepec. Women in Tehuantepec (4.70) are closer in

their average number of symptoms to men of Tehuantepec(3.56) than comparable low-income women of Mexico City (7.27) are to low-income men of Mexico City (5.18). The mean difference between men and women in Tehuantepec is 1.14 symptoms, while in Mexico City it is 2.09 symptoms. While the difference between these mean differences is not quite statistically significant at the 5 per cent level, this was due to the small number of cases in Tehuantepec. The direction of the data is clear and supports the original hypothesis. The Tehuanas are about twice as close to the level of male symptomatology as the women of Mexico City. The Tehuanas are one symptom "worse off" than the Tehuanos, while the women of Mexico City are two symptoms "worse off" than the men of Mexico City.

The mere counting of symptoms (without regard for their patterning) may seem highly oversimplified as a method of assessing psychiatric impairment. The reader is reminded, however, that in the studies mentioned previously, people who reported more symptoms exhibited more impairment when examined individually by psychiatrists. The number of symptoms, then, is a crude but helpful index of impairment.

Do women report fewer symptoms in cultures where they command respect? It is my impression that the women of Midtown and other areas of New York City enjoy much greater status than the women of other countries I have visited. It is in line with the status hypothesis that although women of Midtown report a larger number of psychophysiological symptoms than Midtown men, they are closer to men in their level of symptomatology (men 2.38, women 3.11) than is the case in the Mexican metropolis (men 4.21, women 6.06).[20]

2. *The lower the income level, the greater the average number of symptoms reported.*

Several findings relative to the Twenty-two Item Score are of interest though they are tangential to the main hypothesis. First, at higher income levels the average number of symptoms was considerably less than at lower income levels. For example, within Mexico City, women of high income averaged 4.80 symptoms, and women of low income averaged 7.27 symptoms. Similarly, men of high income had fewer symptoms (3.66) on the average than men of low income (5.18) (see Table XI-4). It can also be seen that the high-income group in Mexico City averages about the same number of symptoms as the Tehuantepec sample, which is much lower in income level.[21]

The Midtown data also show this trend. Midtowners of high income average fewer symptoms than Midtowners of low income. If the Midtown income distribution had been divided in half (instead of into the lowest one-eighth against the other seven-eighths) the differences between income groups might have been even larger.

3. *Cross-cultural comparisons of symptomatology are difficult to interpret.*

The Tehuantepec respondents report approximately the same average number of symptoms as the low-income group in Midtown.[22] Even though their weekly income level is roughly comparable (under $32 and under $50), the meaning of identical income is quite different in the two communities. There are two reasons for this. First, there is the problem of relative income. Since almost every Tehuantepec family earns under $32 a week, no one is considered poor simply by virtue of being within that income range. Where Midtowners are concerned, only one-eighth of the sample has a family income of under $50 a week. This segment of the metropolitan population is quite poor relative to its geographic neighbors who constitute a reference group. Second, it is questionable to utilize cash income as an index of wealth when comparing a rural and an urban area. Cash income does not indicate overall access to goods in a rural agricultural area, where many people raise and eat their crops and livestock. Barter rather than cash may be the predominant form of exchange. Kinship may determine access to goods rather than the open market. Thus $32 in Tehuantepec is easily the equivalent of $50 in Mexico City.

As a whole, Mexico City residents report about two more psychophysiological symptoms than their fellow metropolitans in Midtown. Actually, the *lowest eighth* income group of Midtowners is on a par with the *higher half* income group of Mexico City dwellers in number of symptoms. Several problems arise in the comparison of Mexico City and Midtown. The first of these may be called the problem of "symptom choice." It should be recalled that the Twenty-two Item Score constitutes a partial measure of only one form or expression of mental disturbance. Do people in Mexico City express mental disturbance through psychophysiological symptoms to the same degree that Midtowners do, or do they utilize other avenues of expression in greater proportion? If psychophysiological symptoms are as good an indicator of overall psychiatric impairment in Mexico as they are in the United States, then we can more confidently make direct comparisons. In order to determine whether this is true or not the symptom checklist would need to be standardized in both cultures against clinical cases and random samples of nonpatients in the community. No effort was made to do this in the present pilot study.

The degree to which psychophysiological symptoms actually reduce role functioning in different nations or environmental settings is also a problem in making direct comparisons. Roles involving manual labor will probably be more affected than those involving interpersonal skills. The predominantly manual labor force of Mexico will perhaps suffer more impairment per given psychophysiological symptom than the more heavily managerial, sales, and clerical labor force of the United States. This may be an oversimplification, however, for a back pain may impair the day laborer, while a headache might reduce the productivity of the executive.

4. *Women generally report more psychophysiological symptoms.*

Women consistently have more aches and complaints than men. This is true even though, as has been shown, there is definite variation in the degree to which the number of symptoms for women exceeds that of men (for example, Tehuantepec compared with Mexico City). The results of surveys in Stirling County and Midtown as well as in Mexico bear this out. Our data show women reporting more complaints than men regardless of income levels in Tehuantepec, Mexico City, and Midtown. This is conveyed in both Table XI-4 and Table XI-5.

These figures suggest a striking consistency in sex differences across nationalities, social strata, and in country and city. The finding that women report more psychophysiological and psychoneurotic symptoms than men is a good example of the cumulative effect of a series of epidemiological studies. The existence of a genuine sex difference in symptoms is given credence when supported by findings from studies of several contrasting cultural groups and when such findings are consistent despite the different techniques of gathering the information, different personnel, translation problems, the variation in meanings of symptoms, and the contrasting cultural modes of expressing mental disturbances. The repeated finding of such relationships in cross-cultural epidemiological studies may thus lead to the development of more universal theories of behavior applicable to a broad range of human types.

There is also evidence, supported by medical study, of basic differences between men and women in *all* types of illness. Hinkle found that women have more complaints (higher morbidity) while men have higher death rates (mortality).[23] In a sample of telephone company employees, more episodes of acute respiratory and gastrointestinal illness, more days of disability, and more visits to the doctor were found among women. Men,

Table XI-5. Complaints reported on Twenty-two Item Score by sex and city (in per cent)

Symptoms	Tehuantepec		Mexico City			
			Low income		High income	
	Male N = 18	Female N = 41	Male N = 38	Female N = 97	Male N = 67	Female N = 100
Feel weak all over	11.1	22.0	15.8	38.1	4.5	7.0
Can't get going	22.2	39.0	44.7	75.3	34.3	46.0
Low and very low spirits	11.1	14.6	15.8	37.1	4.5	15.0
Hot all over	11.1	26.8	36.8	44.3	29.9	28.0
Heart beats hard often	0.0	9.7	2.6	11.3	3.0	3.0
Appetite poor	5.6	4.9	2.6	8.2	0.0	3.0
Restlessness	22.2	31.7	39.5	41.2	37.3	32.0
Worrying type	66.7	68.3	63.2	73.2	44.8	68.0
Shortness of breath often	0.0	4.9	2.6	10.3	0.0	3.0
Nervous often	5.6	12.2	21.1	22.7	11.9	20.0
Fainting (more than a few times)	0.0	0.0	5.3	6.2	0.0	4.0
Trouble getting to sleep often	16.7	12.2	10.5	10.3	7.5	8.0
Sour stomach	5.6	31.7	26.3	39.2	29.9	26.0
Memory not all right	0.0	22.0	26.3	27.8	9.0	22.0
Cold sweats often	16.7	14.6	31.6	19.6	11.9	9.0
Hands tremble often	0.0	0.0	5.3	11.3	7.5	4.0
Clogging in nose	16.7	24.3	15.8	48.5	17.9	27.0
Personal worries get me down physically	33.3	26.8	26.3	43.3	10.4	29.0
Feel somewhat apart even among friends	16.7	17.1	13.2	29.9	11.9	16.0
Nothing turns out right	38.9	36.6	36.8	46.4	22.4	25.0
Headaches often	5.6	2.4	2.6	26.8	4.5	15.0
Wonder anything worthwhile, agree	50.0	48.8	73.7	64.9	61.2	61.0

on the other hand, had more days of disability for chronic illness though they had fewer total days of disability.

If women tend to have more minor ailments, it is not surprising that they also have more psychophysiological complaints. There may well be a physiological basis for the female proneness to these psychophysiological disturbances. Men, however, seem prone to choose psychiatric symptoms which can roughly be described as "acting-out." More men than women are alcoholics. More men are involved in assault and battery, gang fights, homicide, stealing, and other antisocial behavior. There is some evidence from the Midtown survey that men are also more prone to character disorders, such as suspiciousness and rigidity. While the Midtown survey found no sex differences in overall psychiatric impairment, there were marked differences between men and women in the types of disorders exhibited.

The fact that women have a larger average number of psychophysiological complaints does not automatically mean, then, that their overall mental health is worse than that of men. Since the Twenty-two Item Score is largely composed of this type of item, we can only say that women, more than men, tend to report these symptoms. Perhaps it is that women react to stress particularly through these symptoms.

5. *Women's attitudes favoring sexual equality are not related to their sexual status or to the number of their symptoms.*

The prestige status of women is high in Tehuantepec. It was originally expected that this high status would be reflected by or conducive to a "positive self-image." I assumed that positive self-image of each woman could be assessed by her attitudes toward women in general, which were thought to be a projective measure of her attitudes toward herself. Statements concerning female equality were therefore taken to indicate a positive self-image.

Moreover, I also hypothesized that women with a more positive self-image (or attitudes favoring female equality) would report fewer symptoms. A positive self-image was assumed to be indicative of ego-strength. Affection and prestige status were mentioned as two important requisites for building and maintaining ego-strength. Ego-strength was broadly defined as ability to resist stress, to adapt, to plan for survival, and to develop conscious control over the self and the environment. Since women with higher prestige status would have a more positive self-image and hence greater ego-strength, it was postulated that they would be more resistant to environmental stress and report fewer symptoms. Thus women with a positive self-image, as evidenced by attitudes favoring female equality, would also report fewer symptoms.

The data turned out contrary to both hypotheses. The women of Mexico City, particularly those of high socioeconomic status, tended to voice equalitarian attitudes. This was in contrast to the Tehuanas. With minor exceptions, the proportion of equalitarian attitudes increased from provincial Tehuantepec to the low-income group in Mexico City, and from low to high income within Mexico City.[24] This can be seen in Table XI-6.

The proportion of women who believe it is proper for an unmarried woman to go out alone with a man increases from 2.4 per cent in Tehuantepec to 18.6 per cent and 46.0 per cent among women of low and high income in Mexico City. Many factors may be involved in this trend. For one, the degree of sophistication and education may account for the increase. Attitudes of "emancipation," however, may not accurately reflect the true status of women. Often with emancipation, as in urban and especially higher income Mexican families, the woman actually loses power and status as she ceases to provide income for the family. Lewis observed that the *casa chica* pattern (which rests on masculine dominance and the cult of *machismo*, or masculinity) is weaker in rural areas than in the cities, and weaker among the lower classes than the middle or upper classes.[25] This may be a function of the proportion of women in the labor force. Almost all the rural Tehuanas are breadwinners. This is less true in the big city, and even less characteristic of the high-income group. The proportion of women favoring equality with men may thus increase as the actual status and prestige of women decrease.

Table XI-6. Attitudes toward female equality by residence, income, and sex (in per cent)

Attitudes *	Women			Men		
	T † N = 41	MC Lo ‡ N = 97	MC Hi § N = 100	T † N = 18	MC Lo ‡ N = 38	MC Hi § N = 67
Do you believe it is proper for an unmarried woman to go out alone with a man? Yes	2.4	18.6	46.0	0.0	35.1	59.7
Do you believe the place for women is the home? No	9.7	2.6	15.0	5.6	2.6	14.9
Do you believe that men should "wear the pants" in the family? No	7.3	7.2	24.0	11.1	7.9	31.3
Do you believe that men are more intelligent than women? No	36.5	49.5	70.2	11.1	56.7	80.6
Do you think it is natural for married men to have lovers? No	83.0	80.4	88.0	55.6	81.0	80.6

* Attitude questions from Díaz-Guerrero, "Neurosis and the Mexican Family Structure," *American Journal of Psychiatry*, vol. 112 (Dec. 1955), pp. 411–417.
† Tehuantepec.   ‡ Mexico City low income.   § Mexico City high income.

It is also of interest that there does not appear to be a relationship between attitudes favoring equality and the number of psychophysiological symptoms reported by women. No single attitude showed a consistent relationship to the average number of symptoms except: "Men are more intelligent than women." Women who disagreed with this statement averaged fewer symptoms. Why did the data fail to support the hypothesis? Perhaps these social attitudes are somewhat superficial and are not closely related to the personality structure or the symptomatology of the Mexican women. They probably do not measure the "self-image" of the individual woman but rather a stereotyped social image of women in general. In other words, the social attitudes reflected in these questions seem to be more a function of traditional versus modern cultural patterns than of personality dynamics. Hence the statements are probably not as "projective" as they were meant to be. If they had tapped the self-image of each woman, they would presumably have been highly correlated with the amount of symptomatology.

Summary and Directions for Future Research

A questionnaire containing psychophysiological symptoms highly indicative of impairment due to psychoneurotic disorders was administered to samples of the population in Mexico City and Tehuantepec. The data suggested that women whose status approaches that of the men in the same community report fewer symptoms. Metropolitan residents tend to report more symptoms than provincial residents, who maintain their traditional customs and language. Within Mexico City the high-income group reports fewer symptoms on the average than the low-income group.

Through the measures used the people of Tehuantepec display about the same number of symptoms as the low-income Midtowners. Mexico City residents average more symptoms than all the Midtowners. These cross-cultural comparisons pose serious problems, because income and other controls are not similar in range or true value. Furthermore, the psychophysiological reaction to stress is only one of a wide range of reaction types or adjustive devices.[26] Modes of meeting stress may vary between cultures. Thus the use of any isolated reaction type is called into question as a comparable indicator of overall impairment or malfunction.

In general, women are found to report more of these symptoms than men. This finding is common to several studies. In this study attitudes favoring sexual equality were not related to the status of women in the communities where they live. These attitudes also seem unrelated to the number of psychophysiological symptoms women report. Education, emancipation, and sophistication are probably better predictors of these attitudes, but these variables do not necessarily reflect true status.

In retrospect, it seems to me that an initial approach to cross-cultural symptom checklists could be improved by trying out multiple scales that would get at different dimensions of mental disorder. Subscales covering anxiety, depression, expression or control of hostility, suspiciousness, and rigidity, for example, could be carefully pretested in several cultural settings to achieve some comparability of meaning. From such data dynamic interpretations of cultural differences would be possible, and the categories would be more meaningful to the diagnostician.

Another valuable addition to the method used here would be the calibration of native disease entities against a symptom checklist. For example, among the Zapotecs, *espanto* (fright) is a traumatic incident followed by unrest, anorexia, lassitude, and often death. *Vergüenza* (shame) involves repressed anger, and is evidenced by colic and headaches, and conjunctivitis (the latter being thought of as shame in the eye). *Silase* (sadness) is a cousin to melancholia. The evil eye is widely believed in, and the effects of its power are signified by fever, vomiting, coughing, or diarrhea. Its curse is presumed to fall on the unwitting object of some individual's unfulfilled sexual desires.[27] Not one of these magic ailments is without its psychophysiological concomitants. This fact seems to offer a simple method of arriving at systematic definitions of the various syndromes in Mexican folk psychiatry. How closely these ailments parallel the major diagnostic categories now used in the United States is a matter of great interest, for it is a measure of the universality of mental disease categories and of mankind's adaptive techniques.

Notes

1. The author wishes to express his deep appreciation to all those who aided the project: for their help in sponsorship and facilitation of field work, Dr. Manuel Martínez-Baez and Dr. Varela of the School of Public Health and Tropical Diseases, Mexico City, Dr. Castellanos, Chief of Health and Welfare Services in the State of Oaxaca, Mrs. Juanita de Glessen, and particularly Dr. Ernesto Medina Ruíz, Director of the Health Department of the Isthmus, who offered the services of the clinic in Tehuantepec, and his chief nurse, Mrs. Regina León Mariscal and assistant nurse Miss Luisa Delaizuno, who volunteered to serve as interviewers. Also helpful were my friend Sr. Javier Uhthoff, and Dr. Ramón Parres and Professor Sara Margarita Zendejas, and the interviewing staff they recommended, in particular Miss Susan Drucker, who also supervised the interviewing in Mexico City and made valuable suggestions; for the use of some published attitude and symptom questions, Dr. Rogelio Díaz-Guerrero; and for their guidance in previous research on which this study is based and their continuing help, Dr. Arthur Weider and Dr. Victor Sanua.

2. See: L. Srole, T. S. Langner, S. T. Michael, M. K. Opler, and T. A. C. Rennie, *Mental Health in the Metropolis: The Midtown Manhattan Study* [Thomas A. C. Rennie Series in Social Psychiatry, Vol. I (New York: McGraw-Hill Book Company, 1962)], ch. 12.

3. Most recently Hollingshead and Redlich in New Haven have found higher rates of *treated* mental disturbance among persons of low socioeconomic status.

4. In the Midtown Study ratings were assigned independently by two psychiatrists. These ratings indicated the degree of psychiatric impairment in life functioning. While these impairment ratings cover the whole range of symptomatology, the psychophysiological symptoms do not. They probably do not assess brain damage, sociopathic behavior, and some psychoses. They are, however, pretty good indicators of psychophysiological and psychoneurotic disturbances.

5. R. Linton, *The Study of Man* (New York: Appleton-Century-Crofts, 1936), p. 114.

6. E. Benoit-Smullyan, "Status, Status Types and Status Interrelations," *American Sociological Review*, vol. 9 (1944), pp. 151–161.

7. See: H. Goldhamer, and E. A. Shils, "Types of Power and Status," *American Journal of Sociology*, vol. 16, no. 2 (Sept. 1939), pp. 171–182, for a discussion of values determining status.

8. M. Weber, "Class, Status, Party," in *From Max Weber: Essays in Sociology*, H. H. Gerth and C. W. Mills, trans. and eds. (New York: Oxford University Press, 1946), pp. 186–187.

9. These individuals, aged 20 to 59, were studied at a point in time. It is only an assumption that those who were in their twenties in 1953

will show a greater proportion of impaired persons as they pass through their thirties, forties, and fifties. It is possible that persons who were 50 in 1953 have been exposed to more stress, more wars, poorer diet, or harsher child-rearing. If this is true, then the present 20-year-olds will show less impairment when they are in their fifties.

10. B. Neugarten, "Social Class and Friendship Among School Children," *American Journal of Sociology*, vol. 52, no. 4 (Jan. 1946), pp. 305–313.

11. E. Fromm, "Individual and Social Origins of Neurosis," *American Sociological Review*, vol. 9 (Aug. 1944), pp. 380–384.

12. M. Covarrubias, *Mexico South* (New York: Alfred A. Knopf, 1954).

13. R. Díaz-Guerrero, "Neurosis and the Mexican Family Structure," *American Journal of Psychiatry*, vol. 112 (Dec. 1955), pp. 411–417.

14. M. Covarrubias, *op. cit.*, pp. 338–339.

15. R. Díaz-Guerrero, *op. cit.*

16. In Mexico City a psychoanalyst, Dr. Ramón Parres, and a psychologist, Professor Sara Zendejas, recommended seven interviewers. A graduate student in anthropology, Miss Susan Drucker, filled the role of survey supervisor. With her help and with suggestions by three other interviewers (there were seven interviewers in Mexico City, only four of whom attended the initial meeting, during which the questionnaire was revised and the sampling design planned), final revisions in questionnaire wording were made. Spanish-speaking professionals (a librarian, a psychiatrist, and a pathologist), who were of course also fluent in English and were acquainted with medical and psychiatric terminology, aided in these initial versions. Grateful acknowledgment for their assistance is made to Miss Miranda and Dr. Borelli of Payne Whitney Clinic and Dr. García of St. Vincent's Hospital.

17. Only four interviewers made judgments of the class level of different areas of the city. Three were native to the city, one a resident.

18. Establishing relationships with the authorities prior to the sampling was more complex in the case of Tehuantepec. Through Dr. Manuel Martínez-Baez and Dr. Varela of the School of Public Health and Tropical Diseases in Mexico City I received an introduction to Dr. Castellanos, Chief of Public Health in the State of Oaxaca. He in turn gave me a letter to Dr. Ernesto Medina Ruíz, Director of the Health Department of the Isthmus. Dr. Medina's nurses, Mrs. Mariscal the chief nurse, and Miss Delaizuno volunteered their services as interviewers.

19. Other studies show a predominance of women in household samples. In a tenement in Mexico City, housing working-class (but not destitute) families, Oscar Lewis found that 58 per cent of *married* people were women. This does not compare with the 68 per cent of all persons aged 20 to 59 who were women in the Tehuantepec sample, nor the 72 per cent among low-income Mexico City dwellers, but it is identical with the 58 per cent among those of "high" income in Mexico City. The in-

clusion of unmarried women and men would probably raise Lewis' proportion of women further, since the young unmarried men would more likely be itinerant farm workers, or *braceros*.

20. While women reported a greater number of psychophysiological symptoms than men in the Midtown Study, there were no sex differences found in impairment rates of men and women. It should be noted that the impairment ratings were made on the basis of psychophysiological symptoms, behavioral and social symptoms, such as withdrawal and "acting-out," and upon the individual's total role functioning in the marital, parental, and occupational spheres. The psychophysiological symptoms, then, formed only one criterion of the overall mental health rating. Men typically were judged more heavily on their job performance, since unemployment or possession of a job not befitting their education was taken as a clear-cut indication of their impairment. It is not surprising then that women, even though they had more psychophysiological complaints, were not given more severe mental health ratings than the men. It was more difficult to judge their role performance, for, as many authors have pointed out, women's roles are often vague or contradictory in the United States. For example, they were less likely to be downgraded for unemployment. It is also possible that their complaints were often discounted by the psychiatrists, just as managerial persons are more likely to accept women employees' medical excuses for short absences, such as headaches, colds, or menstrual cramps, as legitimate, that is, nonpsychiatric.

21. The variations due to sex, residence, and income are all of the same general order of magnitude. Analysis of variance shows, for example, that the variation in mean number of symptoms due to sex is almost identical with variation due to residence (Tehuantepec versus Mexico City).

22. The Tehuanas report somewhat more symptoms than low-income Midtown women, but the difference is not noteworthy.

23. L. E. Hinkle, Jr., R. Redmont, N. Plummer, and H. G. Wolff, "An Examination of the Relations Between Symptoms, Disability and Serious Illness in Two Homogeneous Groups of Men and Women," *American Journal of Public Health*, vol. 50 (1960).

24. The exception was that about 85 per cent of *all* the Mexican women interviewed did not think it natural for married men to have lovers, indicating a rejection of the *casa chica*.

25. O. Lewis, *Five Families* (New York: Basic Books, 1959), p. 17. The relative unanimity of all the women on the *casa chica* issue seems to call Lewis' impressions into question, however.

26. See: K. Menninger, "Regulatory Devices of the Ego under Major Stress," in *A Psychiatrist's World* (New York: The Viking Press, 1959), pp. 497–515.

27. M. Covarrubias, *op. cit.*, pp. 381–386.

Concluding Note

By *Alexander H. Leighton and Jane M. Murphy*

THIS volume has been concerned with cause in psychiatric disorders. More specifically, it has focused on the ways in which variations in social and cultural configurations may affect the origins, patterning, course, and outcome of such disorders and influence their frequency in populations. Throughout, special attention has been given to this problem in a comparative frame of reference across major sociocultural differences. The reason for interest in this topic is its relevance to the human condition in the enormous variety of sociocultural groups in which human beings live. Our emphasis on peoples of the non-Western world stems in part from a basic theoretical orientation regarding the value of comparative investigations in human research. More important, it indicates recognition of the vastness of this sector of the world's population and the difficulties now shared around the globe in rapid economic development, automation, persistent poverty, space exploration, and the resolution of conflict. In these, it is hoped psychiatry may be able to play a role ameliorative to human distress.

Thus, the attractiveness of the field lies in the excitement of the questions asked, the possible solutions that lie ahead, and the chance of ultimate contribution to knowledge and to the improvement of the human condition. Scientific neatness, however, is not one of the features. The field is exceedingly primitive and disorderly, and we are still largely at the stage of walking around it, examining it descriptively, and considering how to apply the tools and methods of science. Immense bodies of theory exist that are very useful in organizing the complex phenomena and intricate relationships so the mind can more readily grasp them. Validity, however, is another matter, and the tough problems for cracking are those that have to do with the development of dependable evidence and the reworking of theories into checkable forms.

This state of affairs is the reason for the word "approaches" in the book's title and in the topics chosen by the various authors. Matters of conceptualization and technique predominate. Although there is orientation rooted in psychodynamic theory, the focus is on defining psychiatric phenomena in behavioral units that can be classified, counted, and compared across varying circumstances. Theories of social process are treated in a similar manner. They are a source of guidance, but the emphasis is on the delineation of human groups with demonstrable properties that are in some sense measurable and of groups that differ widely along a range so as to permit comparison.

Thus attention is given to cultural difference, but also to cultural change, and to the processes of group integration and disintegration. This is a fairly broad level, calling for research that will yield refinement in successive approximations. It seems a useful starting point, since it takes up at once some of the most pervasive trends and contrasts in modern society the world over. The more specific sociocultural factors can then be understood in relation to their places in larger configurations. A given child-rearing practice or the role of family head, for example, may have very different implications for psychiatric disorder depending on whether they are part of an integrating or disintegrating social system.

Several chapters of the book are devoted to the matter of gathering and categorizing of information. These point to a consideration which underlies theory revision and hypothesis checking, that is, the need for more data at the purely descriptive level. This is best exemplified in psychiatric epidemiology, where a beginning has hardly been made in the mapping operation necessary to provide basic figures on the frequency and distribution of psychiatric disorders. An extremely large task of sheer compilation lies ahead, one that is vital to providing an adequate descriptive base for theory development, and one that may, when it is done, force changes on many of our current ideas. It is important, we believe, to think of this as a scientific task of fact gathering required by the present status of the field even though it is not in many instances immediately relevant to hypothesis testing.

The final point we wish to make looks beyond the contents of the book but is, nevertheless, germane to its approaches. This is the effect of psychiatric disorder on society and culture. In her study in Ghana, Field has raised the question of the influence of schizophrenic thought on religious ideology and the role of depression in witchcraft belief systems, suggesting that many self-confessed witches and warlocks were actually persons suffering from psychiatric disorder.[1] Numbers of writers have pointed out how psychiatric disorder in persons of key importance may have had enormous influence on subsequent history. Guttmacher's account of the illness of George III and its part in bringing about the American Revolution is a case in point.[2]

What we have in mind, however, is something different. It is suggested by the findings thus far produced in epidemiological surveys, namely that there is a high frequency of psychiatric disorder, especially in groups that are poor and socially and culturally disintegrated. It can hardly be doubted that there is a causal interplay here in both directions between psychiatric and sociocultural conditions. Hence the question is raised not only about how noxious sociocultural conditions create and perpetuate psychiatric disorder, but also how such disorders that are manifest in symptoms of depression, apathy, hostility, and paranoid thinking may play a part in perpetuating social pathology. This is particularly apposite in the problem of lifting the standard of living in underdeveloped countries and in economically disadvantaged sections of the Western world.

It has been noted, for instance, that in successful development projects innovation and acculturation often exhibit a quality or process which might be called an "upward spiral," that is, change occurs in a series of stages in which the community or group goes through alternating phases of equilibrium and disequilibrium. If a "steady state" is reached after the first round of introduced change so that the new becomes articulated with the old owing to the interplay of rewards, congruence with the pre-existing values, or any of the other mechanisms that foster receptivity to change, then readiness is likely to be available for a second upward thrust. After the second, there can be a third, and so on. It can easily be seen, however, that fatalistic, paranoid, or hostile tendencies of people in the disadvantaged areas are the very attitudes and orientations most likely to resist the upward spiral all along the way. More than this, even when resistance is overcome and readiness engendered, these same attitudes can promote such unrealistic expectations that the slow and steady gathering of momentum, usually necessary, is impossible to achieve. In this case the stresses and failures of cultural change are likely to begin pouring back to reinforce the apathy and depression and make more remote the possibility of breaking out of the vicious cycle.

The point is that where the greatest need exists, there is also the greatest challenge. It is the kind of challenge for which, we believe, psychiatry has a responsibility to aid in research and service aimed at release from binding symptoms and attitudes, in prevention, and in social planning. The approaches discussed in this volume are concerned with some of the foundations of concept and method that need to be laid for responsible contribution.

Notes

1. M. J. Field, *Search for Security: An Ethno-psychiatric Study of Rural Ghana* (London: Faber & Faber, 1960).

2. M. S. Guttmacher, *America's Last King: An Interpretation of the Madness of George III* (New York: Charles Scribner's Sons, 1941).

Index